Veterinary Dentistry

A Team Approach

Veterinary Dentistry
A Team Approach

Fourth Edition

Matthew S. Lemmons, DVM, Dipl. American Veterinary Dental College

Veterinary Dentist
Dentistry and Oral Surgery
MedVet
Carmel, Indiana;
Visiting Instructor
Veterinary Clinical Sciences
Purdue University College of Veterinary Medicine
West Lafayette, Indiana

ELSEVIER

Elsevier

3251 Riverport Lane
St. Louis, Missouri 63043

VETERINARY DENTISTRY: A TEAM APPROACH ISBN: 978-0-443-11710-7

Content Strategist: Melissa Rawe/Samantha Hart
Senior Content Development Specialist: Ambika Kapoor
Publishing Services Manager: Deepthi Unni
Project Manager: Haritha Dharmarajan
Design Direction: Patrick Ferguson

Working together
to grow libraries in
developing countries

www.elsevier.com • www.bookaid.org

Printed in India
Last digit is the print number: 9 8 7 6 5 4 3 2 1

I dedicate this text to three great people who had the greatest influence on my growth as a dental specialist.

First, I would like to thank Dr. Steven Holmstrom, the original author of this text. He and his talented wife Laurie created this book as a guide to help elevate the entire veterinary team and spent their careers continuing to improve the care our patients receive. Dr. Holmstrom has been a rudder for the AVDC nearly since its inception. His practical approach to the specialty has a major influence on my style of practice. While he is well accomplished, his interactions with the community demonstrate a humility that all specialists should strive for. Yet he is not hesitant to course-correct a mentee when the mentee is in error. I have benefited greatly from his leadership. As he steps out of the captain's role in our specialty, I am still grateful I can call on him for advice.

Second, I would like to recognize Dr. Gary Lantz, who is responsible for not only introducing me to dentistry but also instilling in me a sense of academic excellence and integrity. Dr. Lantz taught both dentistry and surgery at the Purdue University School of Veterinary Medicine. He always focused on student training, and although he expected a lot, he also gave a lot of himself to students who were dedicated to their training. After graduating, while I was pursuing a residency, he implanted in me the importance of high academic standards, pushing me to a higher level.

Finally, I owe a debt of gratitude to Dr. William Gengler. Dr. Gengler was my mentor during my residency, and I still consider him a mentor as I strive to be a better professional. His practical approach to medicine and his philosophy to provide our pets with the same level of treatment we would receive ourselves still influence my approach to patient care. I am fortunate he took a chance on me and had the patience to develop me into a veterinary dentist. Thank you, "G".

CONTRIBUTORS

Ana C. Castejon-Gonzalez, DVM, PhD
Assistant Professor
Dentistry and Oral Surgery Service
Department of Clinical Sciences and
    Advanced Medicine
University of Pennsylvania School of Veterinary
    Medicine
Philadelphia, Pennsylvania

**Matthew S. Lemmons, DVM, Dipl. American
    Veterinary Dental College**
Veterinary Dentist
Dentistry and Oral Surgery
MedVet
Carmel, Indiana;
Visiting Instructor
Veterinary Clinical Sciences
Purdue University College of Veterinary Medicine
West Lafayette, Indiana

**Alexander M. Reiter, Dipl. Tzt., Dr. med. vet.,
    Dipl. AVDC, Dipl. EVDC, FF-AVDC-OMFS**
Professor of Dentistry and Oral Surgery
Department of Clinical Sciences and Advanced
    Medicine
University of Pennsylvania School of Veterinary
    Medicine
Philadelphia, Pennsylvania

The fourth edition of *Holmstrom's Veterinary Dentistry, A Team Approach* has updates as per the latest information available. Since the previous edition, the specialty of veterinary dentistry has entered a "golden era" of research, leading to an exponential increase in our understanding of veterinary oral pathology. It is likely that at the time of publication, some of the information will need to be updated yet again. This text provides a foundation for the veterinary practice to understand dental care and improve overall patient outcomes.

Of note, the current nomenclature established by the American Veterinary Dental College has been used. Nomenclature is consistently being updated to describe pathology and improve medical communication most accurately. As well, the currently accepted abbreviations for AVDC case logs have been updated and noted in bracketed bold terms.

Regarding communication, a chapter dedicated to medical communication has been added. This topic is of great importance according to the author as great communication is a cardinal characteristic of great teams, and failures in communication are a major cause of medical errors. Additionally, one may find that open and consistent communication may improve patient well-being and medical team morale.

CONTENTS

Introduction to Veterinary Dentistry

LEARNING OBJECTIVES

When you have completed this chapter, you will be able to:

- Differentiate between the terms mesaticephalic, brachycephalic, and dolichocephalic.
- Identify the anatomic components that comprise the mandibles and maxilla.
- Describe the structure of the teeth and supporting tissues.
- List the dental formulas for dogs and cats.
- Identify the terms used to designate position and direction in the oral cavity.
- Describe the anatomic and Triadan numbering systems.
- Describe the method for recording pathology on a dental chart.

KEY TERMS

Alveolar mucosa	Dolichocephalic	Occlusion
Alveolar process	Enamel	Odontoblasts
Ameloblasts	Four-handed dental charting	Palatal
Anatomic system	Furcation	Palatine rugae
Apical	Gingiva	Periodontal ligament
Apical delta	Interproximal area	Periodontium
Brachycephalic	Labial	Pulp
Buccal	Lingual	Sublingual
Cementoenamel junction	Mandible	Sulcus
Cementum	Mandibular symphysis	Temporomandibular joint
Coronal	Maxilla	Triadan system
Dentin	Mesaticephalic	Vestibular
Diastema	Mesial	
Distal	Mucogingival junction	

SPECIALTIES OF DENTISTRY

As veterinary medicine advances, the need for specialty medicine has increased. As of the writing of this book, there are 22 specialty organizations recognized by the American Veterinary Medical Association, some of which have several subspecialties. The American Veterinary Dental College (AVDC) was founded in 1988, and the subspeciality of equine dentistry was recognized in 2014.

Currently within the AVDC, there are three focused groups that can be thought of as a subspecialty. These are oral and maxillofacial surgery (focusing on oral surgery beyond extractions), zoo and wildlife certification, and equine dental specialty.

Other subspecialties do not currently exist within the AVDC. There are categories that the specialty of dentistry is separated into. These are oral medicine, periodontics, endodontics, restorative dentistry and prosthodontics, oral and maxillofacial surgery, and orthodontics.

DENTAL ANATOMY AND DENTAL TERMINOLOGY

In all aspects of veterinary medicine, communication is vital. This includes communication between members of the healthcare team, with clients, and between hospitals. Communication is so crucial that a chapter has been added to this edition. Good communication begins with all parties having a common language. In the scope of this text, that language is proper medical terminology, including appropriate dental terminology.

GENERAL ANATOMY

To be able to recognize oral disease, technicians and veterinarians must first understand normal oral anatomy, function, and physiology. After establishing this baseline, technicians and veterinarians can recognize the changes that occur as an oral disease progresses and select the appropriate techniques to prevent and treat the disease. For example, without knowing the number of roots that a tooth has, the practitioner cannot extract the tooth.

OSTEOLOMY AND OCCLUSION
Types of Heads

Three types of skulls are common: mesaticephalic, brachycephalic, and dolichocephalic. These words have a common root, cephalic, which means head.

Mesaticephalic

Mesatic means medium. *Mesaticephalic* is the most common head type. Poodles, corgis, German shepherds, Labrador retrievers, and domestic shorthair cats are typical examples (Fig. 1.1).

Brachycephalic

Brachy means short. *Brachycephalic* animals have short, wide heads. This characteristic commonly results in crowded and rotated premolar teeth, a condition that may lead to periodontal disease. Boxers, pugs, bulldogs, and Persian cats are common examples of the brachycephalic type (Fig. 1.2).

Dolichocephalic

Dolicho means long. *Dolichocephalic* animals have long, narrow heads. Collies, greyhounds, borzois, and seal point Siamese cats are common examples of this type (Fig. 1.3).

Maxilla

The upper jaw is made up of the paired incisive and maxillary bones (Fig. 1.4) that are collectively

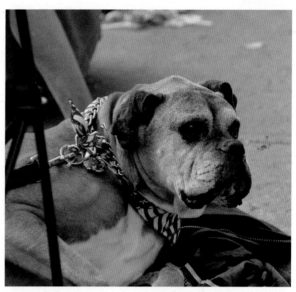

Fig. 1.2 The boxer is an example of a brachycephalic head type.

known as the *maxilla* when referring to the jaws. The roof of the mouth is composed of hard and soft palates. The hard palate is the portion of the roof of the mouth that consists of hard bone (palatal process of maxillae and the palatine bones) and separates the oral cavity from the nasal sinuses. The hard palate is covered with mucosa that has irregular ridges, called the *palatine rugae*. The incisive papilla (Fig. 1.5) lies behind the maxillary first incisors. The incisive ducts

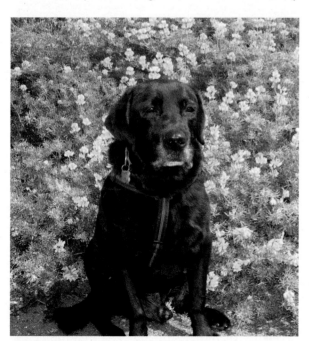

Fig. 1.1 The Labrador is an example of a mesaticephalic head type.

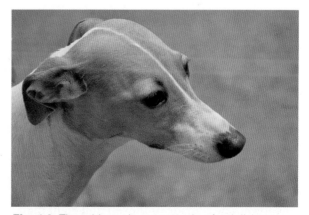

Fig. 1.3 The whippet is an example of a dolichocephalic head type.

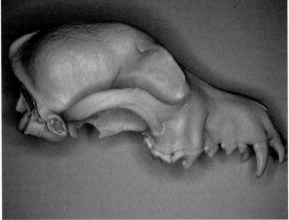

Fig. 1.4 Maxilla or upper jaw.

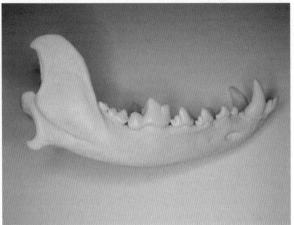

Fig. 1.6 Mandibles or lower jaw.

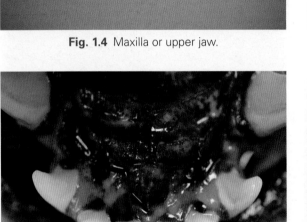

Fig. 1.5 Incisive papilla located palatal to the maxillary first incisors.

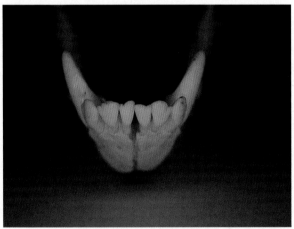

Fig. 1.7 Mandibular symphysis.

exit on each side of the incisive papilla. The incisive ducts communicate with the vomeronasal organ, which is separate from the remainder of the olfaction apparatus. This organ allows dogs to respond emotionally to molecules such as pheromones that travel up the incisive canal. The soft palate is the caudal portion of the roof of the mouth, which does not have an underlying bone. The soft palate separates the nasopharynx from the oropharynx.

Mandibles

The lower jaw is made of the left and right mandibles that are collectively known as the *mandible* (Fig. 1.6). The two mandibles join at the mandibular symphysis. The *mandibular symphysis* (Fig. 1.7) is a fibrocartilaginous joint with cruciate ligaments that provide some flexibility This structure is radiolucent, so radiographs of the rostral mandibles in dogs and cats will always show a lucent line running between. Mobility within the symphysis that results in the occlusal level of the incisors of one side to be more coronal than the other may be abnormal. This could be due to periodontal bone loss, trauma, or laxity, secondary to age. The mandibles are connected to either side of the base of the skull

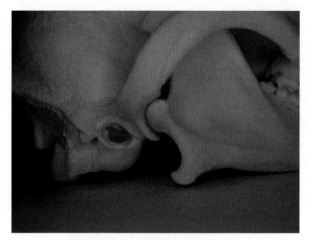

Fig. 1.8 Temporomandibular joint.

by a hinge joint called the *temporomandibular joint* (TMJ) (Fig. 1.8).

NORMAL OCCLUSION

Occlusion refers to the way the teeth fit together. Humans have true occlusal surfaces in which the premolars and molars directly oppose each other. Dogs and cats have sectorial occlusion, whereby chewing occurs on the sides of the teeth, excluding the distal aspect of the mandibular first molar and the mandibular second molar in relation to the maxillary molars in the dog.

Normal occlusion in dogs and cats is a *scissors bite*, in which the mandibular (lower) teeth meet the palatal side (inside) of the maxillary (upper) teeth (Fig. 1.9). Normally, the incisal edge of the

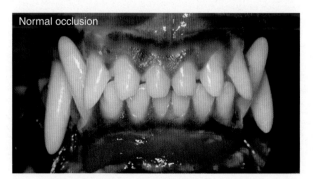

Fig. 1.9 Normal occlusion of the incisors.

mandibular incisors rest on a ledge on the palatal side of the maxillary incisors known as the *cingulum*. The mandibular canines fit within the diastema (space) roughly equidistant between the lateral incisor and maxillary canines. The cusp of the mandibular first premolar fits midway between the maxillary canine and first premolar. The remainder of the premolars are intermeshed in a similar fashion. The lower teeth are approximately one-half a tooth in front of their maxillary counterparts. The maxillary premolar teeth do not contact the mandibular premolar teeth. The cusps of the mandibular premolar teeth are positioned lingual to the arch of the maxillary premolar teeth. The distal one-third of the mandibular first molar in the dog is occlusal in shape and occludes against the maxillary first molar. The mandibular second molar occludes with the maxillary second molar, and there is minor occlusion of the mandibular third molar with the maxillary second molar.

Tongue

The tongue is a fleshy, muscular organ in the mouth used for tasting, licking, swallowing, articulating, grooming, and thermoregulation. The tongue lies between the two mandibles; the structures and surfaces beneath the tongue are referred to as *sublingual.* The surface of the tongue is covered by specialized oral mucosa that includes lingual papillae.

TOOTH AND PERIODONTIUM
Tooth Anatomy

The tooth may be divided into the crown and root (Fig. 1.10). The tip of the crown is known as the *cusp*

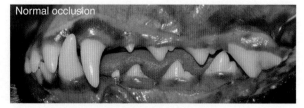

Fig. 1.10 Normal occlusion of the premolars.

if it comes to a peak. The same area of the maxillary first and second incisors and the mandibular incisors is known as the incisal edge, and in regard to most molars, it is known as the occlusal surface. The crown is covered with *enamel*, which is the hardest substance in the body. However, it may fracture in patients who chew bones and other hard substances. Normally, enamel is present only above the gumline. Enamel is produced by cells called *ameloblasts* when the tooth is developing. The junction, where the enamel and cementum (see Periodontium section) meet, is known as the *cementoenamel junction*. In the dog, the two substances typically meet at an abutment or have a small gap between them. Less commonly the cementum overlaps the enamel, and infrequently the enamel overlies the cementum. Just coronal to the cementoenamel junction is a thickening of the crown that is typically called the "enamel bulge," where the crown widens slightly. The enamel does not become thicker in this area.

The tooth root should be completely covered by periodontal tissues. The part of the root furthest from the crown is known as the apex. The area where roots meet near the crown is called the *furcation*.

The bulk of the tooth consists of dentin. *Dentin* is a hard tissue deep to the enamel and surrounds the pulp. It is produced by *odontoblasts*, which are cells that line the periphery of pulp. Throughout the life of the tooth, the odontoblast continues to produce dentin. The innermost portion of the tooth is the *pulp*. The pulp is housed in the pulp cavity, which is further divided into the pulp chamber (portion within the crown) and root canal (portion within the root). As previously mentioned, the pulp is lined by odontoblasts. The remainder of the pulp chamber consists of nerves, blood vessels, and a variety of different types of cells and fibrous tissue. The pulp communicates with the surrounding tissues via blood vessels and nerves entering the tooth through a series of small channels known as apical foramina, collectively known as the *apical delta*. Occasionally, other channels exist coronal to the apex called lateral canals.

Root Structure of the Adult Dog

An understanding of the root structure is important. When extracting teeth (with a few exceptions discussed later), all roots should be removed to prevent further complications. To remove all the roots, the practitioner must know the number of roots and understand the anatomy. In the dog, the incisors, canines, first premolar, and mandibular third molar have one root each. The maxillary second and third premolars; the mandibular second, third, and fourth premolars; and the mandibular first and second molars have two roots each. The maxillary fourth premolar, first molar, and second molar have three roots each. One key to remembering the number of roots is to recall that the mandibles do not have any three-rooted teeth (Figs. 1.11 and 1.12).

It should be noted that variations in the root structure are often present. These variations include fused roots and supernumerary roots. For example, often the maxillary second molar has fusion of the palatal and distobuccal roots, and not uncommonly, the maxillary third premolar has a supernumerary root. These are summarized in Table 1.1.

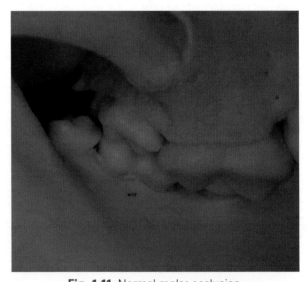

Fig. 1.11 Normal molar occlusion.

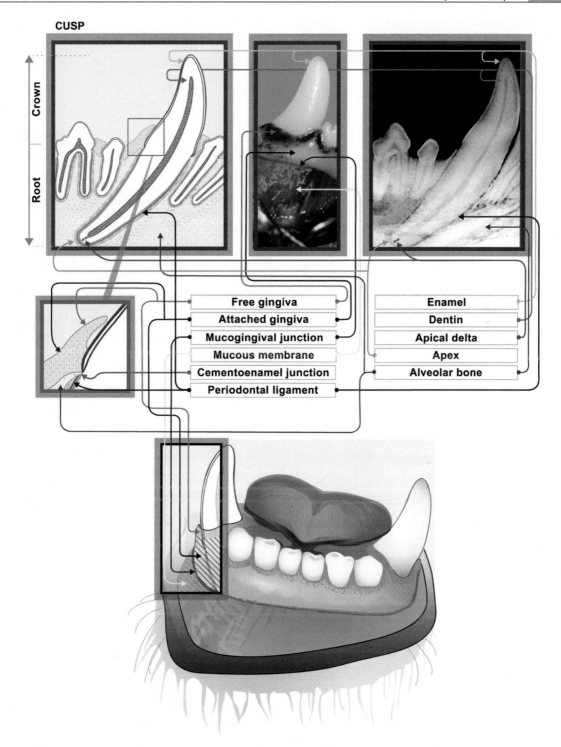

CUSP

Crown

Root

Free gingiva	Enamel
Attached gingiva	Dentin
Mucogingival junction	Apical delta
Mucous membrane	Apex
Cementoenamel junction	Alveolar bone
Periodontal ligament	

Fig. 1.12 Diagram of the general anatomy of the tooth. (Courtesy Veterinary Information Network [VIN].)

TABLE 1.1   Teeth of the Dog, Including Numbers of Roots

Tooth Type	Number in Each Maxillary Quadrant	Number of Roots
Maxillary Quadrants		
Incisor	Three	One
Canine	One	One
Premolar	Four	First: one
		Second and third: two
		Fourth: three
Molar	Two	Three. The palatal and distobuccal root of the second molar may be fused

Tooth Type	Number in Each Mandibular Quadrant	Number of Roots
Mandibular Quadrants		
Incisor	Three	One
Canine	One	One
Premolar	Four	First: one
		Second, third, and fourth: two
Molar	Three	First and second: two
		Third: one

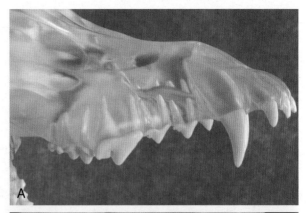

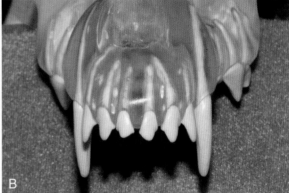

Fig. 1.13 (A) Root anatomy of the maxillary teeth of the dog. (B) Facial view of root anatomy of the maxillary incisors.

Root Structure of the Adult Cat

In the cat, the incisors and canines have one root each. The maxillary third premolars, mandibular third and fourth premolars, and mandibular first molar have two roots each. The maxillary fourth premolar has three roots. The maxillary second premolar and molar may have one single root, two fused roots, or two separate roots (Figs. 1.13 and 1.14). These are summarized in Table 1.2.

Gingiva

The *gingiva* (gums in lay terms) is a special form of oral mucosa that surrounds each tooth and is connected to the tooth and alveolar bone. The gingiva is separated into attached gingiva and free gingiva. Attached gingiva is keratinized stratified mucosa. This keratinization makes the gingiva more durable and therefore better able to withstand the forces of chewing. Attached gingiva is more closely associated with the tooth and alveolar bone through connective tissue, making it less mobile. Free gingiva is the portion of the gingiva that is not directly attached to the tooth or supporting structure. It reflects to face the tooth, creating the gingival *sulcus*. The sulcus is lined by nonkeratinized mucosa and connects to the tooth via a junctional epithelium. The sulcus should be less than 3 mm deep in a dog and less than 1 mm deep in a cat. A slight groove exists between the free and attached gingiva, which is known as the free gingival groove.

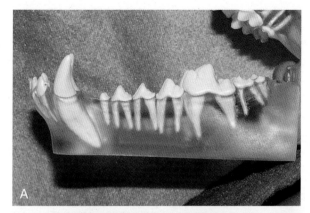

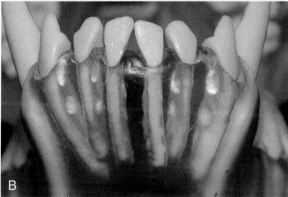

Fig. 1.14 (A) Root anatomy of the mandibular teeth of the dog. (B) Facial view of root anatomy of the mandibular incisors.

TABLE 1.2	**Teeth of the Cat, Including Numbers of Roots**	
Tooth Type	**Number in Each Maxillary Quadrant**	**Number of Roots**
Maxillary Quadrants		
Incisor	Three	One
Canine	One	One
Premolar	Three (missing first premolar)	Second: one or two fused roots Third: two Fourth: three
Molar	One	One root, two fused roots, or two separate roots
Tooth Type	**Number in Each Mandibular Quadrant**	**Number of Roots**
Mandibular Quadrants		
Incisor	Three	One
Canine	One	One
Premolar	Two (missing first and second)	Two each
Molar	One	Two

Alveolar Mucosa

The *alveolar mucosa* is the nonkeratinized soft tissue covering the bone. Its decreased keratinization increases the susceptibility of the tissue to trauma caused by chewing and periodontal inflammation. This tissue appears smoother and is thinner. It tends to have less collagen and more elastin than the gingiva, which allows it to stretch slightly. The border between the alveolar mucosa and the gingiva is called the *mucogingival junction* (Fig. 1.15).

Periodontium

The *periodontium* is the attachment apparatus and structures that support the tooth. Separately, these structures are the alveolar process, periodontal ligament, cementum, and gingiva. Gingiva was discussed above. The tooth root is housed in the *alveolar process*, which is the bony socket within the jaws. This bone is a specialized form of cortical bone called bundle bone. Together with the surrounding trabecular bone and alveolar crest, this bone is called the alveolar bone. The *periodontal ligament* connects the alveolar process to the root cementum. *Cementum* is the external covering of the tooth root and unlike the enamel, is a vital substance. Sharpey's fibers are found where the periodontal ligament attaches to the cementum and alveolar process. These fibers are mineralized and are interlaced in cementum and bone.

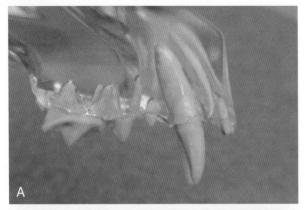

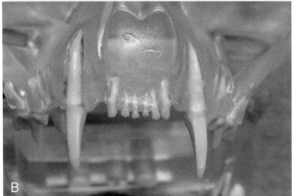

Fig. 1.15 (A) View from the side of the feline maxillary tooth model showing all of the teeth. (B) The view from the front of the feline maxillary model showing the incisors and canines.

DENTAL FORMULA FOR THE PUPPY

The deciduous dentition period is the period during which only deciduous teeth are present. Deciduous teeth (DT) (sometimes called primary or baby teeth by laypeople) are the first generation of teeth in diphyodont species. During maturation, the deciduous teeth are exfoliated when the permanent teeth erupt into the oral cavity.

The permanent dentition period is the period during which only permanent (adult or secondary) teeth are present. The mixed dentition period is the period during which both deciduous and permanent teeth are present.

The puppy is born without teeth. The deciduous canine dentition of a puppy consists of 28 teeth. Its

	DECIDUOUS (PRIMARY)		PERMANENT (ADULT)	
Teeth	Puppy	Kitten	Dog	Cat
Incisors	4–6	3–4	12–16	11–16
Canines	3–5	3–4	12–16	12–20
Premolars	5–6	5–6	16–20	16–20
Molars	–	–	16–24	20–24

TABLE 1.3 Approximate Ages (in Weeks) When Teeth Erupt in Dogs and Cats

deciduous incisors normally erupt at approximately 3 to 4 weeks of age, the canines at 3 weeks, and the deciduous premolars at 4 to 12 weeks of age. The age at which the teeth erupt varies among breed lines. On each side, upper and lower, an adult dog has three incisors, one canine, and three premolars. Puppies do not have deciduous molars. The dental formula for the puppy is as follows:

$$2 \times \left(3/3i, 1/1c, 3/3p\right) = 28$$

Generally, deciduous teeth fall out (exfoliate) 1 to 2 weeks before the eruption of permanent teeth. What triggers a tooth to exfoliate is not fully understood. One theory is that as the permanent tooth develops, it puts pressure on the deciduous tooth, stimulating a resorptive process. Once the tooth root is resorbed, the crown loosens from the gingival attachment and falls off.

The approximate ages at which deciduous and permanent teeth erupt are listed in Table 1.3.

DENTAL FORMULA FOR THE ADULT DOG

The permanent canine dental formula on each side of the mouth, upper and lower, consists of three incisors, one canine, and four premolars. On each side, the upper jaw has two molars and the lower jaw has three molars. The incisors are used for gnawing and grooming. The canine teeth are used for holding and tearing. The arrangement of the premolars, which are used for cutting and breaking up food, resembles pinking shears. The molars are used for grinding. The permanent incisor teeth erupt at 3 to 5 months of age, the canine and premolar teeth at 4 to 6 months, and the molars at 5 to 7 months. The dental formula for the adult dog is as follows:

$$2 \times (3/3I, 1/1C, 4/4P, 2/3M) = 42$$

DENTAL FORMULA FOR THE KITTEN

The kitten's dentition is similar to that of the puppy except that two, rather than three, deciduous premolars are present in the lower jaw. The kitten's deciduous teeth erupt earlier than those of the puppy. The incisors erupt at 2 to 3 weeks of age, the deciduous canines erupt at 3 to 4 weeks of age, and the deciduous premolars erupt at 3 to 6 weeks of age. The dental formula for a kitten is as follows:

$$2 \times (3/3i, 1/1c, 3/2p) = 26$$

DENTAL FORMULA FOR THE ADULT CAT

On each side of the mouth, upper and lower, the adult cat has three incisors, one canine, and one molar. On each side the cat has three premolars on the upper jaw and two premolars on the lower jaw. The permanent incisors erupt at 3 to 4 months of age, the canines at 4 to 5 months of age, premolars at 4 to 6 months of age, and molars at 4 to 5 months of age. The dental formula for the adult cat is as follows:

$$2 \times (3/3I, 1/1C, 3/2P, 1/1M) = 30$$

POSITIONAL TERMINOLOGY

The reference point for anatomic terms in the mouth is the teeth. The term *vestibular* indicates the direction toward the outside of the teeth. *Labial* (toward the lips) and *buccal* (toward the cheeks) are alternative terms.

Palatal and *lingual* refer to the direction toward the middle of the mouth—palatal describes the maxillary teeth and lingual the mandibular teeth. Although these terms are often used interchangeably, they are properly used specifically for upper and lower dentition, respectively. If a line is drawn along the dental arch and a mark is placed representing the center of the line between the first incisors, *mesial* is the side of the tooth closest to the center of the line, and *distal* is the portion farthest from the center of the line (Fig. 1.16).

Line Angles

Line angles represent the "corners" of the tooth. Each line angle will indicate either mesial or distal and either buccal or palatal/lingual, and the

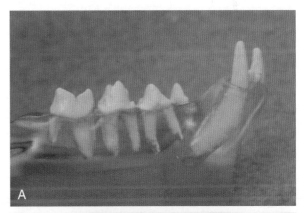

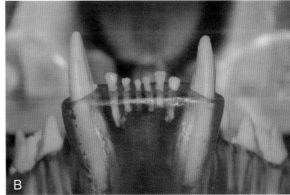

Fig. 1.16 (A) View from the side of the feline mandibular tooth model showing all of the teeth. (B) The view from the front of the feline mandibular model showing the incisors and canines.

words are contracted to make a single word. For example, the corner where the mesial and buccal sides of a tooth meet is the mesiobuccal line angle. Line angles and sides of the tooth are important in describing fractures and tooth defects.

Coronal-Apical Directions

Coronal refers to the direction toward the crown, and *apical* means the direction toward the root of the tooth. For example, a fracture at the tip of the crown could also be described as a fracture in the coronal third of the tooth.

The area in between two teeth is known as the *interproximal area*. A gap between teeth, such as between the maxillary third incisor and canine, is known as a *diastema*.

ANATOMIC AND TRIADAN NUMBERING SYSTEMS

In human dentistry, the universal nomenclature system is standard. In the nomenclature system, the numbering starts with the upper right third molar (#1) and proceeds around the arch to #16. The lower left third molar is #17 and the counting proceeds around the arch to the lower right third molar, #32.

Because the veterinary profession treats a variety of species with different numbers of teeth, the use of the universal nomenclature system is impractical and would result in the same tooth being identified by a different number, depending on the animal being treated. For this reason, the veterinary profession has adopted the anatomic and Triadan systems. By using the anatomic or Triadan system, veterinary team members can easily annotate medical records. Currently, both the anatomic and Triadan systems are acceptable. Each system has its advantages and disadvantages.

Anatomic System

The *anatomic system* is a way to name each tooth based on its location (left vs. right and maxilla vs. mandible) and the tooth type. The full anatomic name of a tooth is written out in order as; left or right,

maxillary or mandibular, tooth number followed by tooth type. Examples include the left maxillary first incisor or right mandibular fourth premolar.

Although not fully recognized by the AVDC, the full anatomic name of a tooth can be abbreviated. Abbreviations for the tooth types are I for incisors, C for canines, P for premolars, and M for molars. To indicate the side of the mouth where the tooth is, a number representing the tooth is written on the left side of the letter for the left side of the patient's mouth or on the right side of the letter for the right side of the patient's mouth. A helpful way to remember this convention is as follows: left side of patient, left side of letter; right side of patient, right side of letter.

The maxillary (upper) teeth are indicated as a superscript number. The mandibular teeth are indicated as a subscript number.

Incisors = I

The incisors are identified by the capital letter I. When writing the tooth type on ruled paper, the veterinary staff member should generally write the letter on the line. A lowercase letter i should be used in reference to a deciduous tooth. The incisor located closest to the center of the mouth is incisor #1, incisor #2 is the intermediate incisor, and incisor #3 is the lateral incisor. The central right maxillary incisor is I^1. The central left mandibular incisor is $_1I$.

Canines = C

The permanent canine teeth are identified by the capital letter C. The deciduous canine tooth is indicated by the lowercase letter c. Because only one canine tooth is present in each quadrant, only the number 1 is used. The left mandibular canine is known as $_1C$. The right maxillary canine tooth is known as C^1.

Premolars = P

The premolars are represented by the capital letter P. Deciduous premolar teeth are represented by a lowercase p. In the dog the premolars are numbered sequentially beginning with 1 and moving back in the mouth. Because the cat does not have a first premolar in the maxilla (upper jaw) or a first or second premolar in the mandibles (lower jaws), premolar numbering starts with 2 in the maxilla and 3 in the mandibles. The left maxillary fourth premolar is called ^{4}P, and the right mandibular fourth premolar is called P$_4$. The cat does not have ^{1}P, P^1, $_1$P, $_2$P, P$_1$, or P$_2$.

Molars = M

The molars are indicated by the letter *M*. Remember that no deciduous molars exist. The first molar is indicated by 1, and successive molars by 2 and 3, if present. The right maxillary first molar is M^1. The left mandibular first molar is $_1$M.

Shortcut

A shortcut in the notation of multiple teeth is to indicate the tooth numbers as a chain. For example, ^{321}I^{123} indicates all the maxillary incisors.

Advantages

The advantage of the anatomic system is that it uses clear anatomic terminology which describe the named tooth clearly.

Disadvantages

Although this is an intuitive system, as electronic records become accepted, entering superscript and subscript input becomes more laborious.

Triadan Numbering System

The *Triadan system* is a method of labeling the teeth based on the quadrant and tooth number, providing a three-digit number unique to each tooth. The many numbers in the Triadan numbering system make it seem confusing at first (Box 1.1). Despite its appearance, the Triadan system is quite simple once the code is memorized. The Triadan system uses three numbers. The first number identifies the quadrant (remember that there are four) of the mouth. The second and third numbers identify the tooth, which is always represented by two numbers.

Quadrant

The quadrants are identified as 1xx for right maxillary, 2xx for left maxillary, 3xx for left mandibular,

BOX 1.1 Triadan System Guidelines

Label quadrant first (add 400 for deciduous teeth)
Right Maxilla: 100 (500)
Left Maxilla: 200 (600)
Left Mandible: 300 (700)
Right Mandible: 400 (800)
Incisors: X01–X03
Canines: X04
Premolars: X05–X08
Molars: X09–X11

Note: Cats do not have first premolar on maxilla or first and second premolar on mandible.
Missing maxillary 05
Missing mandibular 05, 06

and 4xx for right mandibular. The quadrant is indicated by the first of three numbers (Fig. 1.17).

Tooth

The numbering of the teeth begins in the front of the mouth. The central incisor is identified as tooth 01, the intermediate incisor as 02, the lateral (or corner) incisor as 03, the canine as 04, the first premolar as 05, and the first molar as 09. Remember, in the Triadan system the type of tooth is always identified by two numbers. Combined with the quadrant, there are three numbers. For example, the left maxillary canine tooth

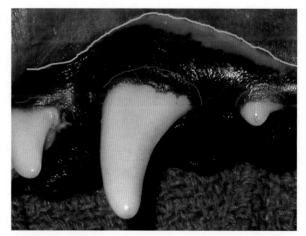

Fig. 1.17 Mucogingival junction is marked in *green*. Free gingiva and attached gingiva border marked in *red*.

is identified as 204. The right maxillary fourth premolar is identified as 108, the left mandibular first molar as 309, and the right mandibular central incisor as 401 (Figs. 1.18 and 1.19).

with the fourth premolar being 08 and the third premolar being 07, as it is in the dog. This convention allows identical teeth to have identical numbers in different species and decreases confusion.

Rule of 4 and 9

For species that have fewer teeth, the rule of 4 and 9 has been developed. This rule states that the canine tooth is always designated by 04 and the first molar by 09. Teeth are counted from 01 to 05. The first molar is counted as 09, and then the count goes backward,

Deciduous Teeth

In the young patient, deciduous teeth are identified as being in quadrants 5 for the right maxillary (upper), 6 for the left maxillary (upper), 7 for the left mandibular (lower), and 8 for the right mandibular (lower).

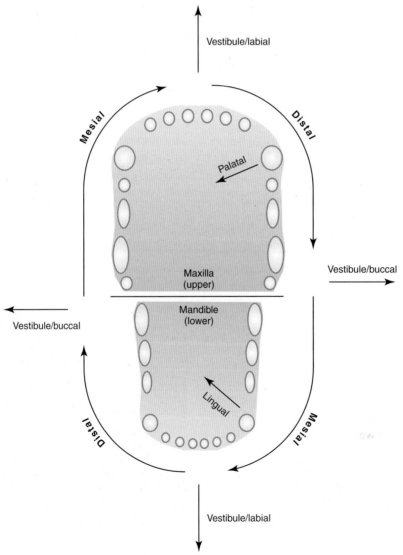

Fig. 1.18 Positional terminology.

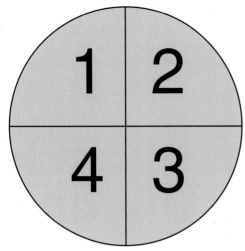

Fig. 1.19 Quadrants used in the Triadan numbering system.

Advantages

The primary advantage of the Triadan system is that it can be used with nonalphanumeric computers. Secondly, referring to the tooth type as "one-o-one" for the right maxillary first incisor or "three eleven" for the left mandibular third molar is convenient.

Disadvantage

The disadvantage of the Triadan system is that it is not intuitive. The team must know the code to understand which tooth is being identified. However, once learned, it is easy to use and therefore its popularity has increased.

DENTAL CHART FOR THE DOG

A dental chart should be used to keep a visual record of the patient's oral health status (Fig. 1.20). The teeth are oriented to the viewer, who is facing the patient. The patient's right side is indicated on the left side of the chart, and the patient's left side is on the right side of the chart. The first row of teeth represents the labial/buccal (outside) of the maxillary (upper) teeth. The second row of teeth represents the palatal (inside) of the maxillary teeth. The third row of teeth represents the lingual (inside) of the mandibular

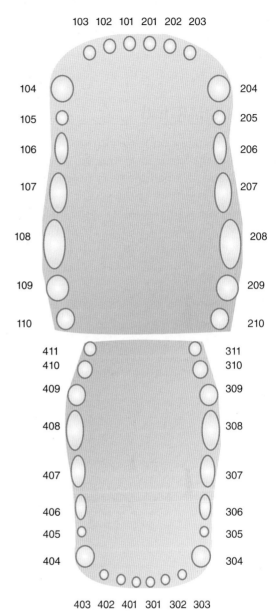

Fig. 1.20 Triadan numbering system in the dog.

(lower) teeth. The lowest row of teeth represents the labial/buccal (outside) of the mandibular (lower) teeth. The boxes indicate the depth of the sulcus, or pocket, at the time of successive dental procedures. The first charted depth is indicated in the row closest to the tooth (date #1). Successive procedures are noted in the next rows.

DENTAL CHART FOR THE CAT

Except for the number of teeth, the dental chart for the cat is identical to that for the dog (Fig. 1.21).

DENTAL CHARTING

Dental charts allow multiple visits to be recorded. Each time the patient is treated, the date is recorded and the pathology is noted. The first number that is written in the square is the pocket depth, and the second number is the total attachment loss. The patient in Fig. 1.22 has a 3-mm pocket with no attachment loss. It is charted as

3/0. The patient in Fig. 1.23 has a 3-mm pocket with 2 mm of additional attachment loss. This is charted as 3/5. The patient in Fig. 1.24 has gingival hyperplasia that is approximately 8-mm deep. The sulcular depth is approximately 2 mm. The 8 mm of pseudopocket and 2 mm of sulcular depth are added together for the first number (pocket depth) of 10, whereas the second number is normally the attachment loss; however, in this case, the 8 mm of pseudopocket is indicated, and thus 10/2 would be written. When the first number is larger than the second, it is a site with hyperplasia; when it is smaller, it is a site with recession; and when there is only one number, there is neither recession nor hyperplasia.

Electronic dental charts are available and have some advantages and disadvantages to handwritten charts. These allow for a cleaner and neater method of charting compared to handwritten charts. In turn, records sent with clients and to referring hospitals are more presentable. They also can be integrated into electronic medical records either directly or as an attached file. Finally, these electronic charts may allow for cloud-based storage, providing access to charts if on-site storage is compromised. However, not all will allow for drawing of lesions, making written descriptions necessary. Additionally, the user is limited to descriptors made by the developer, which may not use correct terminology or may not be updated with current terminology.

FOUR-HANDED DENTAL CHARTING

Dental examination, including periodontal probing and use of the dental explorer, requires the use of both hands. This makes recording dental pathology challenging. In the past, using dictation tools such as microcassette recorders and similar technology has been proposed. This still requires the operator to record the dictation

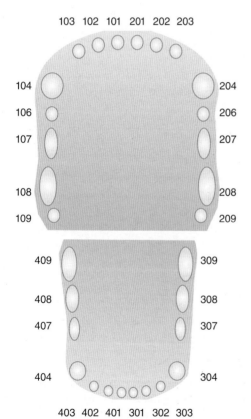

103 102 101 201 202 203

104   204
106   206
107   207
108   208
109   209

409   309
408   308
407   307
404   304

403 402 401 301 302 303

Fig. 1.21 Triadan numbering system in the cat.

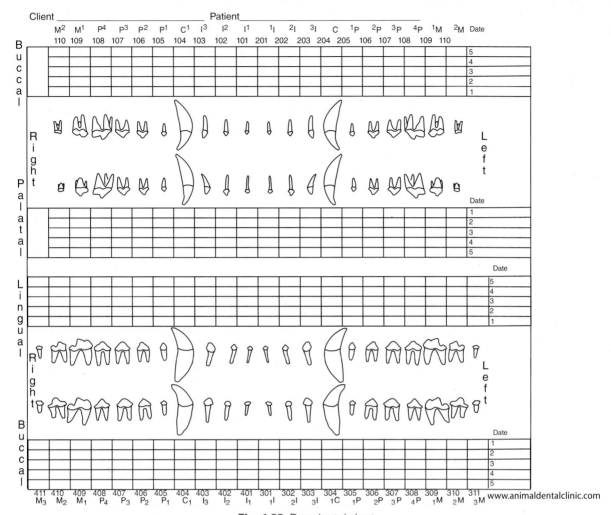

Fig. 1.22 Dog dental chart.

onto the dental chart later. Using a technique called *four-handed charting*, the examiner can dictate in real time to the assistant who then records findings in the dental chart. This allows for efficient charting and reduces the time spent transcribing records later. The experienced team can also record procedures including details of materials used at that time. The operator is ultimately responsible for confirming that the charting is accurate.

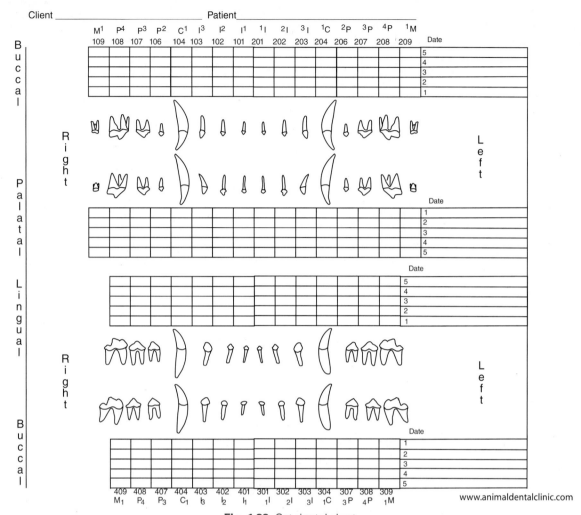

Fig. 1.23 Cat dental chart.

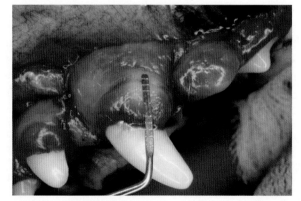

Fig. 1.24 Gingival hyperplasia with probe out of pocket, over hyperplastic area.

CHAPTER 1 WORKSHEET (ANSWERS ARE ON PAGE 294)

1. The three types of skull shapes are _____, _____, and _____.
2. The area where the two mandibles join in the oral cavity is known as the _____, and they are connected to the base of the skull by the _____.
3. The puppy has _____ teeth, whereas the adult dog has _____ teeth.
4. _____ is the hardest substance in the body and covers the crown of the tooth.
5. Dentin is produced by _____, which are cells that line the pulp chamber.
6. Of what four components is the periodontium is made?
7. The area between the free gingiva and the tooth when the tooth is healthy is known as the _____.
8. The tooth is held in place in the alveolar process, or socket, by the _____.
9. The dental formula for the adult dog is: _____.
10. The dental formula for the adult cat is: _____.
11. The following maxillary teeth have one root in the dog (anatomic system): _____.
12. The following mandibular teeth have two roots in the dog (anatomic system): _____.
13. The following maxillary teeth have three roots in the cat (anatomic system): _____.
14. In the Triadan system, adult quadrants are identified as _____ for right maxillary, _____ for left maxillary, _____ for left mandibular, and _____ for right mandibular.
15. The rule of 4 and 9 states that 04 is always the _____ tooth and the _____ is always tooth 09.
16. The left maxillary first premolar in the dog would be listed as tooth #_____, whereas the right mandibular third premolar in the cat would be listed as tooth #_____.
17. The process of having the examiner dictate charting findings to an assistant is called _____.
18. The ridges of the hard palate are called the _____.

FURTHER READING

Crossley DA. Tooth enamel thickness in the mature dentition of domestic dogs and cats—preliminary study. *J Vet Dent*. 1995;12(3):111–113.

Hernández SZ, Negro VB, de Puch G, Saccomanno DM. Morphology of the cementoenamel junction in permanent teeth of dogs: a scanning electron microscopic study. *J Vet Dent*. 2020;37(3):159–166. doi:10.1177/0898756420973482.

Verstraete FJ, Terpak CH. Anatomical variations in the dentition of the domestic cat. *J Vet Dent*. 1997;14(4):137–140. Erratum in: *J Vet Dent*. 1998;15(1):34.

2

The Oral Examination and Disease Recognition

LEARNING OBJECTIVES

When you have completed this chapter, you will be able to:

- Describe the four classes of malocclusion and discuss the various clinical presentations seen with these conditions.
- List and describe the classifications of oropharyngeal inflammation.
- Describe possible abnormal conditions of the tooth surface, including abnormalities in enamel formation.
- List and describe the various dental fracture classification schemes that apply to veterinary dentistry.
- List structures that may be associated with maxillofacial fractures and the goals of treating these injuries.
- List and describe common oral medical diseases, including neoplastic conditions of the oral cavity.

KEY TERMS

Abrasion	Dentigerous cyst	Oronasal fistula
Acanthomatous ameloblastoma	Distoversion	Osteomyelitis
	Enamel hypomineralization	Palatitis
Alveolar mucositis	Enamel hypoplasia	Pericoronitis
Amelogenesis imperfecta	Endodontics	Periodontitis
Anodontia	Fibrosarcoma	Periostitis ossificans
Attrition	Fusion	Peripheral odontogenic fibroma
Avulsion	Gemination	
Buccoversion	Gingival hyperplasia	Persistent deciduous teeth
Caries	Gingivitis	Pharyngitis
Caudal crossbite	Glossitis	Preventative orthodontics
Caudal mucositis	Hypodontia	Pyogenic granuloma
Cheilitis	Interceptive orthodontics	Rostral crossbite
Class I malocclusion	Labial/buccal mucositis	Squamous cell carcinoma
Class II malocclusion	Labioversion	Stomatitis
Class III malocclusion	Linguoversion	Sublingual mucositis
Class IV malocclusion	Malignant melanoma	Supernumerary teeth
Contact mucositis	Mesioversion	Tonsillitis
Craniomandibular osteopathy	Odontoma	Tooth luxation
Crossbite	Oligodontia	Tooth resorption

This chapter is devoted to the overview of oral examination and the recognition of veterinary dental diseases. The treatment of veterinary dental conditions is covered in subsequent chapters.

All the members of the veterinary team play important roles in healthcare. Although the diagnosis of the disease should be left to the veterinarian, the technician and other team members assist the veterinarian by recognizing conditions that appear abnormal and alerting the veterinarian to them. This chapter discusses various disease conditions that the team might observe.

Given the variety in species, breed, genetics, and size of our patients, we must be aware of which patients are more commonly affected by certain diseases and how these diseases may manifest.

ORAL EXAMINATION

The complete oral examination is both a structured and unstructured exercise. It is structured as a complete physical examination that should be a systemic review of the entire patient, organized in such a manner that no body system is neglected. The complete oral examination is performed in the same manner, assuring that every surface of each tooth and the related structures are examined.

During the dental cleaning process (intubation, cleaning, and making of radiographs), there is an opportunity for each person involved not to observe and report the disease or symptom of the disease to the examining veterinarian. No opportunity to assess disease should be neglected.

The oral examination should always be conducted in a systematic manner. The order of events may vary between practices. Regardless of the order, the following should be a part of every anesthetized oral examination, including periodontal probing and examination of each tooth, visual and tactile inspection of the tongue sublingual tissues and cheeks, visual inspection of the hard and soft palate, oropharynx and tonsils, and tactile inspection of the bones of the jaws and associated joints. In addition to these steps, the patient's occlusion and examination of the related extra-oral structures (masticatory muscles, zygoma, and ocular structures) should be performed before intubation.

These findings should be recorded in the dental chart as discussed in Chapter 1.

PEDODONTICS

Puppies and kittens exhibit a variety of dental conditions, both genetic (inherited) and acquired. The diseases discussed in this section are those diseases that are present at birth (congenital) or occur during the juvenile period of life. Because our patients do not always have appropriate veterinary care at this stage due to various reasons, these diseases are sometimes diagnosed later in life.

Missing Teeth

It is not uncommon for dogs, and less frequently, for cats to not develop a full complement of permanent teeth. Most commonly this is in the form of *hypodontia* (HYP), which is a lack of just a few teeth, such as missing the mandibular fourth premolars. *Oligodontia* (OLI) also occurs, which is a lack of development of several teeth. This is more commonly seen in toy breed dogs and dogs with epithelial mutations, such as the Xolo or Chinese Crested. Rarely, *anodontia* (ANO) or a complete lack of tooth development is present.

Teeth may be truly missing, formed and have not erupted, or erupted and all or part of the tooth was lost. Dental radiographs must be taken to evaluate the area of the missing tooth. In dental charts, a circle around the tooth indicates that it is missing.

Teeth may fail to erupt and be trapped under soft tissue or impacted by bone or an adjacent tooth. This most commonly affects the mandibular first premolar in brachycephalic dogs but can happen with any tooth in dogs and cats. This may lead to the formation of a *dentigerous cyst* (DTC) or a cyst lined by epithelial cells derived from the enamel epithelium of the tooth-forming organ. Fig. 2.1 shows a radiograph of a DTC and a photograph of an unerupted tooth exposed for extraction. If not treated, these cysts may compromise the associated bone and surrounding structures.

Persistent Deciduous Teeth

A *persistent deciduous tooth* (DT/P) is a deciduous tooth that does not exfoliate when the permanent tooth erupts. DT/P (sometimes called

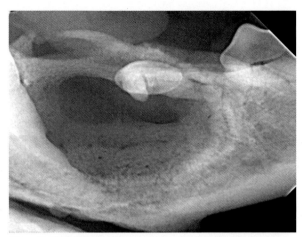

Fig. 2.1 This radiograph shows a dentigerous cyst as a result of the left mandibular first premolar not erupting.

the deciduous canine tooth is displacing the maxillary canine. In addition to causing the possible displacement of the adult canine, the abnormal periodontal border may cause periodontal disease resulting from plaque being trapped between the deciduous and adult teeth. The general rule applies: there is no room for two teeth of the same type in the same mouth at the same time. Unless they are extremely loose, retained deciduous teeth should be extracted as soon as possible after the adult tooth starts to erupt. The patient in Fig. 2.2 has a persistent left maxillary deciduous canine that should be extracted. The patient in Fig. 2.3 has a left maxillary deciduous third incisor where the other teeth are all permanent teeth. It is unknown if the permanent tooth is present. Intraoral radiographs are indicated to see if the adult tooth never formed

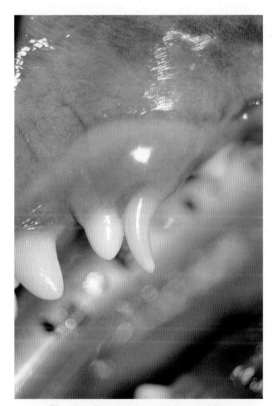

Fig. 2.2 Persistent deciduous 604.

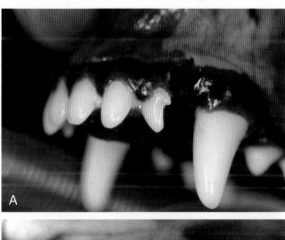

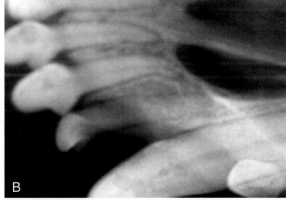

Fig. 2.3 (A) A persistent deciduous third incisor. (B) Radiograph showing that the adult tooth never formed.

retained deciduous teeth by lay people) may cause orthodontic and periodontic abnormalities. The extraction of these teeth may help prevent such complications. In the patient shown in Fig. 2.2, or if it is impacted and has the potential to cause a DTC. In this case, radiographs demonstrated the permanent tooth did not form and immediate treatment is not necessary.

Orthodontic pathology will be discussed in more depth later in the chapter. Due to the association with deciduous teeth, preventative orthodontic measures are within this section.

The term *preventative orthodontics* describes the process of extracting deciduous teeth to prevent orthodontic malocclusions (MALs). This includes the extraction of deciduous teeth that have not been exfoliated as the permanent tooth begins to erupt. *Interceptive orthodontics* describes extractions performed to treat an established MAL. This includes the extraction of a DT/P whose permanent counterpart has fully erupted in MAL. The extraction of a mandibular deciduous canine tooth of patients with mandibular distoclusion (overbite) is certainly interceptive orthodontics, as it prevents trauma secondary to MAL. In some cases, it may be considered preventative orthodontics if the goal is to allow the mandibles to reach their full growth potential without impedance from MAL. In these cases, if left untreated, further potential forward growth of the mandible cannot occur. Additionally, the deciduous mandibular canine teeth cause trauma to the hard palate, causing pain and potentially leading to damage to the bone of the hard palate and the developing permanent maxillary incisors and canine teeth. Extraction of these teeth does not cause the jaw to grow correctly or longer. Rather, it removes any possible obstruction to the full development of the jaw and eliminates trauma. To be effective, this type of orthodontic treatment should be performed before the patient reaches 12 weeks of age, preferably much earlier. It should be noted that there is a high likelihood that the permanent dentition will still erupt in MAL, and the client should prepare for additional procedures in the future.

Abnormalities of Enamel Formation

Cells called *ameloblasts* create enamel. *Amelogenesis imperfecta* includes genetic and/or developmental enamel formation and maturation abnormalities, such as enamel hypoplasia (E/H) and enamel hypomineralization (E/HM). *Enamel hypoplasia* refers to inadequate deposition of the enamel matrix. This can affect one or several teeth and may be focal or multifocal. The crowns of affected teeth can have areas of normal enamel next to areas of hypoplastic or missing enamel.

Enamel hypomineralization refers to inadequate mineralization of the enamel matrix. This often affects several or all teeth. The crowns of affected teeth are covered by soft enamel that may be worn rapidly.

The causes of these lesions include genetic, infectious (due to fever), and localized injuries. The patient in Fig. 2.4 has E/H of multiple teeth, the result of an infection while the teeth were being formed.

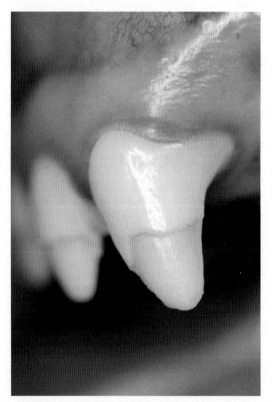

Fig. 2.4 The production of enamel was interrupted at a very young age but then resumed.

Pericoronitis

Because the gingiva does not typically attach to enamel, partially erupted teeth have a gap between the gingiva and crown of the tooth, allowing impaction of debris and bacteria. The lack of eruption is often secondary to a physical barrier such as another tooth, as seen in Fig. 2.5. When the eruption of a tooth is impeded by a physical barrier, this is known as an impacted tooth (T/I). This can lead to *pericoronitis* (PEC) or inflammation of the gingiva of a partially erupted tooth. Treatment is

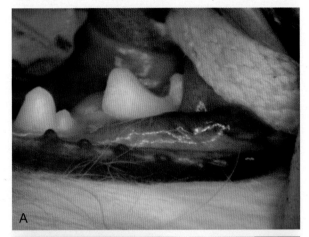

A

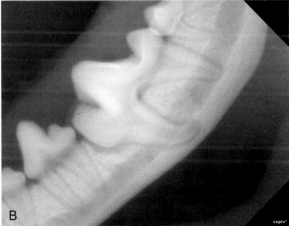

B

Fig. 2.5 (A) Pericornitis: a partially erupted mandibular first molar that has been trapped by the mandibular fourth premolar. (B) Pericornitis radiograph: the mesial portion of the mandibular first molar was trapped by the fourth premolar. Extraction of the fourth premolar allowed the eruption of the first molar.

generally extraction; however, orthodontic movement or gingival surgery can be performed in specialty practices (Fig. 2.5A and B, PEC). In this case, it may be possible to extract the tooth causing impaction to allow the other tooth to erupt fully. This will only occur if the patient is young and there is still eruptive potential.

Developmental Diseases of the Jaws
Craniomandibular Osteopathy

Craniomandibular osteopathy (CMO), known in lay terms as lion jaw, is a suspected inherited condition that occurs primarily in West Highland white terriers and occasionally in other breeds in which a proliferative nonneoplastic bone forms in the bones of the jaw, often associated with the temporomandibular joint. Patients with CMO are treated symptomatically for pain, which usually lessens as the patient gets older. In some cases, this can lead to a restricted opening of the jaws. Fig. 2.6 shows nonneoplastic bone produced in the region of the TMJ.

Periostitis Ossificans

Periostitis ossificans (PEO) typically occurs in immature large-breed dogs. It causes a unilateral swelling of the ventral portion of the mandible. It is diagnosed radiographically by a two-layered (double) ventral mandibular cortex. This is periosteal new bone formation, which is thought to be an inflammatory condition that spontaneously disappears (Fig. 2.7).

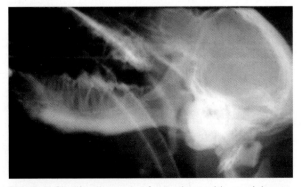

Fig. 2.6 Skull radiograph of a patient with cranial mandibular osteodystrophy.

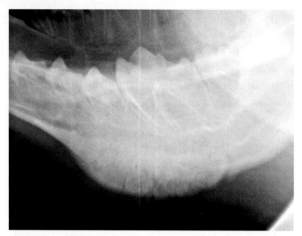

Fig. 2.7 Radiograph of a young dog with periostitis ossificans.

Ankylosis and Pseudoankylosis of the TMJ

If the bones of the TMJ (temporal bone, condylar process of mandible) or adjacent bones (zygomatic bone, zygomatic process of temporal bone, ramus of mandible) are fractured when a patient is young, there is potential for a malunion of the bones that can ankylosis the TMJ (TMJ/A) or cause abnormal bone contact, preventing full extension of the TMJ. This can prevent the patients from being able to fully open their mouth and can lead to MAL. These patients may have extreme difficulty in eating. Often these patients need specialized surgery to allow the mouth to fully open. Juvenile cats are the most frequently affected by this, but dogs can be affected as well. This CT of a juvenile cat demonstrates the abnormal anatomy of the TMJ with the contralateral side for comparison (Fig. 2.8).

Fractured Deciduous Teeth

Fractured deciduous teeth occur fairly frequently. They may be caused by running into objects, catching rocks or other hard substances, or overzealous playing of games such as tug-of-war. If left untreated, fractured primary teeth may result in abscessation, which can cause a defect in enamel production of the developing permanent tooth or nearby permanent teeth, known as *enamel hypoplasia* and may or may not form a fistula in the

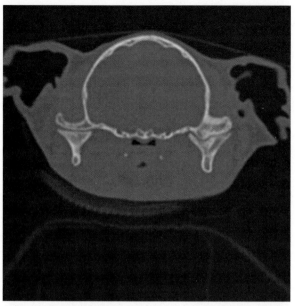

Fig. 2.8 Computed tomography images of TMJ ankylosis of the left TMJ. This resulted in the patient being unable to open the mouth.

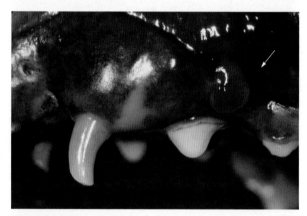

Fig. 2.9 A fractured deciduous canine tooth has caused a fistula (*arrow*) in the mucous membrane.

soft tissue. Fig. 2.9 shows a fractured left maxillary canine. Note the fistula formation (*arrow*) above the premolar as an extension of the fracture and subsequent abscess. This tooth should be extracted.

Supernumerary Teeth

Supernumerary teeth (T/SN) are extra teeth in addition to the species normal dentition. These are typically incisors or maxillary first premolars, although all types of teeth may be supernumerary. One problem that T/SN may cause is crowding. The patient in Fig. 2.10 has a supernumerary left mandibular fourth premolar ($_4$P, 308). The patient in Fig. 2.11 has a supernumerary canine tooth. Typically, these are seen as a single supernumerary incisor, which may be positioned palatally/lingually or facially. T/SN can cause malpositioning and noneruption of other teeth and/or severe plaque accumulation and predispose to periodontal disease owing to the lack of normal cleaning action. T/SN that contribute to MAL or crowding should be extracted only after intraoral radiographic evaluation to differentiate between deciduous and permanent teeth and to confirm the tooth is not a gemination tooth

(T/GEM). This is important to prevent extracting permanent instead of deciduous teeth. Deciduous teeth are smaller than their permanent counterparts and the roots of deciduous teeth are relatively long in relation to the crown. It should be noted that T/SN may not erupt and can form a DTC.

Fusion and Gemination Teeth

Fusion (T/FUS) is the joining of two developing teeth that have different tooth buds. A *gemination tooth* is one in which a tooth bud is partially divided in an attempt to form two teeth. The left maxillary first incisor in Fig. 2.12 is a T/GEM. A

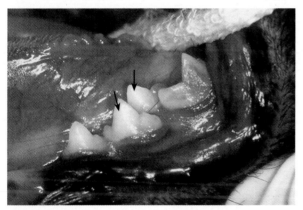

Fig. 2.10 Supernumerary left mandibular fourth premolars in a cat (*arrows*).

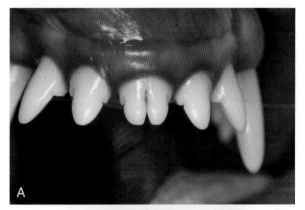

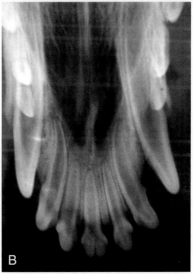

Fig. 2.12 (A) This patient has a gemination tooth, as demonstrated by the radiograph (B).

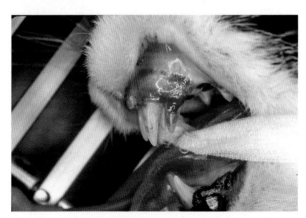

Fig. 2.11 Supernumerary canine tooth in a cat.

radiograph is necessary to differentiate between the two. Two complete roots (or root sets) will be seen with T/FUS teeth, whereas only one root (or a shared root) with twin crowns will be seen with gemination teeth (T/GEM).

Tooth Dilaceration

Tooth dilaceration is an abnormally formed root or crown in which the root or crown has an abrupt abnormal bend. This may be caused by trauma during the tooth's development or by genetic conditions. It may be an unusual finding discovered while taking dental radiographs without pathology or it may be accompanied by severe pathology. The patient in Fig. 2.13 has dilaceration of the left

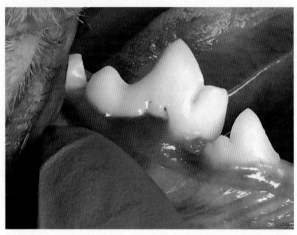

Fig. 2.14 Gross appearance of a right mandibular first molar with dens invaginatus.

mandibular first molar. In this form of dilaceration, there is often a concurrent condition called dens invaginatus (T/DEN), in which the exterior of the tooth enfolds into the interior (Fig. 2.14). This can lead to pulpitis and subsequent infection, necessitating extraction of the tooth. In extreme cases, severe osteomyelitis (OST) can occur. Dilaceration is not uncommonly seen in the mandibular molars and premolars of toy-breed dogs. This is not necessarily pathologic but can lead to difficulty during extraction.

MALOCCLUSION

Orthodontic disease is oral disease caused by the malalignment of teeth that is called *malocclusion*. MAL can be caused by dental MAL or skeletal MAL. There are four classes of MAL. Dental MALs with a normal relationship between the upper and lower jaws are class I malocclusion (MAL1), whereas skeletal MALs would cause class II, III or IV malocclusions and are all summarized in Box 2.1. Skeletal MALs occur when the upper and lower jaw relationship is abnormal, which generally leads to abnormal tooth alignment. Unless these MALs are causing abnormal tooth on tooth or tooth on soft tissue trauma or may lead to periodontal complications, treatment is not necessary.

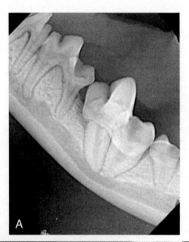

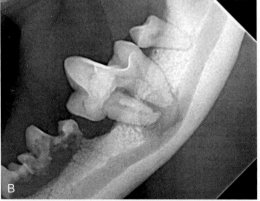

Fig. 2.13 Dilacerated first molar and persistent deciduous teeth. Initial (A) and 4 years later (B) with tooth resorption of the retained deciduous teeth.

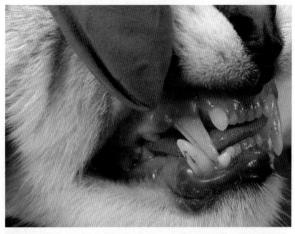

Fig. 2.15 Mesioversion of the right maxillary canine in a cat. This was initially misdiagnosed as a TMJ luxation.

Class I Malocclusion

Patients with *class I malocclusion*, also known as neutroclusion, have overall normal occlusion except that one or more teeth are out of alignment. The jaws are of normal length and width. MAL1 occurs in several disease conditions.

Mesioversion

Mesioversion (MV) is when a tooth is in its normal position and tipped with the cusp directed abnormally toward the mesial line. This is most commonly seen with the maxillary canine teeth. This may be referred to by breeders as spearing canines, lanced canines, or tusk teeth. The condition appears to be genetic and is most prevalent in shelties and Persian cats. This results in a portion of the tooth being unerupted, which leads to periodontitis.

Additionally, the mandibular canine teeth cannot fit into the diastema between the maxillary third incisor and canine and are typically tipped buccally. Treatment includes orthodontic correction and extraction. The cat in Fig. 2.15 has MV of the right maxillary canine tooth.

Base-Narrowed Canines

Base-narrowed canines may be caused by a structural narrowing of the mandible or by the eruption of the canines in an overly upright position. The mandibular canines normally diverge from each other. Base-narrowed canines may cause indentation into and ulceration of the hard palate, or even perforation of the palate. A base-narrowed canine is a *linguoversion* (MAL1/LV), which describes a tooth that is in its anatomically correct position in the dental arch but is abnormally angled in a lingual direction.

The patient in Fig. 2.16A was not treated for this condition and developed an oronasal fistula that has perforated into the nasal cavity. Fig. 2.16 demonstrates the fistula with a gutta-percha point. This type of MAL is common in all breeds but is most seen in standard poodles and dogs with standard poodle genetics.

Linguoversion can also be secondary to mandibular distocclusion or class II malocclusion (MAL2)

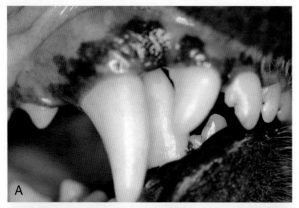

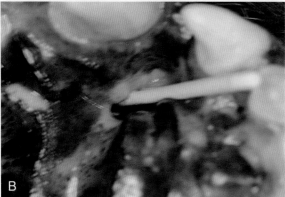

Fig. 2.16 (A) This patient has a base-narrowed canine that was not treated. (B) Gutta-percha has been used to demonstrate the fistula.

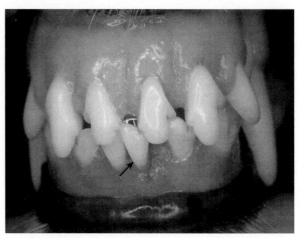

Fig. 2.17 Anterior crossbite (*arrow*).

(described below) where the mandibular canine teeth are distal to the normal position and subsequently trapped by the maxillary canine teeth, thus directing the mandibular canine teeth toward the hard palate. This specific type of MAL may be best treated by crown reduction and vital pulpotomy.

Crossbite

Crossbite (CB) describes a MAL in which a mandibular tooth or teeth have a more buccal or labial position than the antagonist maxillary tooth. It can be classified as rostral or caudal.

In *rostral crossbite* (CB/R), which is like anterior CB in human terminology, one or more of the mandibular incisor teeth is labial to the opposing maxillary incisor teeth when the mouth is closed. In this case, the relationship between the mandibles and

maxillae is normal, and only the incisors are in an abnormal relationship (see Class II Malocclusion). In the patient in Fig. 2.17, the maxillary central and intermediate incisors are displaced palatally and the mandibular central, intermediate, and lateral incisors are displaced labially. Untreated, these teeth (usually the mandibular incisors) may fall out because of chronic trauma. Several treatment options exist, including extraction of the misaligned teeth and placement of an orthodontic appliance to move the maxillary teeth labially and the mandibular teeth lingually. This type of CB is seen in all breeds but more frequently in retrievers, bird dogs, and bully breeds. It should be noted that many of these are truly MAL2 with secondary CB.

In *caudal crossbite* (CB/C), which is like posterior CB in human terminology, one or more of the maxillary premolars are lingual to the mandibular premolars or molars when the mouth is closed. The left mandibular first molar is occluding buccal to the left maxillary fourth premolar in Fig. 2.18. One may see more calculus accumulation on the mandibular first molar in these cases. This type of CB is most common in Collie dogs.

Other Forms of Class I Malocclusion

Additional class 1 occlusions include *labioversion* (MAL/LABV), which describes an incisor or canine

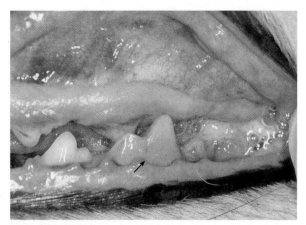

Fig. 2.18 Posterior crossbite causing left mandibular first molar (*arrow*) to occlude buccal to the maxillary fourth premolar.

tooth that is in its anatomically correct position in the dental arch but abnormally angled in a labial direction. *Buccoversion* (MAL/BV) describes a premolar or molar tooth that is in its anatomically correct position in the dental arch but is abnormally angled in a buccal direction.

In truth, teeth can be abnormally tipped in any direction and can also be rotated.

Class II Malocclusion

A *class II malocclusion* occurs when the mandibles occlude caudal to their normal position. This is also known as mandibular distoclusion. This may cause the mandibular canine teeth and incisors to penetrate the hard palate, causing trauma to the palate and maxillary canine teeth. Additionally, an oronasal fistula may result. The patient in Fig. 2.19 is in mandibular distoclusion. Treatment options for these MALs include selective extractions, crown reduction with appropriate endodontic therapy, and in some cases, orthodontic movement.

Class III Malocclusion

Class III malocclusion (MAL3) occurs when the mandibles occlude rostrally to their normal position. With MAL3, the mandibular incisors occlude labially to the maxillary incisors. With time, this

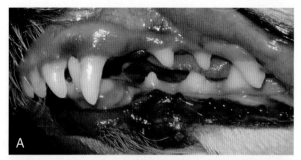

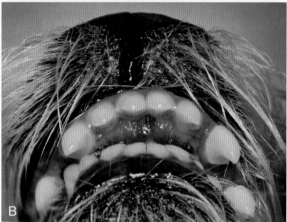

Fig. 2.19 (A) The mandible in this patient is much shorter than the maxilla (B). (With permission from AVDC https://avdc.org/avdc-nomenclature/.)

may cause excessive wear and injury to both teeth. The maxillary incisors may contact the gingiva of mandibular incisors, leading to inflammation of the periodontal tissues. The shortened maxilla may cause crowding of the teeth and subsequent rotation of teeth. The mandible may be "bowed." In Fig. 2.20, the left mandibular canine is occluding against the left maxillary third incisor.

Class IV Malocclusion, Maxillomandibular Asymmetry

Asymmetric skeletal MAL in which the first incisors of the mandible and maxilla do not align evenly is known as *Class IV Malocclusion* (MAL4). This was once known as a wry bite. MAL4 may be caused by uneven mandibular lengths or by the failure of the maxilla to develop evenly. The origin

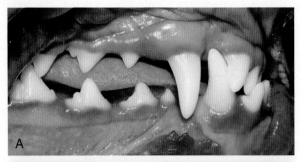

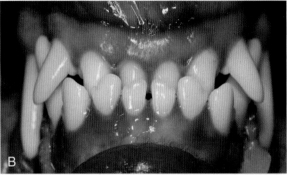

Fig. 2.20 (A and B) The mandible of this patient is longer than the maxilla. (With permission from AVDC.)

of asymmetric skeletal MAL may be genetic (inheritance of uneven jaw lengths) or the condition may be caused by trauma to the bones during the development of the facial structure. Treatment ranges from extraction of teeth to placement of orthodontic appliances.

Types of asymmetric skeletal MAL include maxillary-mandibular asymmetry, which can occur in a rostrocaudal, side-to-side or in a dorsoventral direction.

- Maxillary-mandibular asymmetry in a rostrocaudal direction (MAL4/RC) occurs when mandibular mesioclusion or distoclusion is present on one side of the face, while the contralateral side retains normal dental alignment.
- Maxillary-mandibular asymmetry in a side-to-side direction (MAL4STS) occurs when there is loss of the midline alignment of the maxilla and mandible.
- Maxillary-mandibular asymmetry in a dorsoventral direction (MAL4/DV) results in an open bite (OB) that is defined as an abnormal vertical space between opposing dental arches when the mouth is closed.

OROPHARYNGEAL INFLAMMATION

The most common cause of oropharyngeal inflammation is periodontal disease. As this disease is the most treated disease in veterinary dentistry and is one of the most commonly seen diseases in small animal practice, its pathogenesis, prevention, and treatment are covered in three additional chapters within this text. The following describes the inflammation of various tissues within the oral cavity and specific inflammatory conditions:

Oropharyngeal inflammation is classified by location as follows:

Gingivitis: Inflammation of the gingiva that is most often caused by bacterial plaque. Gingivitis may only affect the free gingiva or the free gingiva and attached gingiva. Fig. 2.21 shows gingivitis. Note that although only gingivitis is seen in this patient, periodontitis cannot be ruled out without further diagnostics.

Periodontitis: Inflammation of friction of teeth against an external object (although gingiva is typically included) (Fig. 2.22). The loss of periodontal tissues secondary to periodontitis leads to periodontal disease, which is staged by the amount of tissue lost.

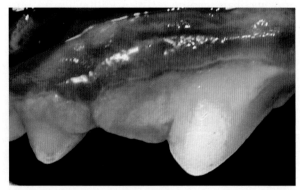

Fig. 2.21 Stage I gingivitis. (With permission from AVDC.)

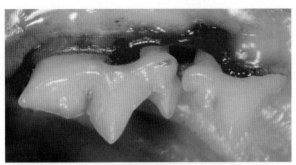

Fig. 2.22 This patient has periodontitis with loss of attached gingiva and pocket formation. (With permission from AVDC.)

Alveolar mucositis: Inflammation of alveolar mucosa (i.e., mucosa overlying the alveolar process and extending from the mucogingival junction without obvious demarcation to the vestibular sulcus and to the floor of the mouth).

Sublingual mucositis: Inflammation of mucosa on the floor of the mouth.

Labial/buccal mucositis: Inflammation of lip/cheek mucosa.

Caudal mucositis: Inflammation of mucosa of the caudal oral cavity, bordered medially by the palatoglossal folds, dorsally by the soft palate, and rostrally by the alveolar and buccal mucosa (Fig. 2.23).

Contact mucositis (CU): Lesions in susceptible individuals that are secondary to mucosal contact with a tooth surface bearing the responsible irritant, allergen, or antigen. They have also been called contact ulcers and kissing ulcers (Fig. 2.24).

Palatitis: Inflammation of mucosa covering the hard and/or soft palate (Fig. 2.25).

Glossitis: Inflammation of mucosa of the dorsal and/or ventral tongue surface (Fig. 2.26).

Cheilitis: Inflammation of the lip, including the mucocutaneous junction area and skin of the lip (Fig. 2.27).

Osteomyelitis: Inflammation of the bone. Bone with an abnormal appearance should be biopsied to understand the cause of inflammation (bacterial vs. fungal) and to rule out neoplasia.

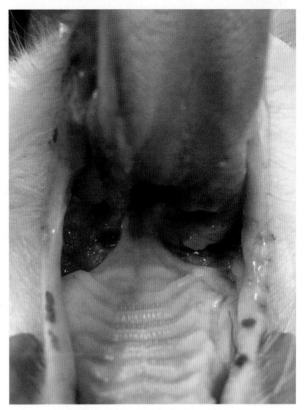

Fig. 2.23 Caudal stomatitis of a cat.

Stomatitis (ST): Inflammation of the mucosal lining of any of the structures in the mouth; in clinical use, the term should be reserved to describe widespread oral inflammation (beyond gingivitis and periodontitis) that may also extend into submucosal tissues. Please note that "stomatitis" is not a diagnosis. Specific diseases associated with ST are discussed later in the book.

Tonsillitis (TON/IN): Inflammation of the palatine tonsil.

Pharyngitis (PHA/IN): Inflammation of the pharynx.

Specific Inflammatory Diseases Other Than Periodontal Disease

Feline stomatitis (FST) A condition in the cat characterized by inflammation of the oral mucosa,

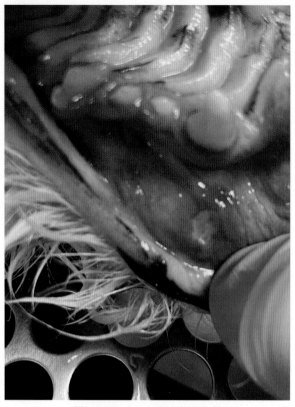

Fig. 2.24 Contact mucositis.

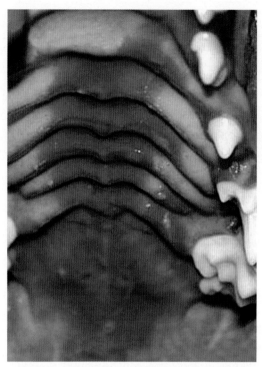

Fig. 2.25 This patient has a palatitis. (With permission from AVDC.)

often affecting the area immediately lateral to the palatoglossal folds with or without inflammation of another oral mucosa (i.e., gingiva, alveolar mucosa, labial/buccal mucosa, sublingual mucosa, and/or lingual mucosa); it commonly presents during the chronic stage, with or without (often proliferative) inflammation extending into the mucosa of the oropharynx. It is currently thought to be related to feline calicivirus. Affected cats tend to have an alteration in the numbers of a specific lymphocyte population (not typically measured on the CBC). The disease can be debilitating as the patients are often anorectic and have been suffering from chronic inflammation.

Canine chronic ulcerative stomatitis (CCUS) is a painful immune-mediated disease of dogs in which there is inflammation of several mucosal tissues of the oral cavity (Fig. 2.28). Previously known as chronic ulcerative paradental stomatitis (CUPS),

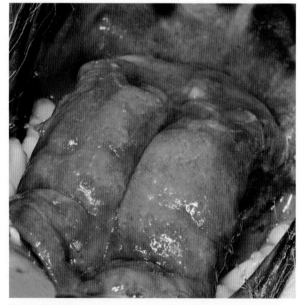

Fig. 2.26 This patient has a severe inflammation of the tongue or glossitis. (With permission from AVDC.)

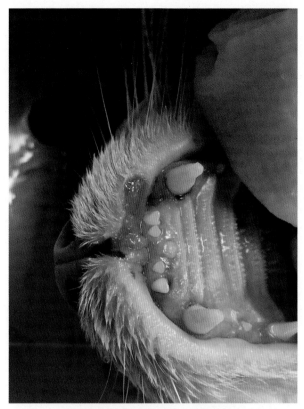

Fig. 2.27 Cat affected by cheilitis.

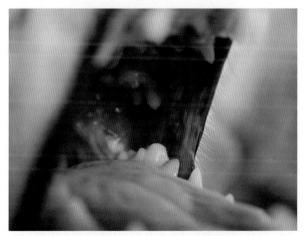

Fig. 2.28 Buccal mucositis associated with canine chronic ulcerative stomatitis.

often CU is present. It shares many similarities to oral lichen planus that affects humans. The cause is unknown.

The result is the development of painful ulcers of the mucosa that are in intimate contact with the accumulations of plaque on the surfaces of the teeth.

Treatment choices vary based on disease severity and the ability to provide daily tooth brushing. In cases with less severe inflammation, daily tooth brushing to minimize plaque accumulation can be effective. In these cases, the usage of sub-antimicrobial oral doxycycline is beneficial. Another treatment protocol is the usage of a combination of metronidazole and cyclosporine. In cases of severe inflammation, full mouth extraction may be recommended.

It is important to state that while both FST and CCUS are forms of stomatitis, the etiology and treatment are very different and, in that sense, it is not appropriate to compare the two diseases.

Immune-Mediated Conditions Affecting the Mouth

Pemphigus vulgaris (PV): An autoimmune disease caused by autoantibodies against components of the protein structures that hold the cells together. As a result, there are oral blisters and/or ulcerative oral and mucocutaneous lesions.

Bullous pemphigoid (BUP): An autoimmune disease caused by autoantibodies against the structures that hold the epithelium to the connective tissue. Clinical findings include erythematous, erosive, blistering, and/or ulcerative oral lesions.

Lupus erythematosus (LE): An autoimmune disease caused by autoantibodies against both the nucleus and cytoplasm. In addition to involving the oral cavity, the skin and multiple organs may be involved.

Masticatory muscle myositis (MMM): MMM (or masticatory myositis) is an autoimmune disease that affects the temporal, masseter, and medial and lateral pterygoid muscles. Acutely, there may be swelling of the jaw muscles (unilateral or bilateral), drooling, and pain on opening the mouth. There may be third eyelid protrusion and exophthalmos. After the acute stage, there is atrophy and fibrosis of the masticatory muscles that may result in an inability to open the mouth (trismus). The sagittal crest becomes pronounced, and the eyes may sink in.

MMM is caused by the body creating antibodies against 2M muscle fibers. These fibers are only found in the above-listed muscles. Diagnostic tests include biopsy, serology, and imaging. Biopsy of the affected muscles is a very sensitive test if performed in the acute phase. During the chronic phase, non-specific fibrosis may be present. Serology testing for antibodies against 2M muscle fibers can be performed. Use of immunosuppressant drugs or testing in the chronic phase may lead to a false negative test. Computed tomography (CT) evaluation with contrast can demonstrate areas of inflammation in the masticatory muscles and can guide where best to perform a biopsy. Treatment is usually with immunosuppressant drugs. In case the mouth will not open, carefully open the mouth manually under anesthesia. Feeding very soft or liquid food during recovery is usually necessary. Ultimately, the degree of recovery will depend on the extent of damage to the muscle tissue. MMM is often misdiagnosed as a retroorbital abscess, which can lead to inappropriate treatment with antibiotics, which in turn just delays proper treatment.

ADVERSE CONDITIONS OF THE CROWN

Surface Conditions

Abrasion

Abrasion (AB) results from the repeated friction of the teeth against an external object such as hair, toys, or housing. Over time, the friction causes the loss of dental hard tissues. Abrasive surfaces such as the fibers on tennis balls and dirt on toys are common culprits. Patients who grasp kennel wires, chain link fences, and other hard surfaces on housing will often cause distal AB of the canine teeth. This can compromise the tooth and make it more

prone to fracture. The patient in Fig. 2.29 suffers from chronic skin disease and chews its hair as a result. Its mandibular incisors and canines show severe wear.

Attrition

Attrition (AT) results from the friction of teeth against each other. AT can occur in mild MAL3, which results in a level bite. As a result, the incisal edges may have worn, owing to direct contact. In more severe Class III Malocclusions, grooves may

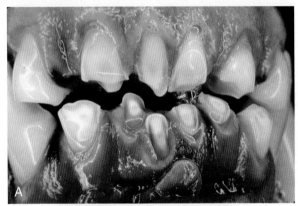

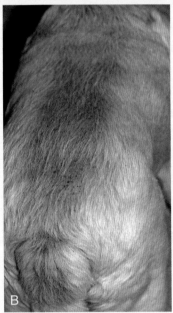

Fig. 2.29 These teeth (A) are worn and the skin (B) is irritated from chronic chewing.

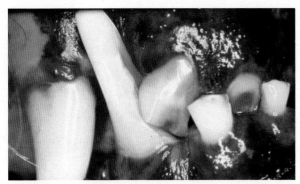

Fig. 2.30 This patient's tooth has worn as a result of abnormal tooth on tooth contac.

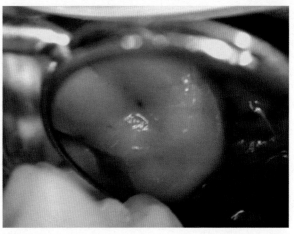

Fig. 2.31 Early carious lesion (cavity) of a maxillary first molar in a dog.

be created in the canine teeth from wear against the opposite canine or incisor. Cases of caudal CB may cause wear of the molars and premolars. Fig. 2.30 shows severe wear of the mandibular canine. The right mandibular canine shows severe wear resulting from friction against the right maxillary third incisor.

Caries (CA), also called cavities, are a breakdown of dental hard tissue caused by acidic byproducts of bacterial metabolism. These infrequently occur in dogs. The G.V. Black classification system denotes cavities by location. This system is less frequently used in veterinary medicine and will not be covered in detail. However, the most common classes found in dogs are class I caries, which are pits and fissures on the occlusal surfaces of teeth, and class V caries, which occur on the buccal and labial surfaces. Treatment options depend on the depth of the lesion and include extraction, simple restorations, endodontic therapy, and crown restorations. Fig. 2.31 demonstrates an early carious lesion of a maxillary first molar. The patient in Fig. 2.32 has advanced CA of the maxillary first molar.

ENDODONTIC DISEASE

Endodontics is the treatment of disease associated with the pulp of the tooth. Endodontic disease may be caused by fractures, trauma, and iatrogenic factors (conditions caused by the healthcare provider) such as overheating the tooth during cleaning procedures.

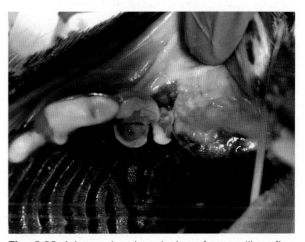

Fig. 2.32 Advanced carious lesion of a maxillary first molar in a dog.

Fracture Classification

Fighting, collisions with automobiles, the catching or chewing of hard objects, and cage/kennel chewing are common causes of tooth fractures (T/FX). T/FX are further subdivided as per the tissue(s) affected and the region on the tooth affected:

Enamel fracture (T/FX/EF): A fracture with loss of crown substance confined to the enamel. Most of these fractures do not require treatment.

Enamel Infraction (T/FX/EI): Damage to the enamel that causes fissures in the enamel, sometimes

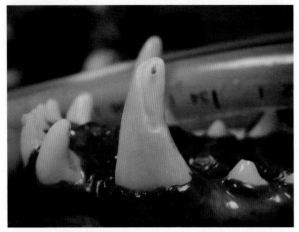

Fig. 2.33 Complicated crown fracture of the right maxillary canine in a dog. Note the pulp is *black/gray* in color that indicates pulp death.

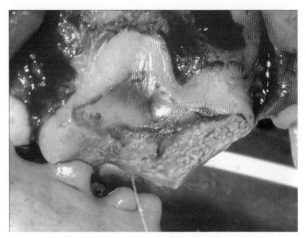

Fig. 2.34 Complicated crown root fracture

called crazing lines, in which the enamel is not lost. Most of these fractures do not require treatment either.

Uncomplicated crown fracture (T/FX/UCF): A fracture of the crown that does not expose the pulp.

Complicated crown fracture (T/FX/CCF): A fracture of the crown that exposes the pulp (Fig. 2.33). These teeth should be treated by extraction or endodontic therapy.

Uncomplicated crown-root fracture (T/FX/UCRF): A fracture of the crown and root that does not expose the pulp.

Complicated crown-root fracture (T/FX/CCRF): A fracture of the crown and root that exposes the pulp (Fig. 2.34).

Root fracture (T/FX/RF): A fracture involving the root.

Fractures of Specific Tooth Types
Incisors

Damage to incisors may be acute fracture or from AT and AB. Fractures of the incisors often result from falls; running into hard objects; catching hard objects; fighting; and chewing enclosures to escape. AB and AT, although not a fracture, can also lead to exposure of the dentin and pulp and are treated similarly to fractures. Fractures of the incisors may be difficult to see as typically the maxillary incisors cover the mandibular incisors (masking trauma to the mandibular) and the damage to maxillary incisors is typically found on the palatal aspect of the tooth (masking trauma to the maxillary incisors). Also, T/FX/RFs are not uncommon, which often go undetected until dental radiographs are made.

Canines

The canines are susceptible to trauma because of their position, use, and length. The canines have several important functions. Primarily, these teeth are used for holding and tearing. Additionally, the maxillary canines serve to hold the superior lip out. Without these teeth, some patients pinch or bite their lips between the mandibular canines and gums, as is seen in some cats that lose their maxillary canine teeth. In dogs with relatively wide tongues, the mandibular canine teeth may keep the tongue centralized and prevent it from protruding. Like the incisors, canines are fractured when patients fight and chew, catch, and run into hard objects.

Premolars

Fractures of the premolars are most often due to chewing inappropriate objects such as hooves, bones, antlers, pressed rawhide products, and hard artificial toys such as hard nylon toys. This list is not exhaustive, and any hard object should not be chewed. The most noted fractured premolar is the maxillary fourth premolar. Often this is seen as a "slab" fracture. This fracture results from the force that is placed on a very small area of the tooth (cusp) when the patient bites down. The sheer force fractures enamel and dentin, exposing the pulp. These "slab" fractures often result in a crown T/FX/RF, compromising the periodontal tissues.

A fractured fourth premolar may also result in a sinus tract below the eye due to the associated inflammation. Fig. 2.35 shows a patient with a chronic draining sinus tract below the left eye. The patient had been unsuccessfully treated with many courses of antibiotics prior to the current treatment. If the condition goes on long enough, the tooth may start to resorb (Fig. 2.36). However, the sinus tract will not resolve until the tooth is treated with complete extraction or successful root canal therapy. Sinus tracts can be associated with other teeth, but the maxillary fourth premolar is the most common.

Molars

Fractures of the molars usually occur in combination with fractures of the maxillary fourth

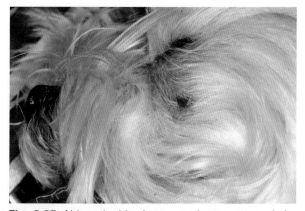

Fig. 2.35 Although this does not always occur, draining fistulas below the eye are often caused by a tooth fracture.

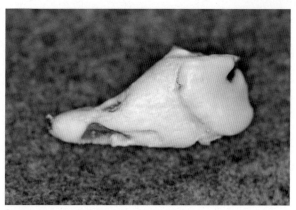

Fig. 2.36 The holes in this root are caused by chronic infection and inflammation.

premolar. When patients chew extremely hard objects, the same forces are applied to the mandibular first molar as to the maxillary fourth premolar. Practitioners may miss these fractures during physical examinations because the tongue overlaps the teeth when the mouth is open, and the maxillary fourth premolars and molars cover them when the mouth is closed.

Tooth Discoloration

The teeth and cusps take on a variety of colors that may indicate a pathologic condition. The normal, healthy tooth is white. If wear has exposed dentin, the center of the exposed portion may appear rust-colored to dark brown. If the pulp has been exposed and has become necrotic, it appears black and the tooth may lose its translucent appear.

Pink, purple, or tan teeth indicate previous irreversible pulpitis. Irreversible pulpitis can occur without pulp exposure due to impact on the tooth. This trauma may result from being hit by a car, running into a solid object, or colliding with another dog's tooth. In the right conditions, the pulp can become inflamed as a result. This may be reversible, and no treatment is required. There are subtle indicators that the patient is in pain, but pain can still be present. In some cases, this may lead to irreversible pulpitis. In this case, the pulp hemorrhages and dies because of the increased internal pressure

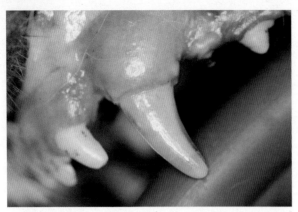

Fig. 2.37 Teeth with pulpal hemorrhage usually start out *pink* and eventually turn tan.

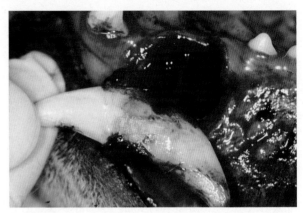

Fig. 2.38 This maxillary canine has been avulsed from the socket.

in the tooth and consequential ischemia. The odontoblasts that line the pulp chamber and guard the dentinal tubules die, preventing new dentin formation. This also causes blood cells to enter the dentinal tubules. Initially, the result is a pink tooth. As the hemoglobin loses oxygen, the tooth changes to purple and later to tan. It is likely that approximately 90% of these discolored teeth have non-vital pulps. This may indicate ongoing inflammation or the potential of future periapical inflammation in the future. The left maxillary canine shown in Fig. 2.37 is purple. The recommended treatment for this tooth is root canal therapy.

TOOTH LUXATION AND AVULSION

Tooth luxation (T/LUX) is partial displacement of the tooth from the socket. The tooth may still be vital. Immediate repositioning and splinting are recommended. Root canal therapy may be necessary.

Intrusive luxation can cause the maxillary canine tooth to enter the nasal sinus. Imaging is necessary to find the missing tooth, which needs to be carefully extracted.

Avulsion (T/A) is complete displacement of the tooth from the socket.

If these teeth are to be saved, they must be replaced quickly. In the case of luxation, as the root

is not exposed, treatment can be delayed for a day or more. In the case of complete T/A, it should be replaced immediately. Special solutions are available to help preserve the lost tooth, but usually, they are not readily available. Clients may place the tooth in cow's milk as a first aid measure. Endodontic therapy is required (see Chapter 12). In Fig. 2.38, the left maxillary canine (204) has been avulsed from the socket. Saving this tooth requires immediate replacement and splinting followed by root canal therapy 6 weeks later.

TOOTH RESORPTION

Tooth resorption (TR) is the odontoclastic uptake of mineralized dental tissue, leading to loss of enamel and dentin and causing potential pain and inflammation, and eventually tooth loss. It was formerly called feline odontoclastic resorptive lesions (FORL). Because this condition occurs in species other than the cat, the name was changed to "tooth resorption." These lesions were first discovered at the neck of the tooth, the area in which the root and crown come together. They were therefore first known as "neck lesions." These lesions have since been given several other names: resorptive lesions, cervical line lesions, and feline cavities. TR is the currently recognized term. The cause of the disease is unknown. What is known is odontoclasts enter the tooth and resorb the mineralized tissues. Given this is more commonly found in cats, the staging and treatment of this disease are discussed in Chapter 10. However, this condition is not uncommon in dogs.

ORAL MEDICAL DISEASE

Oronasal Fistulas

A fistula is an abnormal communication between two structures. *Oronasal fistulas* (ONF) is a communication between the nasal sinus and oral cavity. These most often result from advanced periodontal disease on the palatal side of the maxillary canines, although other maxillary teeth can be involved. As the plate of bone between the involved area and the nasal cavity breaks down secondary to periodontitis, fistulas develop. They are often present but not diagnosed before the extraction of the canine. Failed primary closure of the soft tissues after the extraction of these teeth will typically result in a larger oronasal fistula. The patient in Fig. 2.39 has lost his left maxillary canine as a result of chronic periodontal disease. A hole exists that opens to the nasal cavity. These can also occur secondary to other inflammatory diseases and injuries and are not always associated with a tooth. These often occur on the midline of the hard palate and may be associated with the soft palate.

Uremic Ulceration

Patients with advanced renal disease may develop ulcerations on the tip of the tongue. This is easily assessed with preoperative biochemistry and urinalysis.

Hyperparathyroidism With Fibrous Osteodystrophy

Hyperparathyroidism can be primary due to overproduction of parathyroid hormone or secondary due to renal disease. This can result in demineralization of the bones, with the alveolar bone being one of the first areas affected (Fig. 2.40), resulting in mobile teeth and often swelling of the jaws, known as fibrous osteodystrophy (FOD). Renal secondary hyperparathyroidism can occur in patients of any age. The changes noted on serum chemistry in these cases are not always remarkable. Primary hyperparathyroidism is typically found in adult animals and is diagnosed through analysis of ionized calcium and parathyroid hormone levels.

ORAL NEOPLASIA

Clinically Nonaggressive Tumors

Although they may grow large locally, clinically nonaggressive tumors generally do not spread deep

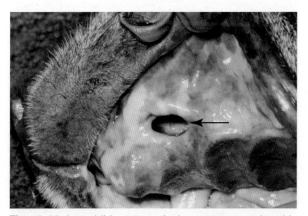

Fig. 2.39 In addition to missing many teeth, this patient has an oronasal fistula (*arrow*) from a previously extracted canine.

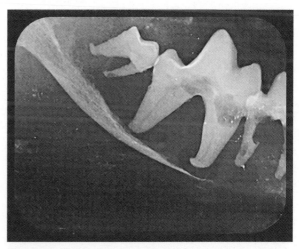

Fig. 2.40 Fibrous osteodystrophy from renal secondary hyperparathyroidism.

into tissue or metastasize to lymph nodes or lungs. Often, they respond well to surgical removal. If left untreated, they can cause discomfort due to ulceration and lead to periodontal complications if the tumor grows over the associated tooth or interferes with normal mastication. These tumors do not typically displace teeth.

Papilloma

Canine oral viral papillomatosis (OM/PAP) occurs in young dogs, frequently less than 2 years of age. There are typically wart-like lesions on the oral mucous membrane, but they also may occur on the lips. This is caused by a virus and generally will go away with time (Fig. 2.41). Occasionally, surgery may be necessary if the warts get large enough to interfere with mastication and swallowing.

Focal Fibrous Hyperplasia

Benign hyperplastic lesions are common and usually result from periodontal disease or other irritation. They respond well to local excision and removal of the originating cause.

Cheek-Chewing Lesion

Oral trauma from cheek chewing (CL/B) may result in lesions that appear thickened and irregular. The histopathologic description for

these is oral fibroepithelial polyp. These may occur in other regions covered by oral mucosa, namely sublingually as a tongue-chewing lesion (CL/T). Excision can be performed if the lesion is interfering with normal mastication, but if the trauma continues, the lesion will return and the offending teeth should be extracted. If these lesions appear ulcerated or discolored, biopsy is recommended.

Pyogenic Granuloma

Pyogenic granuloma (PYO) is an inflammatory lesion found in cats, often secondary to traumatic occlusion. Often confused on first appearance as a cancerous lesion, these can occur due to MAL or after dental extraction. The patient in Fig. 2.42 is a cat with a PYO caused by trauma from the opposing

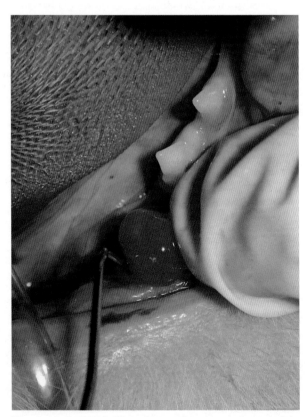

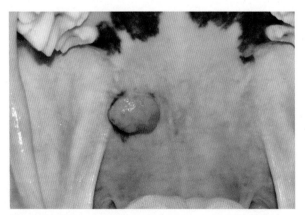

Fig. 2.41 This young patient has an oral viral papilloma, which is in the process of resorbing.

Fig. 2.42 Pyogenic granuloma after extraction of right mandibular molar.

maxillary fourth premolar after extraction of the mandibular molar. Extraction of the left maxillary fourth premolar and removal of the lesion provided relief. As these lesions resemble neoplasia, biopsy is recommended.

Gingival Hyperplasia

Gingival hyperplasia (GH), the proliferation of normal gingival cells, is common among some breeds, particularly the collie, boxer, and cocker spaniel. Pocket formation and periodontal disease may result from this hyperplastic tissue. Fig. 2.43 shows GH of the entire left maxilla. The first premolar and supernumerary first premolar are completely covered. This can also occur secondary to certain drugs such as cyclosporine and amlodipine. In the case of drug-induced GH, the tissue often appears more friable than that with the familial form.

Peripheral Odontogenic Fibroma

Peripheral odontogenic fibroma (OM/POF) (previously known as fibromatous epulis) is characterized by the presence of a tumor associated with the gingiva containing primarily fibrous tissues that resemble periodontal ligament tissue typically with odontogenic epithelium and often bone-like tissue. Generally, OM/POF (Fig. 2.44) responds well to excision; however, it may return if the excision

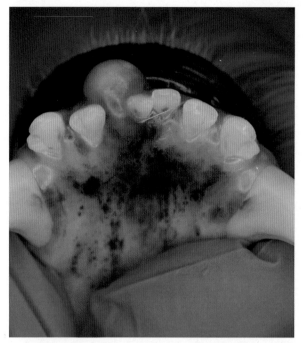

Fig. 2.44 POF of rostral mandibles of a dog.

is incomplete. Typically, if the associated tooth is extracted at the time of tumor removal, the tumor will not return. Enough bone-like mineralization may be present to give the lesion a hard texture. This variation had previously been called an ossifying epulis.

Odontomas

Odontomas (OM/OD) are a mass of cells that have enamel, dentin, cementum, and small tooth-like structures. Masses with characteristics resembling normal teeth are considered compound OM/OD. Complex odontomas (OM/ODX) have a more disorganized arrangement. Although these can be fairly extensive and invasive, conservative excision is usually successful. Fig. 2.45A shows a complex odontoma that involves the lower mandible and its radiograph (Fig. 2.45B).

Ulcerative Eosinophilic Stomatitis

Ulcerative eosinophilic stomatitis is a disease of King Charles Spaniels. The lesions tend to be focal

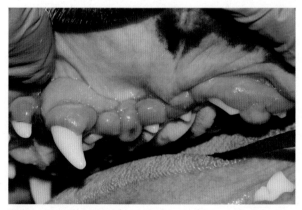

Fig. 2.43 Gingival hyperplasia tends to run along familial lines.

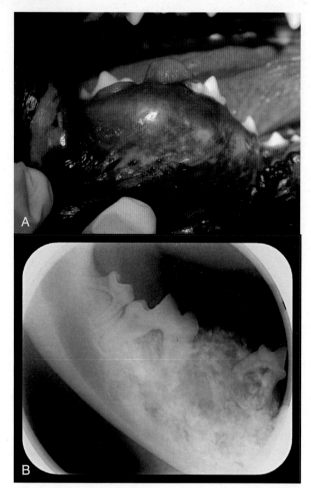

Fig. 2.45 (A) and (B) Compound odontoma of the right mandible in a young dog. Note the presence of "denticles" in the radiograph.

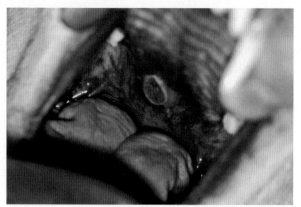

Fig. 2.46 Eosinophilic palatitis in a King Charles spaniel.

raised areas on the palate, but histologically they do not exhibit granuloma formation. The cause of the lesions is unknown (Fig. 2.46).

Clinically Aggressive Tumors
Acanthomatous Ameloblastoma

The *acanthomatous ameloblastoma* (OM/AA) is primarily composed of proliferating epithelial cells of suspected dental origin associated with the tissue. Although they are classified as benign, these tumors tend to invade bone, which makes dental radiographic evaluation and aggressive surgery important. Fig. 2.47 is an OM/AA that has formed in the region of the left maxillary fourth premolar and first molar. This tumor is seen somewhat frequently in dogs and rarely in cats. The most common location to find this in the dog is the rostral mandibles, particularly the incisor region.

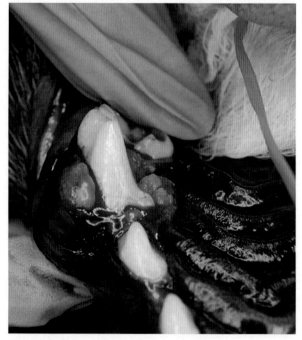

Fig. 2.47 Acanthomatous ameloblastoma of the left maxillary fourth premolar in a dog.

Acanthomatous ameloblastoma had previously been called acanthomatous epulis. This term is no longer used. Some pathologists will separate OM/AA into conventional ameloblastoma and canine OM/AA. This is based on certain microscopic features and does not necessarily change treatment recommendations.

Plasma Cell Tumor

Plasma cell tumor (OM/PCT) is a locally aggressive tumor. A CT scan will help to delineate the tumor; wide excision is indicated (Fig. 2.48). It is not known to be metastatic in dogs (not reported in cats). In humans, it is associated with multiple myeloma, and urine protein electrophoresis is recommended to rule out a monoclonal gammopathy that could indicate multiple myeloma. If an increase in total proteins or globulin is noted in serum chemistry, it may be prudent to assess urine in canine patients for a monoclonal gammopathy.

Malignant Tumors

Squamous cell carcinoma. Squamous cell carcinoma (OM/SCC) is a tumor of the epithelial tissue and can arise in a variety of locations in the mouth. SCCs can occur in tonsillar crypts and the gingiva. Tonsillar SCC generally has a poor prognosis.

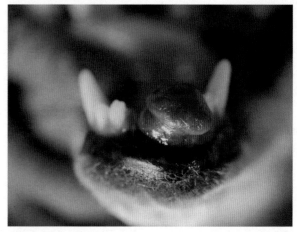

Fig. 2.49 Squamous cell carcinoma of the rostral left mandible of a dog.

Gingival SCC can have a good prognosis in dogs if completely excised. The appearance is typically smooth to irregular and ulcerated with pink to red tissue. The tumor in Fig. 2.49 is an SCC of an adult dog. On complete excision, the long-term prognosis is good.

SCC can affect young dogs as well. Fig. 2.50 demonstrates an SCC of the right maxilla in a juvenile dog. Papillary OM/SCC is a variant of SCC, which was once thought to be limited to young dogs. Although it often occurs in dogs under

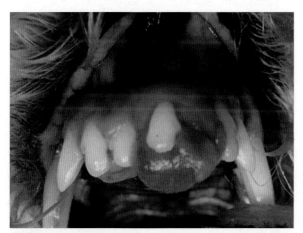

Fig. 2.48 Plasmacytoma. This patient has an extramedullary plasmacytoma, which required surgeries to resolve. (Courtesy Dr. Dae Hyun Kwon.)

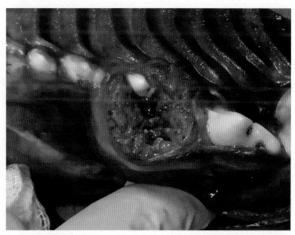

Fig. 2.50 Papillary squamous cell carcinoma of a juvenile dog.

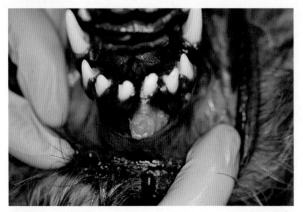

Fig. 2.51 Papillary squamous cell carcinoma of a mature dog.

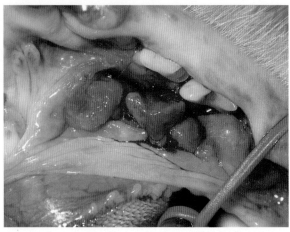

Fig. 2.53 Sublingual squamous cell carcinoma of a cat.

9 months of age, it has also been noted in mature patients. The patient in Fig. 2.51 is a mature dog with a papillary SCC. With aggressive surgical treatment, it can still be completely excised in the dog with a low risk of recurrence.

Squamous cell carcinoma of the cat generally has a poor prognosis as local recurrence is typical. Fig. 2.52 shows a radiograph of OM/SCC of the right mandible of a cat. The prognosis is poor. It is not uncommon to find lingual and sublingual SCC in the cat as shown in Fig. 2.53.

Fibrosarcoma

Fibrosarcoma (OM/FS) is a tumor of the fibroblasts occurring in the mandible or maxilla (Fig. 2.54). They may create fleshy, protruding, and firm masses that sometimes are friable. As the masses grow, they

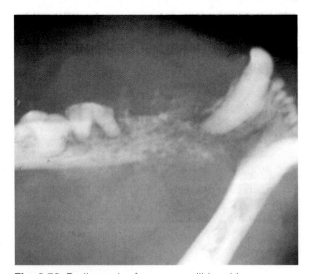

Fig. 2.52 Radiograph of a cat mandible with squamous cell carcinoma.

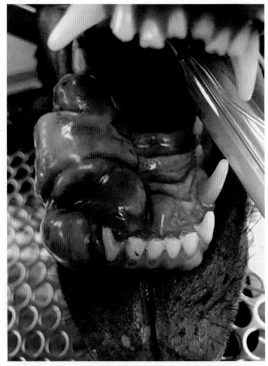

Fig. 2.54 Fibrosarcoma of left maxilla of a dog.

can become ulcerated and infected. Typically, it is the local growth that becomes the problem rather than the spreading of this tumor to the lymph nodes or lungs. Recurrence after excision is common and often postsurgical radiation is warranted. A variation called a high biologic grade low histologic grade OM/FS exists and can appear histologically benign while behaving as a malignant neoplasm.

Malignant Melanoma

Malignant melanoma (OM/MM) is a malignancy of the melanocytes and occurs on any site in the oral cavity: gingiva, buccal mucosa, hard and soft palates, tonsils, and tongue. They are locally invasive and highly metastatic to the lungs, regional lymph nodes, and bone. As with many malignancies, clients may first notice a minor change such as bad breath oral bleeding. These can appear darkly pigmented or nonpigmented. The prognosis is guarded because recurrence and metastasis are common. With advances in special histopathologic staining, such as Ki-67 immunolabeling, a clearer picture of prognosis may be available. Fig. 2.55 shows a OM/MM of the maxilla. The Oncept vaccine may help extend the lifespan of canine patients who have had successful surgical excision of oral melanoma. The available data is not consistent across studies.

Lymphoma/Lymphosarcoma

In the dog, cutaneous epitheliotropic T-cell lymphosarcoma (OM/LS) occurs in patients over 10 years of age, but it may or not be associated with dermatalogic disease (Fig. 2.56). In the mouth, there is inflammation, increased blood flow, and an irregular surface. Differential diagnoses include autoimmune diseases, such as PV, LE, and periodontal disease. Diagnosis is made by histopathology of the affected site, which may be the gingiva, lip, or tongue.

Lymphoma can also manifest in the tonsil as it is a lymphoid tissue. This appears more as a solid tonsillar mass or tonsillar enlargement.

Mast Cell Tumor

Mast cell tumors (OM/MCT) are the most common cutaneous tumors of dogs; however, they are rarely found in the oral cavity. MCT in the oral cavity can demonstrate an aggressive clinical course. They have a high incidence of lymph node metastasis at the time of diagnosis that results in a poor prognosis. Despite a more aggressive clinical course, treatment can result in remission.

Multilobular Tumor of Bone

Multilobular tumor of bone (OM/MTB) may produce bone and/or cartilage. There are several

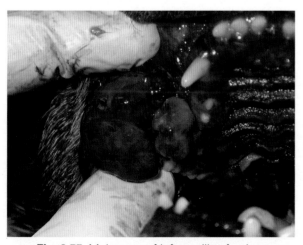

Fig. 2.55 Melanoma of left maxilla of a dog.

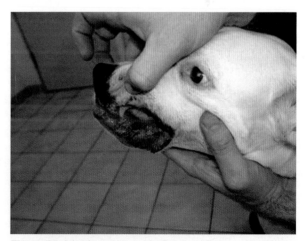

Fig. 2.56 Multicentric epithelial lymphoma. A 13-year-old neutered Pitbull, the tumor had been present for 1.5 years. (Courtesy Dr. David Miller.)

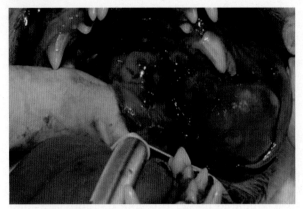

Fig. 2.57 Maxillary multilobular osteochondroma bellows. A 4-year-old dog with a left-sided swollen orbit unable to open its mouth.

names for this type of tumor and OM/MTB is the currently recognized name by the AVDC. It is a slowly progressive neoplasm that compresses adjacent structures. Metastasis is rare but can occur. Local recurrence can be expected in about 50% of surgically excised cases (Fig. 2.57).

Salivary Gland Adenocarcinoma

Salivary gland adenocarcinomas (SG/ADC) are rare in cats and dogs; by the time they are diagnosed, they have already metastasized to the lymph nodes. Treatment may include surgical excision, radiotherapy, and chemotherapy. Even with these treatments, the prognosis cannot be predicted.

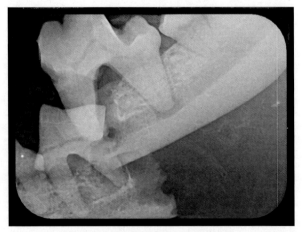

Fig. 2.58 Fracture of left mandible.

Other Traumatic Oral Conditions
Fractures of the Jaws

Facial trauma from fights, motor vehicle accidents, falls, and other miscellaneous traumas lead to pain, inability or difficulty eating, and without successful treatment, chronic pain and discomfort. These may present as fractures of the mandible (MN/FX) (Fig. 2.58), fractures of the maxilla (MX/FX), symphyseal separation (SYM/S), luxation of the TMJ (TMJ/LUX), or a combination of any of these conditions. The goal of treating these conditions is extraction of compromised teeth, re-establishing the patient's normal occlusion, and maintaining fixation until the tissues heal. Treatment methods vary based on location and the operator's experience.

Separation of the mandibular symphysis is not a fracture but a tear in the fibrocartilage and ligaments between the rostral portion of the right and left mandibles. This most often occurs in the cat.

Temporomandibular joint luxation can present as the inability to close the mouth or MAL. This often occurs secondary to trauma. It is rare in the dog and more common in the cat. These can be diagnosed by very well-positioned radiographs, but CT assessment is preferred as it may reveal other pathology not obvious on the radiographs. Differential diagnosis includes neoplasia, MAL, and fracture of the mandibles or temporal bone. Note that TMJ luxation is much less common than fractures of the ramus in the cat, which often mimics a luxation clinically. To that point, a definitive diagnosis must be made before attempting repair of a TMJ luxation as the standard treatment of a luxation will not treat a fracture and may lead to additional trauma to the patient. These conditions are summarized in Box 2.2.

BOX 2.2   Conditions Which Mimic TMJ Luxation
Ramus fracture
Symphyseal separation
Luxation of maxillary canine tooth
Mesioversion of maxillary canine tooth

Ballistic Trauma

Ballistic oral trauma (TMA/B) is typically due to missile projectiles such as air rifles and firearms and less commonly due to other ranged weapons such as bow and arrow. The extent of the trauma may be minimal (such as low-powered bird shot) or severe that is often the case with many handguns and rifles. Affected oral tissues include oral mucosa, teeth, and bone and often can extend to adjacent structures such as the sinuses and periorbital and orbital structures. Patient triage in the acute presentation is extremely important to rule out adjacent trauma to vital structures that may take priority over oral tissues. Often these are incidental findings if low velocity/low power ballistics are the cause. Treatment of oral trauma includes soft tissue repair, treatment of fractured teeth, and stabilization of maxillofacial fractures. Removal of lead remnants is not typically necessary.

Electric Cord Shock

Trauma caused by chewing electric cords (TMA/E) may not be discovered for days or even months after the injury. Soft tissue injury to the palate, jaws, cheeks, and lips often occurs as does injury to the nearby bone. Affected teeth typically become necrotic. In an emergent situation, the patient should be monitored for the development of noncardiogenic pulmonary edema. The treatment of the oral wounds is typically delayed for 2 to 3 weeks to allow the full extent of the injuries to present. While delaying treatment, supportive care in the form of broad-spectrum antibiotics and pain control is recommended. The final treatment may be as simple as the extraction of the compromised teeth to involve soft tissue and bone debridement with soft tissue reconstruction.

Foreign Bodies

Foreign bodies (FB) are sometimes caught on the tooth or trapped in the oral cavity. Rubber bands may be wrapped around teeth, and bones may become lodged between teeth. The retention of this foreign material can cause infection and even tooth loss.

Mandibular Lip Avulsion

Traumatic lip T/A injuries occur because of caudal force applied to the lip and gingiva. This can be caused by automobiles, falls, bite wounds, trauma from objects, and several other causes.

CHAPTER 2 WORKSHEET (ANSWERS ON PAGE 294)

1. _____ orthodontics is the process of extracting primary teeth when it appears that they will cause orthodontic malocclusions and _____ is the extraction of teeth to treat an established malocclusion.
2. In what breed does craniomandibular osteopathy occur primarily?
3. A class _____ malocclusion is said to occur when the jaws are of normal length but teeth are abnormally aligned.
4. _____ is inflammation of the gingiva.
5. The inflammation of the periodontal tissues other than the gingiva and the loss of the tissues is known as _____.
6. _____ results from the friction of teeth against an external object such as hair or a tennis ball.
7. _____ occurs as the result of the friction of teeth against each other.
8. _____ is the result of inadequate deposition of the enamel matrix and can result from conditions that cause a temporary debilitation of the patient, such as high fever.
9. _____ is the treatment of disease associated with the pulp of the tooth.
10. A fracture that has penetrated enamel and dentin and exposed the pulp chamber should be treated by _____ or _____.

11. Purple discoloration indicates _____.
12. A _____ is the partial displacement of the tooth from its socket.
13. _____ is a condition common to cats (but occurs rarely in dogs) in which the mineralized dental tissue is resorbed by odontoclasts, leading to pain and inflammation.
14. _____ is a communication between the nasal sinus and oral cavity.
15. Boxers commonly develop a lesion known as _____, which is a proliferation of normal gingival cells.
16. Formerly known as a fibromatous epulis, _____ is a benign tumor of the gingiva that can have mineralization within the tumor.
17. _____ is a painful inflammatory condition in dogs, which was once known as CUPS.
18. A locally aggressive lesion of the jaws that is often found in the rostral mandibles of the dog and is not malignant is the _____.
19. _____ has a good prognosis if present in the gingiva of the dog and is completely excised but has a poor prognosis in cats.
20. A tear in the fibrocartilage of the connection of the rostral portion of the mandibles is known as _____.

FURTHER READING

Hale FA. Localized intrinsic staining of teeth due to pulpitis and pulp necrosis in dogs. *J Vet Dent.* 2001;18(1):14–20. doi:10.1177/089875640101800102.

Feigin K, Bell C, Shope B, Henzel S, Snyder C. Analysis and assessment of pulp vitality of 102 intrinsically stained teeth in dogs. *J Vet Dent.* 2022;39(1):21–33. doi:10.1177/08987564211060387.

Ford KR, Anderson JG, Stapleton BL, et al. Medical management of canine chronic ulcerative stomatitis using cyclosporine and metronidazole. *J Vet Dent.* 2023;40(2):109–124. doi:10.1177/08987564221148755.

Dental Instruments and Equipment

LEARNING OBJECTIVES

When you have completed this chapter, you will be able to:

- List the hand instruments used in veterinary dentistry and describe the structure and purpose of each.

- Describe the materials used for sharpening hand dental instruments and explain the technique used to sharpen them.
- Explain the principle utilized by the ultrasonic scaler and differentiate between magnetostrictive and piezoelectric devices.

- Differentiate between sonic and rotary scalers.
- Differentiate between electric-powered and air-powered dental polishing units.
- Discuss the types of air-compressor systems used in veterinary dentistry and describe the care of the systems.

- Differentiate between the uses and care of low-speed and high-speed handpieces.
- List and describe the types and uses of burs available for low-speed handpieces.

KEY TERMS

Arkansas stone
Calculus removal forceps
Conical stone
Curette
Dental bur
Explorer
Flat stone
Handle
High-speed handpiece

India stone
Low-speed handpiece
Periodontal probe
Piezoelectric ultrasonic scalers
Pigtail explorer
Power scaler
Rotary scaler
Scaler
Shank

Sonic scaler
Terminal shank
Three-way syringe
Torque
Turbine
Ultrasonic ferroceramic rod
Ultrasonic instrument
Ultrasonic stacks
Working end

Many instruments used in general surgery are also used in veterinary dentistry. Nonetheless, there is a plethora of dentistry-specific instruments and equipment as well as modifications of common surgical instruments. This chapter is devoted to the use and maintenance of instruments and equipment required for the prevention and treatment of periodontal disease and basic oral surgery. The equipment and materials required for dental radiology and advanced procedures are discussed in subsequent chapters.

ORGANIZATION OF THE DENTAL DEPARTMENT

Given the variety and number of instruments each dental procedure necessitates, a comprehensive organization system is required. Organizing the dental equipment into trays that can be pulled from the shelf as needed is a very efficient method of organizing dental equipment (Fig. 3.1A and B). Cassettes, kidney pans, and other containers that can be steam-sterilized are

also useful (Fig. 3.2A and B). Keeping packs of similar use identical instruments will not only aid in assuring all items are within the pack or tray but also aid the operator as he or she will always know what items are available and will not have to use mental energy to ask for additional instruments. To this part, using coded stickers or bands with each instrument pack will aid in making sure all packs are reassembled correctly. When using bands, keep in mind that band placement may affect the operation of the instrument, such as if the band is placed near the box lock of hinged instruments.

Photographs of each instrument, its name, use, and location can be kept in a binder to allow for quick identification. Alternately, this information can be kept electronically. The latter method allows for easy updating when including current inventory and equipment currently out for repair or maintenance. Labeling cabinets by contents and keeping materials and equipment grouped by use can help the team find instruments quickly.

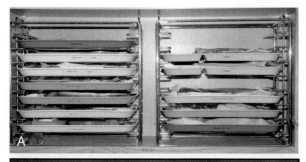

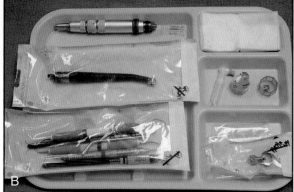

Fig. 3.1 (A) Trays are organized in racks on a shelf in the operatory. (B) Prophy tray set up for use.

PERIODONTAL INSTRUMENTS

Hand Instruments

Veterinary technicians and practitioners use four main types of hand instruments during cleaning and prophylaxis; the periodontal probe, explorer, scaler, and curette (Fig. 3.3). Most instruments have four specific parts: handle, shank, terminal shank, and working end. *Handles*, the parts that are grasped, come in a variety of round, tapered, and hexagonal shapes. The best handle shape for the procedure depends on individual preference. The *shank* joins the working end with the handle. The length and curvature of the shank determines the teeth that the instrument will be able to access. The *terminal shank* is the part of the shank that is closest to the working end. The *working end* of the instrument is the portion that comes in contact with the tooth.

Explorers

Although explorers and periodontal probes are two different types of instruments, they are usually

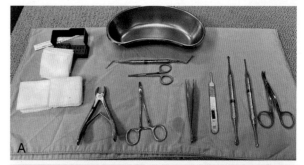

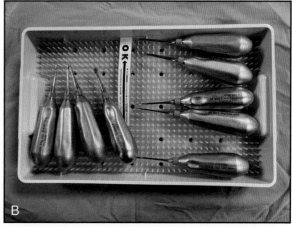

Fig. 3.2 (A and B) Feline elevator/luxator set in sterilizable cassette.

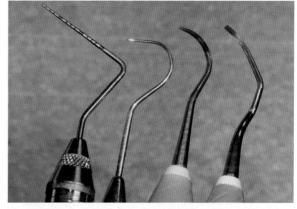

Fig. 3.3 Types of hand instruments: periodontal probe, Shepherd's hook, scaler, and curette.

manufactured as double-ended instruments. One end is the periodontal probe, and the other end is the explorer. *Explorers* are sharp instruments used to detect plaque and calculus. They are also used to explore cavities and check for exposed pulp chambers. The design of the explorer increases the operator's tactile sensitivity.

No. 23 Explorer

The No. 23 explorer, commonly called the shepherd's hook (or crook), is the most commonly found explorer (Fig. 3.4). It is typically found in combination with the periodontal probe.

Pigtail Explorer

A *pigtail explorer* is a curved explorer that allows the operator to glide along the tooth surface in search of irregularities and magnifies the user's tactile sense (Fig. 3.5). Pigtail explorers usually come hooked to the right on one end and to the left on the other, allowing for a greater range of exploration.

Periodontal Probes

Periodontal probes are used to measure the depth of the gingival sulcus or periodontal pocket (depending on the case) and to measure oral lesions of a diameter of less than a centimeter. Many types of periodontal probes are available. Box 3.1 lists some commonly used probes. The probes shown in Fig. 3.6 are two commonly used probes with different measurements. One is the Marquis color-coded probe (Fig. 3.6A), which is marked in 3-mm graduations.

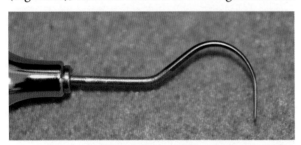

Fig. 3.4 Shepherd's hook explorer.

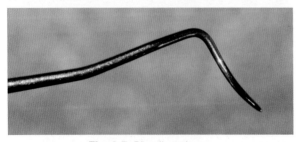

Fig. 3.5 Pigtail explorer.

> ### BOX 3.1   Periodontal Probes and Markings (mm)
>
> Marquis Color Coded Probe: 3, 6, 9, 12
> UNC 15 Probe: 1, 2, 3, 4, 5, 6, 7, 8, 9, 10, 11, 12, 13, 14, 15
> Williams Probe: 1, 2, 3, 5, 7, 8, 9, 10

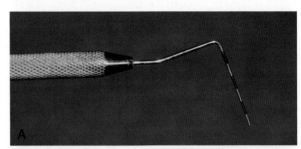

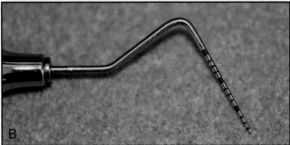

Fig. 3.6 (A) Banded periodontal probe. (B) Notched periodontal probe.

The other is the Williams probe which is marked in 1, 2, 3, 5, 7, 8, 9 and 10 mm (Fig. 3.6B). This probe allows for more precise measurement in the cat.

HAND MIRROR

A hand mirror should be kept in every basic prophylaxis kit and advanced periodontal pack (Fig. 3.7). These are necessary for complete visualization every dental surface and are useful for retracting tissues during scaling and polishing. Often the operator will be frustrated due to mirror fogging during use. A simple solution is to warm the mirror against the buccal mucosa for ten seconds before use.

Calculus Removal Forceps

The calculus removal forceps allows for quick removal of large pieces of calculus (Fig. 3.8). The

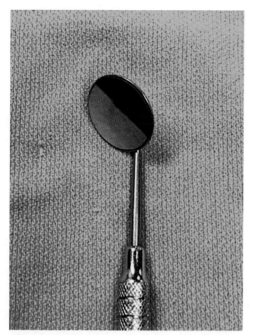

Fig. 3.7 A hand mirror is used both for diagnostic purposes and as a retraction device.

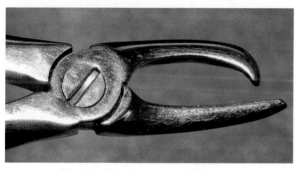

Fig. 3.8 Calculus removal forceps.

instrument has tips of different lengths and shapes. The longer tip is placed over the crown, and the shorter tip is placed under the calculus. Calculus is sheared off the tooth when the two parts of the handle are brought together. When using this instrument, the technician or practitioner must be careful not to damage the enamel surface or gingiva.

Hand Scalers

Scalers are sharp instruments used to remove supragingival calculus (calculus above the gumline). These have two sharp sides and a sharp tip on the working end and generally have two working ends. They are particularly useful in removing calculus from narrow but deep fissures such as those located on the buccal surface of the fourth premolar. Because they may damage the gingiva and periodontal ligament, scalers should not be used subgingivally.

Scalers have a sharp point or a tip (T). The face (F) is the flat side of the instrument between the two cutting edges. The cutting edge (C), the working portion of the scaler, is the confluence of the face and the sides (Fig. 3.9). To be effective, scalers must be sharpened regularly.

Several types of scalers exist (Fig. 3.10). The scaler in the middle of Fig. 3.10, generally called a *sickle scaler*, is most commonly used. The ends

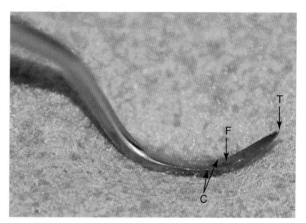

Fig. 3.9 Parts of a scaler: *F*, face; *C*, cutting edge; and *T*, tip.

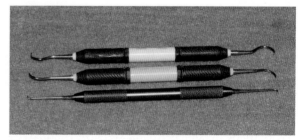

Fig. 3.10 The scaler at the top has a sickle scaler on one end and a 33 on the other. The scaler in the middle is a sickle scaler, with each end being a mirror image of the other. The instrument on the bottom is a fine scaler for extremely small teeth. It is known as Morris 0-00.

of this scaler are mirror images of each other. Depending on the manufacturer, sickle scalers are denoted H6/7, S6/7, or N6/7. The scaler at the top of Fig. 3.10 has a sickle scaler on one end and a #33 scaler on the other. The instrument on the bottom of Fig. 3.10 is a fine scaler for extremely small teeth. It is known as Morris 0-00.

Hand scalers may be universal or area-specific. Universal scalers have the face of the instrument perpendicular to the terminal shank, allowing both sides of the working end to be used for scaling. Area-specific scalers have the face offset, and usually, the two working ends are mirror images of each other, allowing adaptation to opposite surfaces.

Curettes

Curettes have two sharp sides and a round toe. They are used to remove calculus subgingivally. The tip of the curette, called the *toe* (T), is rounded. The *face* (F) of the curette is the concave side. The *cutting edge* (C) is the confluence of the sides and the face. Curettes have a round back (Fig. 3.11). A comparison of the rounded toe of the curette to the pointed tip of the scaler is shown in Fig. 3.12.

Like some scalers, curettes are designed so that each end is a mirror image of the opposite end. This allows adaptation to the curved dental surface. If one end does not appear to be adapting to the curvature of the tooth, the instrument can be rotated. As with hand scalers, curettes may be universal or area-specific such as the Gracey curette. Curettes may be purchased as individual instruments or as a set.

Curette and Scaler Care

The best practice is to sharpen each instrument after cleaning and disinfecting and before every use. Heavy-duty industrial gloves should be used while cleaning instruments. Alternatively, ultrasonic instrument cleaners may be used. Ideally, the operator should have several instrument packs to clean, sharpen, and sterilize the instruments between uses. Although dental procedures are not sterile, sterilization reduces the risks of cross-infection among patients and from patients

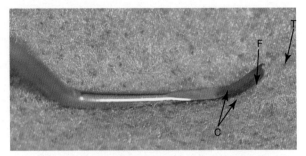

Fig. 3.11 The point of the curette, called the toe (*T*), is rounded. The face (*F*) of the curette is the concave side. The cutting edge (*C*) is the confluence of the sides and the face. Curettes have a round back.

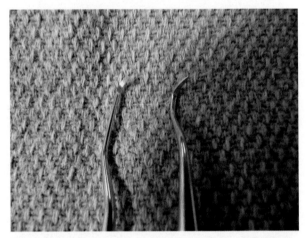

Fig. 3.12 Dental curette on left and scaler on right.

to staff members (e.g., if staff members accidentally injure themselves with the instrument).

Testing for Sharpness

Visual inspection. The edge of the instrument can be visually inspected with a bright light. The instrument is held and rotated toward the light source. If the instrument is dull, the edge is rounded and reflects light. If the instrument is sharp, the edge does not reflect light.

Sharpening stick. A sharpening stick is an acrylic or plastic rod (Fig. 3.13). A syringe casing may also be used to check for sharpness. To test, the edge of the instrument is drawn across the rod. A dull blade glides over the surface without catching

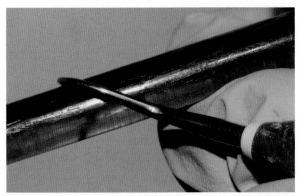

Fig. 3.13 An acrylic rod may be used to check for sharpness. The instrument should "catch" when dragged along the rod.

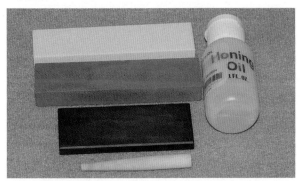

Fig. 3.14 A variety of stones and oil are necessary to sharpen instruments. *Top*, Arkansas stone; *Top middle*, India stone; *Lower middle*, ceramic stone; *Bottom*, conical stone.

at it. Conversely, a sharp blade easily catches as the instrument is drawn against the surface of the sharpening stick.

Sharpening Equipment

Stones. Several types of stones are available for sharpening (Fig. 3.14). An *India stone* is made of aluminum oxide and used for the "coarse" sharpening of an overly dull instrument or for changing the plane of one or more of the sides of the instrument. The *Arkansas stone* is a natural stone used for the final sharpening of an instrument that is already close to sharpness. Sharpening with the India stone is followed by the Arkansas stone. Both the Arkansas and the India stones require oil for effective use.

The ceramic stone may also be used for fine sharpening. With ceramic stones, water is generally used as the sharpening medium instead of oil. A conical stone is a round Arkansas stone. It is used to provide a final sharpening to the instrument by working on its face.

Sharpening Technique

Flat stone. A *flat stone* is a rectangular-shaped stone that can be hand-held or kept flat on the workbench. With the first technique, the instrument is held motionless and the stone is moved. Because the edge of the instrument is stationary, the blade is highly visible during sharpening. The second method is to move the instrument against a stationary stone (Fig. 3.15A and B). Because the moving instrument technique is less difficult, it is the method demonstrated in this text.

A few drops of sharpening (or mineral) oil are placed on the sharpening stone (Fig. 3.16). The oil is spread out evenly over the stone with tissue paper (Fig. 3.16). The stone must be lightly coated with oil.

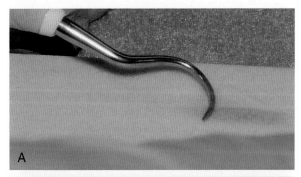

A

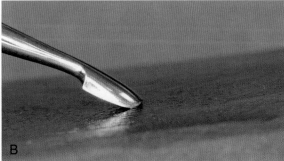

B

Fig. 3.15 (A) Curettes and hands scalers may be sharpened with a flat stone (B) dental elevators may be sharpened with a flat stone as well.

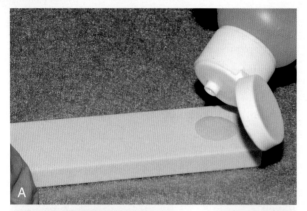

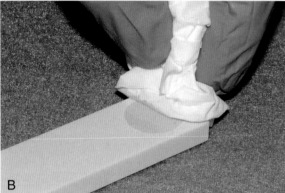

Fig. 3.16 A drop of oil is placed on the stone (A); the oil is then wiped off the stone (B).

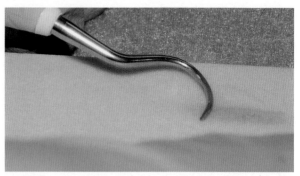

Fig. 3.17 The stone is held firmly against the edge of a table.

The technician must be careful not to wipe off the oil while attempting to spread it. The first step in sharpening the instrument is to hold it firmly against the edge of a table, with the tip facing the operator. The instrument is rotated so that the face is parallel to the ground. This position provides a reference point for the adaptation of the stone (Fig. 3.17).

The stone is held with the thumb and index finger at the top and bottom of the stone (Fig. 3.18).

The operator should exercise caution; the instrument is sharp and can easily cause injury. The stone is first placed at a 90-degree angle to the face of the instrument or straight up and down (Fig. 3.19A).

The upper portion of the stone is rotated approximately 10 to 15 degrees away from the instrument or to the 11 or 1 o'clock positions (Fig. 3.19B). This creates a 75- to 80-degree angle at the edge of the instrument.

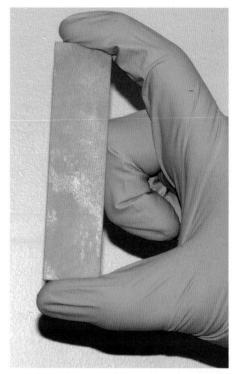

Fig. 3.18 The stone is held with the thumb and index finger at the top and bottom of the stone.

The stone is moved up and down approximately 1 inch. As the stone is moved down, a "flashing" should be observed on the face of the instrument. The flashing consists of stone oil, stone particles, and instrument particles (Fig. 3.20).

As the stone moves up, the flashing should recoat the stone. If the stone is tipped too much (e.g.,

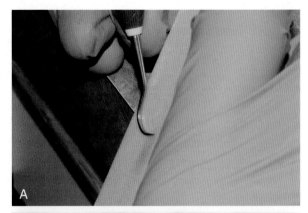

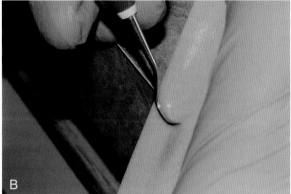

Fig. 3.19 (A) The instrument is placed so that the face is 90 degrees to the stone. (B) It is then rotated outward 10 to 15 degrees.

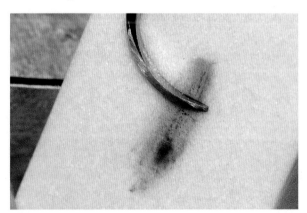

Fig. 3.20 If held at the proper angle, a flashing will be noted on the up stroke.

the top of the stone is before 11 o'clock or past 1 o'clock), the stone will miss the convergence of the face of the instrument and the side, and the blade

will not be sharpened. If the stone is tipped too little (e.g., the top is toward 12 o'clock), the blade may become dull. The sharpening should end on the down stroke, which helps prevent the formation of a bur on the sharpened edge.

A Gleason guide is a jig that can be placed on a flat stone and aids in maintaining the proper angle for sharpening both universal and area-specific instruments (Fig. 3.21). Resting the terminal shank on the guide and moving the instrument in a pendulum motion will sharpen the instrument on a consistent angle. One must pay attention to use the correct side (universal vs. area-specific).

Conical stone. The conical stone is rolled over the face (Fig. 3.22). Overuse of this technique shortens the life of the instrument, the strength of which lies in the direction from the face to the back. If the face is removed, the instrument becomes weaker. The advantage of sharpening with a flat stone is that the strength of the instrument is maintained even as the sides of the instrument become worn.

Rx honing machine. This unit simplifies sharpening. It consists of the following: a diamond disk to sharpen extremely dull instruments; a carbide disk used to maintain an edge with the removal of a minimal amount of metal; a round hone to sharpen explorers and spoons; a U-shaped hone to round off the edge of curettes and keep them sharp.

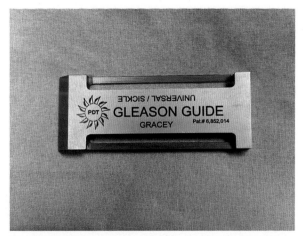

Fig. 3.21 Gleason guides can be used as a jig to keep the proper angle during sharpening scalers and curettes.

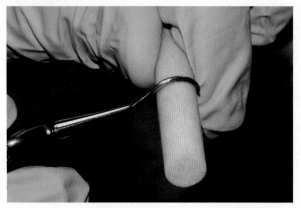

Fig. 3.22 Conical stones may be used for light sharpening of a curette.

A Perio & Scissors Guide is used to establish the angle at which the instruments should be sharpened (Fig. 3.23). With practice, it can be used to maintain instruments of exodontia as well.

Sharpening resources and practice. As sharpening is not thoroughly taught in veterinary or technician school, visual resources are often needed to understand the techniques. Fortunately, with internet services such as YouTube, dozens of videos are available to help the new student. It is recommended to watch several videos on the same subject.

One may keep older instruments to practice with. It is not recommended to practice on valuable instruments that are still in operatory circulation.

Powered Instruments for Periodontal Care

Power scalers. *Power scalers* convert electric or pneumatic energy into mechanical vibration

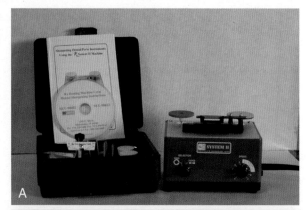

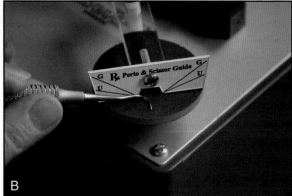

Fig. 3.23 A, The Rx Honing Machine system sharpening unit, with manual and DVD. B, Universal sharpening device. The terminal shank of the Universal curette is lined up with the "U Line" of the Universal scaler. (Courtesy Rx Honing. Mishawaka, Indiana.)

(Table 3.1). Pneumatic scalers are both rotary scalers and sonic scalers, which are rarely used and have been largely removed from this edition of the

TABLE 3.1	**Comparison of Mechanical Scalers**			
Instrument Type	**Cycles per Second**	**Amplitude (mm)**	**Active Tip (mm)**	**Motion**
Magnetostrictive: metal strips	18,000, 25,000, 30,000	0.01–0.05	5–7	Elliptic
Magnetostrictive: ferroceramic rod	42,000	0.01–0.02	13	Circular
Piezoelectric	25,000–45,000	0.2	3	Linear (back and forth)
Sonic	6000	0.5		Elliptic
Rotary			Depends on tip	Circular

text. When the power scaler is placed against calculus, the vibration shatters it, freeing it from the tooth surface. Power scalers operate in the range of 6000 to 50,000 cycles per second. There are three types of power instruments: ultrasonic, sonic, and rotary. Rotary scalers are not recommended for the reasons covered ahead. The ultrasonic and sonic scalers both use irrigation, which in addition to aiding in cooling the working end of the instrument, also affects bacteria and biofilm in a way to decrease bacterial accumulation.

Ultrasonic Instruments

Ultrasonic instruments work by converting electric energy into kinetic energy. Two types of devices in the handpiece can pick up the sound wave and turn it into a vibration: *magnetostrictive* and *piezoelectric*. Magnetostrictive devices use either a ferroceramic rod or metal strips.

Magnetostrictive

Ultrasonic metal strips/stacks. Ultrasonic stacks are metal stacks welded at one end with the working end at the other. When activated, the metal stacks vibrate, creating a kinetic movement of the tip of the working end. The movement is an elliptical pattern. The amplitude of tip movement in these units is between 0.01mm and 0.05 mm, which is an extremely narrow motion. Generally, lower amplitudes are better because they cause less damage to the tooth. Two lengths of inserts are available, which is important to remember when ordering and inserting them into the handpiece (Fig. 3.24). Over time, the stacks separate, necessitating replacement (Fig. 3.25).

Ultrasonic ferroceramic rod. Magnetostrictive ferroceramic rods vibrate and create a circular-type motion at the tip with an amplitude of 0.01 to 0.02 mm. All sides of the tip are equally active (about 13 mm of the tip). The rods are prone to damage if not handled carefully and should be kept protected when not in use.

Inserting ultrasonic inserts. If an ultrasonic stack unit is used, the unit must be turned on and

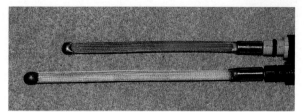

Fig. 3.24 The upper shorter metal strip unit is 30K (30,000 cycles per second), and the lower longer unit is 25K (25,000 cycles per second).

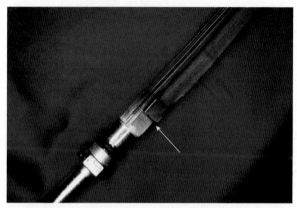

Fig. 3.25 Because of use, this ultrasonic tip has fractured at the weld (*arrow*) and should be replaced.

the handpiece filled with water before insertion. However, with ferroceramic rod units, the handpiece should be drained before insertion of the insert. Forcing the insert into a handpiece that contains water may prevent it from vibrating or cause the tip to fracture.

Piezoelectric

Piezoelectric ultrasonic scalers use crystals in the handpiece to pick up the vibration (Fig. 3.26).

The amplitude of these units is approximately 0.2 mm, which results in a wide, linear-tip motion. The motion of the piezo tip is not uniform. The tip moves farther in one direction than in the other, which means that during use the most active side of the tip must be placed on the part of the tooth where the calculus is to be removed. These tips do wear over time and need to be replaced. The amount of wear should be checked regularly (Fig. 3.27).

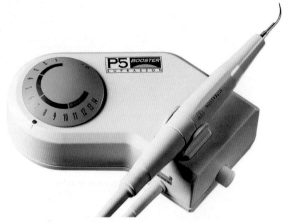

Fig. 3.26 Piezoelectric scaler. (Courtesy Dentalaire, CA, USA.)

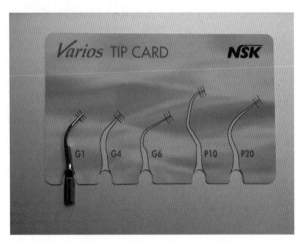

Fig. 3.27 Gauges can be used to check for excessive wear of piezo tips. Once the tip is worn past its recommended length, it should be replaced.

Power settings. The vibrational energy of the ultrasonic scaler can be adjusted through the power settings. Generally lower settings are used subgingivally and higher settings supragingivally. The operator should adhere by the manufacturer's guidelines for each unit.

Irrigating Solutions

Piezoelectric and magnetostrictive units have reservoirs for irrigation during operation. Irrigation not only serves to reduce the heat of the scaler tip, but may also help decrease bacterial load. Most commonly, distilled water is used. A variety of solutions may be placed in the reservoir. The most popular and effective solution is 0.12% chlorhexidine.

When using distilled water, there is potential for the contamination of the waterlines within the equipment. This contamination can affect performance over time and serves as a reservoir for pathogenic transmission to patients. Colloidal silver tablets can be placed in the water reservoir each time it is filled to decrease this risk.

The water flow can be adjusted on these units. It should be set to allow a fine mist of irrigation spray at the tip (Fig. 3.28).

Ultrasonic Tips

As shown in the tip on the top in Fig. 3.29, the beaver-tail tip is relatively wide. This tip was the first type of tip developed, and it is used for supragingival cleaning. The bottom tip is thin and can be used subgingivally on a lower power setting. Furcation tips hook to the left or right, which allows them to gain access to furcations around crowns and be used subgingivally.

Sonic and Rotary Scalers

Sonic scalers are powered instruments that use air to activate the working end and remove calculus. These operate at 6000 cycles per second and have a 0.5-mm amplitude. Their motion is elliptic—a

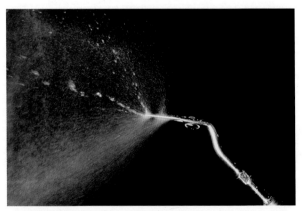

Fig. 3.28 Piezo tip showing the energy nodes.

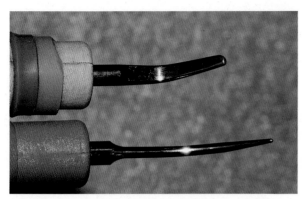

Fig. 3.29 Ultrasonic tips. Top, Beaver-tail insert; bottom, periodontal insert.

figure-of-eight motion. All sides of these tips are active during cleaning, although the cleaning action may not be even. One feature of these units is that the compressed air has a cooling effect. They are less likely to cause heat-related damage to teeth than the ultrasonic scalers.

Air enters the sonic scaler, passes through the shaft, and exits from small holes on the shaft that are covered with a metal ring. The air exits the holes at an angle and causes the ring to start spinning. Because the ring does not fit the shaft tightly, it begins to wobble. This wobbling sets off a vibration that is transmitted down the shaft to the tip (Fig. 3.30).

Rotary scalers are highspeed (see discussion regarding highspeed handpieces later in this chapter) burs that remove calculus as they rotate. The use of rotary scalers is discouraged for two reasons. First, rotary scalers can easily damage the tooth.

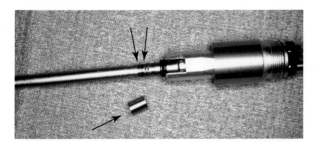

Fig. 3.30 The small metal ring (*arrow*) has been removed from the shaft of the sonic scaler. Air blows out of the small holes (*double arrows*).

Second, burs must be replaced often because they become dull extremely quickly. For proper functioning, a new bur must be used for each patient, which is prohibitively expensive.

DENTAL UNITS FOR POLISHING, CUTTING TEETH, AND REMOVING BONE

Two driving mechanisms exist: electric power and air power. Electric-powered units are generally the least expensive, although some sophisticated electric systems, used for specialized procedures such as implantation and endodontics, rival the price of compressed-air systems.

Electric-Powered Systems

Electric-powered systems operate at lower speeds than air-powered systems and have higher *torque*, which is the ability to overcome resistance to movement. Water or irrigating systems cannot be used with electric-powered systems, except with expensive models. Generally, air-powered systems are preferable to electric-powered systems.

Air-Powered Systems

Two types of air-powered systems exist. One uses compressed gas from a cylinder; the second uses an air compressor. The air compressor pumps air either directly into the dental unit or into a storage tank for slow release to the dental unit. The compressed gas is either room air or nitrogen. Because of associated hazards, oxygen and carbon dioxide should not be used. Oxygen is explosive, and carbon dioxide may be toxic.

Compressed gas systems require a regulator between the tank and the dental unit to maintain a pressure around 60 pounds per square inch (psi) (Fig. 3.31).

Air-Compressor Systems

Compressors take the room air and compress it to drive the handpieces. Most units work by pumping

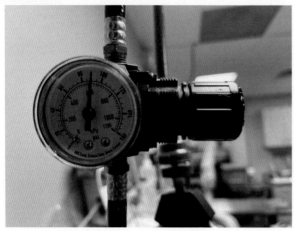

Fig. 3.31 Regulator to govern air pressure from compressed air tank to dental machinery.

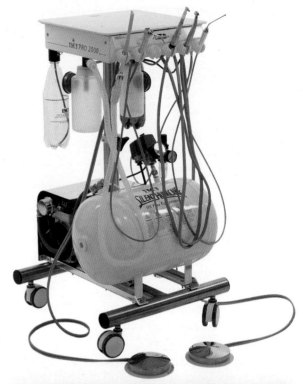

air into an air-storage tank. The compressor pumps air into the tank until the pressure inside the tank reaches between 80 and 100 psi. At this point, the compressor turns off. Air is bled from the tank as it is used by the handpiece at a lower pressure, usually 30 to 40 psi. When the pressure drops below the minimum pressure in the tank, approximately 60 psi, the compressor turns on again, filling the tank back up to 100 psi.

Newer compressors are quieter than traditional air compressors. To reduce noise, refrigerator compressors were converted so that they pump air rather than refrigerator coolant. The single-unit compressor rate is approximately 5½ hp. If a multistation or sonic-scaler handpiece is to be used, a double-unit, 1 hp compressor should be considered. These units are available in portable carts, portable cabinets, and countertop units. They can be custom-built to the practitioner's needs.

Counter or tabletop units allow the unit to be stored in cabinets and other areas remote from the place the procedure is performed. They are self-contained and require only a power source to function.

Dental carts with switches, handpiece holders, and suction are available. The compressor may be mounted on the cart or stored in a remote location. The air is connected by hoses (Fig. 3.32). Dental

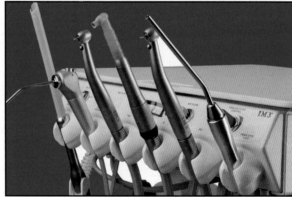

Fig. 3.32 Dental cart. This iM3 unit has low and high speeds, air-water syringe, suction, fiberoptic light, and multiple water bottles. (Courtesy iM3 Vancouver, WA, USA.)

units may also be mounted on walls with the compressor in a remote location, connected by hoses.

Compressor Care

Most air-compressor systems use oil for lubrication. The oil level must be monitored frequently because insufficient oil could cause the compressor to cease functioning. Some systems use a dipstick, like that of an automobile, for checking the oil. Others have a porthole in the side of the oil reservoir. When adding oil, the technician should always use the type of oil recommended by the compressor manufacturer. The oil should also be changed on a schedule recommended by the manufacturer. This is typically yearly.

The compression of air into the storage tank may cause condensation. Air-storage tanks have a drain cock that can be turned to let the water out of the tank (Fig. 3.33). Failure to do so allows water to fill the tank, decreasing the effectiveness of the system, and possibly, ruining the compressor. These should be opened to drain

based on the manufacturer's recommendations. If the drain cock is not closed before the next use, appropriate pressure may never build, causing the compressor to constantly run and damage the motor. Note that this process is loud and can produce a mess.

Low-Speed Handpieces

Different types of handpieces can be attached to compressed-air systems. High-speed handpieces are discussed later in the section on instruments of exodontia. All handpieces use a rubber gasket to ensure a water- and air-tight seal. The practitioner should make sure the gasket is connected when connecting the handpiece (Fig. 3.34). *Low-speed handpieces* are used for polishing with prophy angles and for performing other dental procedures

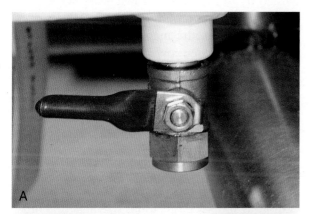

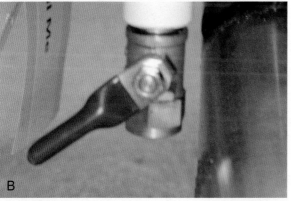

Fig. 3.33 If the compressor has an air-storage tank, it must be periodically drained. (A) Valve closed. (B) Valve open for drainage.

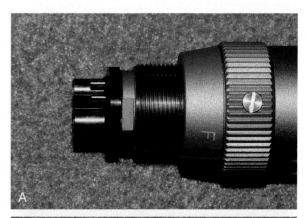

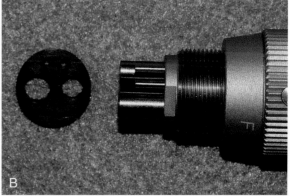

Fig. 3.34 (A) Check to make sure the gasket is on. (B) Gaskets may come off of the handpiece.

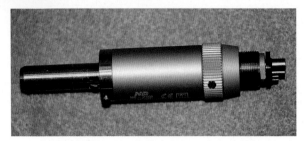

Fig. 3.35 Low-speed handpiece engine.

with contra-angle. They have a high torque and a slow speed of 5000 to 20,000 revolutions per minute (rpm) (Fig. 3.35).

Low-speed attachments. A prophy angle is an attachment that allows the use of a prophy cup for polishing teeth during cleaning. It is a type of contra-angle that is an attachment used to change either the direction or the speed of rotation (Fig. 3.36). These may be reusable with pop-on or screw-on prophy cups or disposable with the cup already attached.

Prophy angles used in human dentistry typically work in a circular motion. The disadvantage of these circular units is that hair can get wrapped in the prophy angle. Disposable nonrotary prophy angles are also available. They oscillate back and forth at 90 degrees. Because they do not rotate 360 degrees, they will not wrap hair around the prophy cup, which is an advantage.

Another advantage of disposable plastic prophy angles is that they are relatively inexpensive and do not need to be cleaned after use; they are simply discarded. They should not be cleaned and used on multiple patients. The rubber in the prophy cup cannot withstand multiple uses. The phrase "prophy cup" has multiple meanings. In this text a *prophy cup* is the rubber cup used on the prophy angle for polishing teeth, and a prophy paste holder is the cup used to hold prophy paste.

Care of low-speed handpieces. The low-speed handpiece must be lubricated at the end of each day of use. The technician must first insert lubricant into the smaller of the two large holes, using the oil or spray that comes with the handpiece. Always use the lubricant recommended by the manufacturer.

Prophy and contra-angles. The specific lubrication of prophy and contra-angles depends on the instrument. Generally, prophy heads must be lubricated weekly with prophy angle lubricant. For many models, the head of the instrument may be twisted off to expose the crown gears that require lubrication. Some prophy angles are self-lubricating. In all cases, the manufacturer's instructions should be consulted for each piece of equipment. Disposable angles by nature do not need maintenance. Table 3.2 lists the maintenance chart.

Three-Way Syringes

Three-way syringes deliver water air or both and are air-powered. These syringes have two buttons. Pressing one button creates a water spray, which can be used to irrigate a tooth surface and clear away prophy paste, tooth shavings, and other debris. Pressing the second button creates an air spray, which can be used to dry the field. The

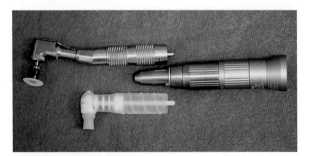

Fig. 3.36 Low-speed attachments. Upper left, contra-angle; right, nose cone; lower left, prophy angle.

TABLE 3.2	**Maintenance Chart**		
Procedure	**Daily**	**Weekly**	**Yearly**
Oil in low speed	√		
Spray in high speed	√		
Check compressor oil level		√	
Drain water out of compressor		√	
Annual compressor maintenance			√

technician must be careful not to flush air into tissues; air can create subcutaneous emphysema or, even worse, enter a blood vessel and create an embolism. Pressing both buttons together creates a mist. The tip of the three-way syringe can be removed for autoclaving.

Suction

Suction units—either combined into a dental cart or separate—are useful in aspirating blood and debris from extraction sites to allow better visualization of retained roots, better visualization of surgical fields, and visualization in performing endodontics.

EXODONTIA INSTRUMENTS

Hand Instruments for Exodontics

The basic hand instruments for extraction include small needle holders, atraumatic forceps, fine scissors, bone curettes, periosteal elevators, dental luxators and elevators, and extraction forceps. Other instruments such as root picks are utilized during surgical complications. The fundamental instruments for extractions are discussed here. The use of these instruments and specialized instruments for procedures beyond general dentistry is discussed later in the text.

In the past, dental elevators and luxators had standard-length handles. These were better suited for operators with hands larger than the average of the profession. The manufacturers have come to understand that a smaller handle and shorter shaft on the instrument are more fitting for the majority of operators. This allows for a more ergonomic grasp of the instrument and safer usage.

Basic Oral Surgery Pack

Oral surgery pack contents vary based on species and operator. Box 3.2 lists minimal needs for oral surgery.

A simple #10 scalpel handle should be in the pack. Appropriate blades for extraction of teeth in dogs and cats are 11 or 15c blades (Fig. 3.37).

BOX 3.2 Basic Oral Surgery Pack

Scalpel Handle
- 11 blade
- 15c blade

Small Needle Drivers
- Derf
- Mathieu
- Castroviejo

Atraumatic Thumb Forceps
Scissors
- LaGrange
- Goldman Fox
- Iris

Bone Curette
- Miller's
- Lucas

Periosteal Elevators (appropriate size for patient)
Dental Luxators
Dental Elevators
Extraction Forceps
Irrigation (saline)
Sponges

Needle drivers should be small enough to allow the operator to access restricted areas, such as when suturing the maxillary second molar extraction site in a small dog. Derf, Mathieu, and Castroviejo are commonly used in oral surgery. Larger needle drivers may prevent easy access.

Thumb forceps should be atraumatic as the oral soft tissues are susceptible to crushing injury. Adson-Brown forceps should be used with caution as there is a great risk of tissue injury (Fig. 3.38).

Several types of scissors are available that are appropriate for use in oral surgery. A popular choice in veterinary oral surgery is the Lagrange scissor. This scissor has a double curve, which allows for easier access to some oral tissues. Simple iris scissors and Goldman-Fox scissors are other common choices. Given the small tissue tags that

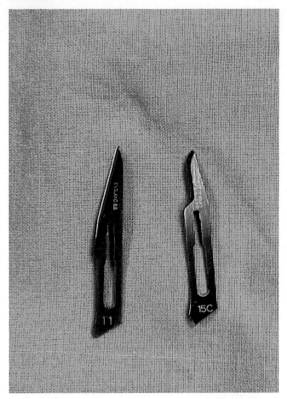

Fig. 3.37 #11 and #15c blades are appropriate for oral surgery.

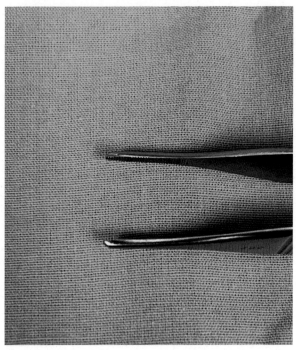

Fig. 3.38 Nontraumatic forceps should be used for handling gingiva.

are being trimmed, using scissors with one serrated blade is useful in gripping tissue while cutting. More advanced procedures may require the usage of Metzenbaum scissors, which have a reduced ability to perforate the mucoperiosteal flap.

Bone curettes are small spoon-like instruments that can be used to debride and excavate the dental alveolus after the tooth has been extracted. Miller and Lucas bone curettes are similar in shape and function. Both are double-ended, providing a mirror image curve (Fig. 3.39). Various sizes are available.

Sterile sponges are excellent for hemostasis and removing debris. All-purpose woven 4 × 4s are the most commonly used sponge in veterinary medicine. Some may find these too large for routine oral surgery and periodontal procedures. Additionally, the weave can become caught on teeth and unravel.

Nonwoven 2 × 2 sponges are an excellent alternative (Fig. 3.40).

When sterilizing, the instruments may be wrapped in a sterile instrument envelope, instrument cassette, or other appropriate container. Sterile envelopes may be penetrated by the instruments, breaking the sterile barrier. Instrument cassettes are an excellent way to organize instruments. Alternatively, instruments which do not fit into a specific cassette can be kept in an appropriate-sized kidney pan.

Periosteal Elevators

Periosteal elevators (Fig. 3.41) are primarily used to raise a mucoperiosteal flap for access to the alveolar bone surrounding a tooth root and for closing extraction sites without tension. Several variations are available, and there is not a consensus on what is the best type for extractions. It is recommended to have various sizes available. A larger periosteal elevator which is appropriate for operating a large dog

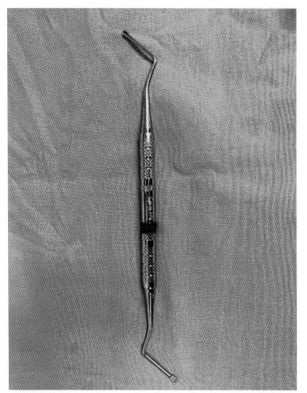

Fig. 3.39 Bone curettes are used to debride the alveolus after extraction.

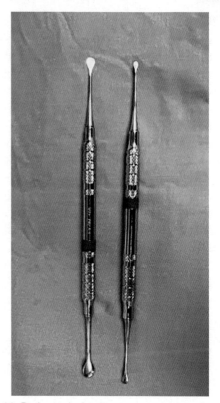

Fig. 3.41 Periosteal elevators are used to raise mucoperiosteal flaps for extractions.

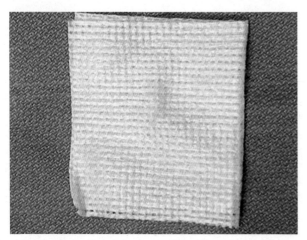

Fig. 3.40 Nonwoven sponges do not snag on bone.

will be too large for a small dog or cat. The Molt No. 9 periosteal is a popular model with a round end and pointed end. The pointed end is excellent for creating a papilla-sparing flap. The novice should be cautious that this pointed end can fenestrate tissue if not used cautiously. Most periosteal elevators used in oral surgery have a sharp (not necessarily pointed) edge.

Luxators

Dental luxators are used as a wedge between the tooth and bone and to sever the periodontal ligament. Luxators have a thin flat blade as compared to the curved thicker blade of the elevator. They may have a straight or curved shaft with the working end being slightly concave to adapt to the tooth. As the working end becomes wider, the corresponding number size increases, typically corresponding to the working width of the instrument. Specialized luxators are available as well. It should be noted that luxators have a thin working end and excessive axial or bending force may break the instrument.

Elevators

Dental elevators are like luxators in that the size corresponds to the working width of the instrument. Often larger sizes (compared to the available sizes of luxators) are available and should be considered when extracting teeth on large and giant breed dogs. The majority of elevators used in veterinary dentistry are winged elevators. Dr. Robert Wiggs developed winged elevators that have the advantage of wedging out teeth with the shaft side of the wing (Fig. 3.42).

These allow for use as a rotational wedge and enable the wheel and axle technique. Specialized elevators such as Cryer elevators are available but used infrequently in veterinary medicine.

Notched elevators are available that have prongs that engage the buccal and lingual or palatal side of a tooth, preventing slippage (Fig. 3.43). These can be very useful when extracting the premolars and molars of cats.

Extraction forceps. Extraction forceps are less consequential in veterinary medicine as they are not typically utilized in the same manner as in humans.

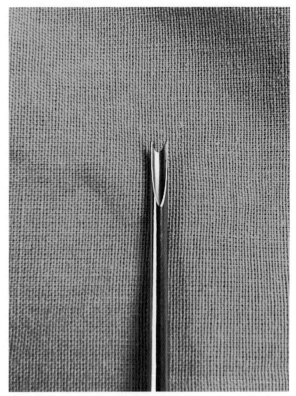

Fig. 3.43 Notched elevators are useful for extracting premolars and molars in cats.

Having regular and smaller forceps available for usage is recommended. Some extraction forceps have a spring between each arm and some do not. This is an operator preference and is dependent on the grasp used to hold the instrument.

Root Tip Picks

Root tip picks are thin and pointed for retrieving root fragments. Root tip picks are used to loosen, then tease root fragments, from the alveolus. They can be used with a second root tip pick or a hypodermic needle to "chopstick" root tips to pick up root fragments. Alternatively, root forceps can be used to grasp the root fragment (Fig. 3.44).

SHARPENING EQUIPMENT

Elevators are sharpened with either a flat stone or an Rx Honing Machine. To sharpen with the Rx Honing

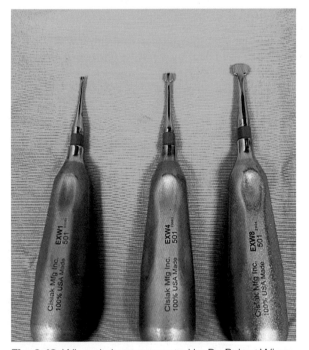

Fig. 3.42 Winged elevators created by Dr. Robert Wiggs.

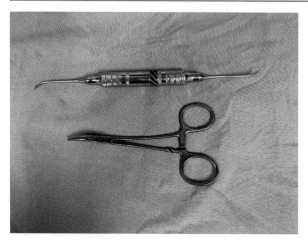

Fig. 3.44 Root pick and forcep.

Machine, the instrument is held at a proper angle and rotated as the disk spins. The angle should follow the manufacturer's edge. A cylindrical attachment can also be used.

Conical stones can be used to sharpen dental elevators when the manufacturer has sharpened the elevator from the concave side (Fig. 3.45).

Professional sharpening services can be hired to aid in maintaining equipment for the hospital. This is an added expense and the hospital needs to have redundant instrumentation to replace any instruments that have been shipped out. Most importantly, the sharpening service should be communicated about what side of the instrument needs to be sharpened as it is not unheard of to have professional services sharpen the wrong surface, creating a second bevel and ruining the instrument.

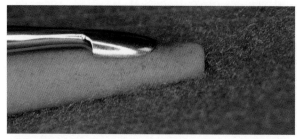

Fig. 3.45 If the elevator was originally sharpened from the inside, a conical stone may be used to sharpen it.

Powered Instruments for Exodontics
High-Speed Handpieces

High-speed handpieces turn at 300,000 to 400,000 rpm. They are used for sectioning teeth, accessing the root canal, removing alveolar bone, and other procedures. Some high-speed handpieces come with fiberoptic lights that are powered either directly by electricity or by converting rotational energy into electricity (Fig. 3.46).

The *turbine* is the portion of the handpiece that collects linear moving air and converts it into rotary movement. Swivel attachments are available that decrease tension on the operator's wrist and allow for more freedom of movement.

Changing high-speed burs. Two styles of high-speed bur heads are available. One uses a push button on the handpiece to open the chuck. The bur may be removed and replaced by simply pressing the button. The second uses a chuck key. The bur may be loosened and removed by twisting the key counterclockwise. The new bur is placed in the handpiece, and the bur key is turned clockwise to tighten (Fig. 3.47).

Burs should be treated as sharps and disposed of in the sharps container. They should be removed from the handpiece when not in use and when the handpiece is covered. If the bur is removed from

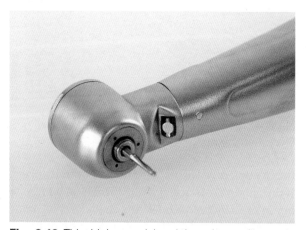

Fig. 3.46 This high-speed handpiece has a fiberoptic light for better visualization of areas being cut. (Courtesy Kruuse/Henry Schein Co., NY, USA.)

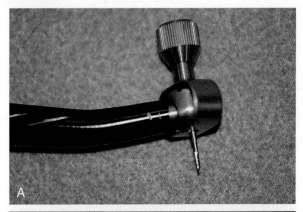

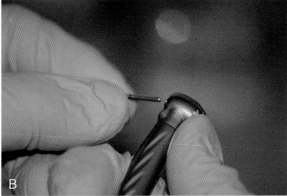

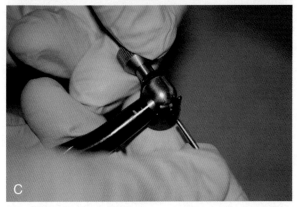

Fig. 3.47 (A) Changing bur. (B) Changing bur push button. (C) Changing bur with chuck key.

the handpiece, a "blank" should be put in its place. If the handpiece is accidentally turned on without a bur in the handpiece chuck, the chuck may be damaged. If a bur does not fit easily into the handpiece or is not easily removed, it should not be forced as this may damage the handpiece.

Bur selection. *Dental burs* are rotary cutting instruments that operate via a handpiece. Burs have a working end, neck, and shank. The shank inserts into the handpiece or contra-angle, and the neck connects the working end to the shank.

There are three types of bur shanks (Table 3.3), HP, RA, and FG (Fig. 3.48). HP stands for "handpiece" and fits directly into the end of the low-speed handpiece. The shank diameter of these burs is 2.35 mm. Burs with HP shanks are typically used for composite trimming and shaping and for trimming teeth of species other than dogs and cats. The shank of these burs is longer than RA and FG burs.

RA stands for "right angle." The shank of HP burs is longer than RA and FG burs. This notch must line up properly with the cylinder of the handpiece to the seat. These burs are designed to be put in a contra-angle (thus sometimes called a CA bur). Many endodontic instruments have RA-type shanks.

The majority of burs used in exodontia have an FG-type shank. FG stands for friction grip and has a diameter of 1.6 mm. These are designed only to be used in high-speed handpieces.

FG-type burs have a working end made of either carbide or diamond coated. Most carbide burs are designed to be single-use. It is likely not financially prudent to attempt to reuse carbide burs, given the overhead in cleaning the burs and the decreased surgical efficiency with repeated usage.

Diamond burs are used for crown preparation and debriding of soft tissue and bone during surgical procedures (Fig. 3.49). A wide variety of shapes and degrees of coarseness is available. These can typically be used five times or more.

Types of FG carbide burs. Fig. 3.50 contains the types of burs and their nomenclature and use are summarized in Table 3.4. Friction grip burs have various lengths of the shank. Longer shanks are useful for accessing structures such as retained roots and short shanks are useful when accessing the caudal teeth in small patients. Typically, the standard shank length is appropriate.

TABLE 3.3	**Dental Bur Shafts**		
Type	**Shape**	**Diameter**	**Examples**
Friction Grip (FG)	Round	1.6 mm	Carbide burs
			Diamond burs
Handpiece (HP)	Round	2.35 mm	Handpiece composite
			Trimming burs
Right Angle (RA)	Round with notch	2.35 mm	Gates Glidden
			Peeso

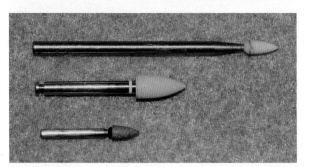

Fig. 3.48 *Top*, Straight-shank bur; middle, right-angle (RA) bur; *bottom*, a friction-grip (FG) bur.

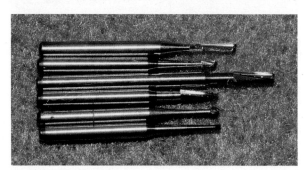

Fig. 3.50 Top to bottom, 331 L (long pear), 330 (pear), 701S (surgical length), 701 (crosscut fissure), 2 (round), 33½ (inverted-cone bur).

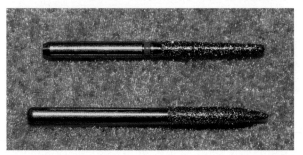

Fig. 3.49 Diamond burs are used for crown preparation.

Round burs. Round burs have a spherical working end. These are numbered $\frac{1}{4}$, $\frac{1}{2}$, 1, 2, 4, and 6. They may be used for access into pulp chambers and for cavity preparations, removing bone, and sectioning small teeth.

Pear-shaped burs. Pear-shaped burs have a pear- or teardrop-shaped working end that tapers toward the shaft. These are numbered in the 320s through 330s. These burs are a cross between the round bur, crosscut bur, and inverted-cone bur. The result is a bur that has a round cutting tip, cutting sides, and a slight taper for undercutting. These burs can be used as a round bur but may provide a better undercut than round burs and can also be used to section small teeth.

Crosscut burs. Crosscut burs are numbered in the 500s through 700s. They are used most commonly for sectioning teeth. The 700 series burs are slightly tapered, and the 500 series burs are cylindrical.

Inverted-cone burs. The inverted-cone burs are given numbers in the 30s (e.g., 33½ $\frac{1}{2}$, 34, 35). The larger the number, the larger the bur. Inverted-cone burs are used for undercutting in cavity preparation. They are wider at the tip than at the shank.

Care of high-speed handpieces

Lubrication. The high-speed handpieces should be lubricated daily with a spray-type cleaner and lubricant or another product recommended by the manufacturer of the handpiece (Fig. 3.51).

Troubleshooting High-Speed Handpieces

Several problems can occur with high-speed handpieces: bur fails to spin, burr falls out, and slow cutting.

Type	Number Series (working end increases in size as number increases)	General Usage
Round	¼–8	Bone removal for extractions
		Access openings for endodontic therapy
		Cavity preparation
Pear	329–332	Bone removal for extractions
		Access openings for endodontic therapy
		Cavity preparation
Inverted Cone	33 ½–36	Cavity preparation
Flat Fissure	55–58	Sectioning teeth
	555–560 (crosscut)	
Taper Fissure	169–171	Sectioning teeth
	699–701 (crosscut)	
Diamond	Several shapes available	Smoothing bone
		Debriding soft tissue
		Crown preparation

TABLE 3.4 Commonly Used FG Burs and General Use

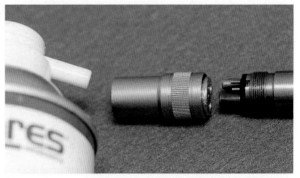

Fig. 3.51 This system has a spray canister with lubricant and a connector that connects with the high-speed handpiece.

A bur that falls out can be caused by reusing dull burs. If the bur is not completely seated, it may fall out when the handpiece is activated. If a longer bur is needed, surgical-length burs are available. Another problem is caused by using inexpensive burs that have inconsistent shank diameters, which results from poor engineering of the bur.

A bad turbine can wear away the inside of the head, particularly the front, where the turbine chuck exits the housing and where the bur is inserted. It may be noticed that the hole is wider than it should be. If that is the case, putting a good turbine in a bad housing will just continue to chew through all future turbines.

Slow cutting is caused by incorrect compressor air pressure setup, a leak in the system, or a defective turbine.

Defective Turbine

The turbine is the internal portion of the high-speed handpiece that spins at an extremely high speed. It is subject to wear over time and must be replaced periodically. Maintenance may be performed in the office. The signs of a defective turbine cartridge include the following: (1) failure of the chuck to tighten around the bur; (2) increased noise or vibration; (3) roughness felt when spinning the bur by hand, with the turbine in or out of handpiece; (4) intermittent stopping of the handpiece; and (5) failure of the handpiece

A bur that fails to spin is likely caused by a defective turbine. Another possible cause is undetected damage cause to the head housing. This may have been caused by dropping the handpiece. Even when the heads are pressed back out when damage is noticed, they are never truly 100% right. It is very easy to knock the handpiece out of the holder or not put it in the holder in the first place.

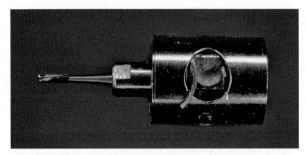

Fig. 3.52 This turbine has fractured from long-term use.

to function. Fig. 3.52 shows a turbine that has fractured.

Changing Turbines

To change the turbine, a "blank" bur is placed in the handpiece. If the bur that is in the handpiece cannot be removed, caution should be exercised to keep from cutting the hands on the bur. Next, the small metal ring (wrench) supplied with the handpiece is placed on the cap of the handpiece. The handpiece cap is unscrewed and removed by rotating the wrench counterclockwise. The turbine cartridge is removed from the handpiece head by pressing on the blank or bur (Fig. 3.53). The new turbine cartridge is placed into the handpiece head. Finally, the new turbine cartridge is aligned with the pin side up. If the pin is not aligned with the slot, the turbine cartridge will not slide completely into the handpiece head. The cap is replaced.

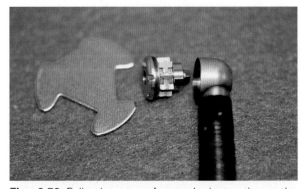

Fig. 3.53 Following manufacturer's instructions, the turbine of the high-speed handpiece can be changed as shown here.

Vet-Tome Powertome

The Vet-Tome is a solenoid-driven periotome with foot pedal operation, designed to cause minimal or no alveolar bone loss and less trauma. Replaceable ultra-thin stainless-steel blades are attached to the handpiece and a mechanical in-and-out action cuts the periodontal ligament similar to a luxator. A thin blade is inserted into the periodontal ligament (PDL) between the tooth and alveolus. The instrument is turned on and the blade is driven into the space. After advancing a few millimeters, the foot peddle is released and a side-to-side movement by the operator is made, cutting the adjacent PDL. Once the blade is freed up, the instrument is turned on again and the blade advances in a similar fashion.

The Vet-Tome will not go through bone and hard tissues, so it may not work for PDLs that are mineralized. It is not a replacement for a good extraction technique, but it makes extraction easier.

LIGHTING AND MAGNIFICATION

With a few exceptions, the following statement holds true for veterinary dentistry: "If you can't see it, you can't do it." Lighting and magnification are two very important aids that allow the technician and practitioner to visualize the structures in the oral cavity. Once used, most ask how they were able to work without them.

Lighting

Lighting is available from a variety of sources. A good surgical light produces wide-ranging and even lighting. Spotlighting is obtained by the use of a light mounted to a headlamp. Focal lighting is achieved by the use of fiber-optic lights built into a handpiece.

There are a number of things to consider when purchasing a light source. Brightness and uniform illumination provide even visualization of the field. Some light sources also have an adjustable spot. The Color Rendering Index (CRI) provides a quantitative measure (up to 100) of a light source that shows colors in comparison to an ideal or natural light source. The higher the CRI, the better the reduction in eye fatigue. There are also cordless and corded LED headlamps. In the cordless versions, the battery is stored on the unit. Whereas it is more convenient not to have a cord attached to a battery pack, three variables to the headlamp include the following: weight, intensity of the light, and battery life. Some will have battery life indicators and some just turn off when out of power. The intensity of the light can also be an important consideration: not intense enough leads to poor visualization; too intense can lead to eye strain.

Magnification

Loupes are available in two types: fixed and flip-up. Fixed has the advantage of being through the lens (TTL) and is the most popular among dentists. They are well-balanced and allow a larger field of view, have lower maintenance, can have prescriptions incorporated into the optics, and retain alignment better than the flip-up type. The flip-up type allows for a greater angle for the loupe optics to be inclined downward. By looking down rather than tilting the head down, less eye strain can be obtained. However, looking down causes greater eye strain.

Binocular eyeglasses produce the best type of magnification. Ideally, they should be adjustable so that the operator's head does not tilt forward; rather, the eyes look down and the head is kept squarely above the shoulders. Two and one-half to three-powered magnification, with a focal length of between 15 and 18 inches, enlarges the subject without excess distortion.

There are a variety of systems available. Some are custom-made for each user—the distance between your eyes called the interpupillary distance (IPD), is fixed. Some have adjustable IPDs, so multiple users can use the same loupe. Loupes can be custom-built for a specific user. Some are attached to lenses that are similar to bifocals or trifocals to allow normal vision or diopter correction. Others have sliding adjustments between the lenses that allow multiple users to use them.

Some have locked adjustments that cannot moved inadvertently.

Another consideration is the ability to disinfect the loupe. Some are completely waterproof so they can be scrubbed. If keeping a loupe clean and sterile is important, some loupes have an autoclavable flip handle so you can move the loupe away from your field of vision when the loupe is not needed and then back in play while remaining sterile (Fig. 3.54). Ideally, have an eye examination to determine if any prescriptions should be incorporated into custom loupes. Wear loupes for short periods each day to let the eyes gradually adjust. There are many choices in loupes, and it is best to try out a few before purchasing. Make sure the frames, nose pads, and other adjustable features are properly adjusted. When using loupes, occasionally take them off and focus on more distant objects. Consider purchasing additional loupes with greater magnification for more delicate procedures. There are also adjustable magnification lenses.

When being fitted for loupes, it is recommended to have a company representative visit the office to assess the surgery table and where the operator will be in relation to the patient. This allows for the best ergonomics.

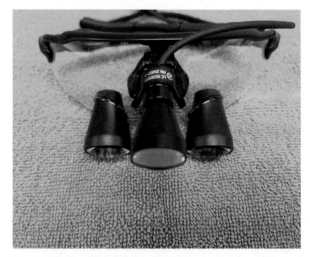

Fig. 3.54 Surgitel fixed surgical loupes with attached light source.

STERILIZATION

All instruments should be cleaned to eliminate gross debris. Whenever possible, dental instruments and equipment should be sterilized via steam or gas. However, there are some instances where this is not possible. Disinfection and sterilization are done to protect the patient as well as every member of the veterinary facility. This is a part of keeping the workplace safe and free of pathogens. Sterility indicators are recommended in oral surgical packs to confirm that the entire pack reached the appropriate temperature.

CHAPTER 3 WORKSHEET (ANSWERS ARE ON PAGE 294)

1. The portions of all instruments are the handle, the shank, the terminal shank, and the _____.
2. Scalers have _____ sharp sides and a sharp tip.
3. Scalers are used to remove _____ calculus only.
4. Curettes and scalers are usually _____; this means that they can adapt to opposite surfaces.
5. Instead of a tip, the curette has a _____ which reduces the risk of trauma to the gingival sulcus.
6. A _____ blade reflects light, whereas a _____ blade does not reflect light.
7. The instrument should be sharpened so that it has a _____ to _____ degree angle.
8. Powered scalers convert _____ or _____ energy into mechanical vibration.
9. The following two types of devices in the handpiece can pick up a sound wave and turn it into a vibration: _____ and _____.
10. The piezoelectric ultrasonic scalers use _____ in the handpiece to pick up the vibration.
11. Handpieces usually operate at _____ to _____ psi.
12. _____ must be periodically drained from air-storage tanks.
13. High-speed handpieces operate at _____ rpm.
14. Low-speed handpieces operate at _____ rpm.
15. Carbide burs should be treated as _____.

4

Personal Safety and Ergonomics

Steven E. Holmstrom, Laurie A. Holmstrom

CHAPTER OUTLINE

LEARNING OBJECTIVES

When you have completed this chapter, you will be able to:

- List the safety equipment required for use when performing veterinary dental procedures.
- Discuss the rationale for use of eye protection, face masks, and gloves when performing veterinary dental procedures.
- Describe proper handwashing techniques.

- List the information that must be included on the label of a chemical container.
- Describe the symptoms of repetitive motion disorders for which a veterinary dental technician is at risk.
- Define ergonomics and discuss methods to address prevention of workplace injuries in the veterinary dental practice.

KEY TERMS

Anionic detergent
Antiseptic
Contact dermatitis
Ergonomics

Eye shields
Material safety data sheet
Neutral position
Repetitive motion disorder

Sharps
Substantivity

HAZCOM

The Federal Hazard Communication Standard (HAZCOM or HCS) is a regulation enforced by the Occupational Safety and Health Administration (OSHA) of the United States Department of Labor. HAZCOM is based on employees' rights and their "need to know" the identities of hazardous substances to which they may be exposed in the work environment. OSHA requires employers to provide workers with preventive safety equipment and ensure that they wear it during dental procedures. To comply with the HAZCOM requirements, employers must also submit a written hazard communication program.

SAFETY REQUIREMENTS FOR VETERINARY DENTISTRY

For the veterinary dentistry practice, OSHA requires that the employers provide safety glasses, masks, and gloves for all employees who perform dental procedures (Fig. 4.1). The employee is responsible for wearing safety equipment during all procedures. After all, it is the employee's health that is at stake and flying debris or other substances can easily cause infections if the employee neglects to wear the safety protection provided. Employees must always be careful to take responsibility for their own safety by wearing the necessary safety equipment and should not expect their employers to remind them before each potentially hazardous procedure.

TYPES OF HAZARDS

Veterinary staff risk exposure to several different hazards. Hazards are classified as follows: chemical, physical, biologic, and ergonomic. Chemical hazards are formulations that can act on the skin, eyes, respiratory tract, alimentary system, and other organs and organ systems. Physical hazards are those that can physically harm. Biological hazards in the veterinary dental practice are

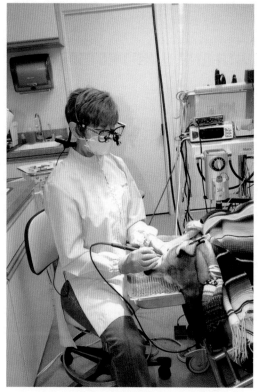

Fig. 4.1 Mask, eye protection, and gloves should be used for every procedure.

organic materials that pose a hazard to the health of practitioners and patients. These hazards include pathogenic bacteria, viruses, toxins, spores, and fungi. Ergonomic hazards are owing to workplace interactions.

EYE PROTECTION

The importance of eye protection cannot be overstated. Infections from a number of sources can cause permanent visual impairment. Unprotected operators are sometimes struck in the eye by pumice while polishing or by a flying piece of tooth during high-speed drilling. Scaling can also send bacteria-laden calculus into the dental technician's eyes or mouth. The calculus almost always scratches the eye and thereby deposits bacteria directly into the wound. Splatter from rinsing acid etch or sodium hypochlorite is potentially devastating to the eyes and can also cause small lesions on the face.

MOUTH AND LUNG PROTECTION

The use of high-speed equipment, such as ultrasonic scalers and high-speed drills, creates a vapor that contains bacteria, blood, saliva, and tooth dust. This vapor extends up to 3 feet from the source and can irritate and infect the respiratory system of people who are not wearing protective masks. The risk extends to nonemployees, such as clients visiting the dental area while a procedure is in progress.

Masks

Respirator masks offer more protection than surgical masks. All masks must fit tightly to function properly. Some allow for adjustments at the upper (nose) and lower (chin) portions of the mask.

HAND AND SKIN PROTECTION

Gloves protect the patient from cross-contamination and the veterinary staff from the toxic materials used in dentistry. Toxins in resins, such as methyl methacrylate, formaldehyde, chloroform, x-ray chemicals, and cold sterilization chemicals, are all absorbed through the skin. Some are carcinogenic and accumulate in the body with repeated exposure. Most affect the liver and kidneys. Because of the critical importance of these organs, all staff members should wear proper safety protection when handling these materials.

HANDWASHING

Proper handwashing is important for disease control. If employees do not wear gloves and are accidentally stabbed by an instrument or bitten by a patient, they may become infected by the organisms on their own skin. Employees should always wash their hands before putting on gloves in case a glove is torn or otherwise penetrated during the course of a procedure.

Handwashing Agents

A number of handwashing agents are available. Simple *anionic detergents* (soaps) help by destroying the cell walls of bacteria. *Antiseptics*, such as alcohol, iodine, iodophors, and hexachlorophene, are also effective. The ability of chlorhexidine, parachlorometaxylenol, and triclosan to stick to surfaces, a property known as *substantivity,* makes these agents superior.

Handwashing Technique

Proper technique in handwashing is important. Rings and other jewelry (e.g., bracelets) should be removed. Hands should be washed for a minimum of 1 minute immediately on arrival to the office and then washed again for 15 seconds between each patient.

Employees should rinse their hands in cold water, making sure to remove all soap. Then, they should dry their hands thoroughly. Many people rinse their hands in hot water, mistakenly believing that if it hurts, it is killing bacteria. In fact, the hot water causes the pores in the hands to open, which draws water from the hands and makes them more susceptible to dermatitis.

GLOVE CONCERNS

Some people develop allergies to latex gloves with time. Three types of hypersensitivity reactions to latex exist. The most common is a *contact dermatitis*, which is a delayed, type IV allergy. It causes a localized rash and develops 24 to 72 hours after exposure. Next frequent is a contact urticaria, which is an immediate, type I allergic reaction that occurs immediately after exposure. Contact urticaria manifests itself as hives, nasal inflammation, general itching, and wheezing. The worst but rarest type is a systemic reaction, also known as a type I reaction, which results in conjunctivitis, asthma, and systemic anaphylaxis. The fact that latex powder remains in the air for a long time if gloves are snapped on complicates the reaction. Because many conditions mimic these hypersensitivities, employees should consult an allergist if they experience problems.

Proper fit in gloves is also important for preventing hand fatigue that can lead to tendonitis in the wrist. Gloves should be loose through the palm of the hand. If they are too tight, the muscles of the palm will cramp with the effort to maintain a relaxed position.

SHARPS

Sharps are materials and equipment which may present a puncture or laceration danger and may transmit infection to the operator. This includes needles, blades, and many endodontic files. To keep from accidentally stabbing themselves, employees should never recap needles with both hands. The needle cover should be scooped up with one hand with the needle (Fig. 4.2) or simply discarded in the sharps container. Sharps containers should be disposed of properly when they reach the full line. To prevent punctures when inserting needles, employees should never continue to pack additional needles in the containers after they are full.

EYE SHIELDS

Light-curing guns use an intense white light to cure resins. Because looking at the light can cause permanent retinal damage, employees should use the approved orange *eye shields,* which help block

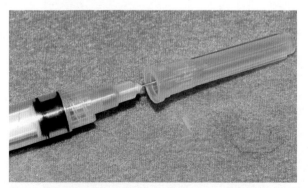

Fig. 4.2 If the cap is placed back on the needle, it should be replaced by scooping the syringe cap.

intense blue light and refrain from looking at the light, except when necessary.

SAFETY WITH PRODUCTS

Employees should always know the materials in the products used for all procedures. Reading the instructions and following them carefully are crucial steps for safety.

Material Safety Data Sheets

Chemical manufacturers and importers must convey hazard-related information to employers by means of labels on containers and *material safety data sheets* (MSDSs) that provide necessary safety information about the product including the type of hazard it presents. In addition, all employers are required to implement a hazard communication program to provide this information to employees. Methods for educating employers include container labeling, MSDSs, and training sessions. Employers must receive sufficient information to design and implement employee protection programs. HAZCOM also provides necessary hazard information to employees so that they can participate in and support the protective measures instituted in their workplaces.

Labels

All hazardous materials in original containers must bear a label from the manufacturer that is legible, in English, and prominently displayed on the container. The following information must be included:
1. Product identity: trade name, product name, or chemical identity.
2. Appropriate hazard warnings: physical and any relevant acute or chronic health hazards.
3. Name and address of the chemical manufacturer, importer, or other responsible party.

Composite Restoration Materials

Most composite restoration materials require an acid etch for maximal adhesion. This solution, which can splatter when rinsed off, is extremely strong and can cause damage if it touches an area other than the enamel. In addition, chemical reactions to the uncured resins are possible. Acid etch should be used with caution. Employees should always wear gloves and glasses and understand the proper way to use this substance.

Toxins

Toxic chemicals, radiographic chemicals, disinfectant surface cleaners, ultrasonic cleaning solutions, and cold-sterilizing chemicals should never be handled without gloves. The toxic substances that cause them to work are absorbed through the skin and can accumulate in the body, causing major health problems in the future. The solutions used in ultrasonic instrument cleaners are not necessarily sterile, and bacteria can enter the hand through small cuts and openings.

REPETITIVE MOTION DISORDERS

Repetitive motion disorders are prevalent in occupations that require repeated small repetitions of a single action. Dental hygienists and computer operators are particularly susceptible to this problem. Veterinary technicians who work exclusively in dentistry are therefore at risk.

Symptoms include stiffness in the neck and shoulders (particularly on the dominant side), soreness in the elbow and/or wrist, hand fatigue, headaches, and tingling or numbness in the fingers of the affected side. Tendonitis may also occur in the elbow and wrist as a result of bad positioning. These symptoms often decrease or disappear completely with increased attention to positioning, stroke and hand placement, ergonomics, and strengthening exercises. Occasionally, the damage to the nerves is so extensive that the technician is no longer able to work in dentistry.

Ergonomics in the Workplace

Prevention of repetitive motion disorders is based on keeping repetitive motions as stress-free as possible. *Ergonomics* is the science of designing the workplace so that operators remain in the most neutral positions possible. It is a good idea to take photographs or videos of practitioners in the operatory to review and improve ergonomics.

Neutral Position

A *neutral position* entails sitting with the knees slightly below the hips, the back straight, the elbow at a 90-degree angle, and the thumb relaxed at the top of the hand. The head points are straightforward, and the shoulders are relaxed. Feet should be flat on the floor or resting on a full footrest on the chair. The back should be as straight as possible, with the head leaning over as little as possible (Fig. 4.3). While working, the employee should be careful to keep the shoulders relaxed (not hunched) and the head level, neither tilted too far forward nor leaning toward either side. (The head weighs 12 pounds and

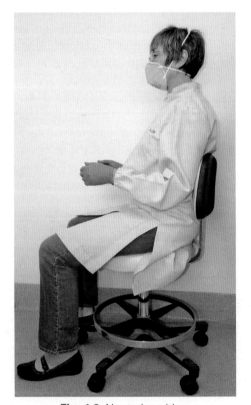

Fig. 4.3 Neutral position.

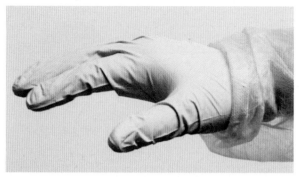

Fig. 4.4 The ambidextrous examination glove pulls the thumb back.

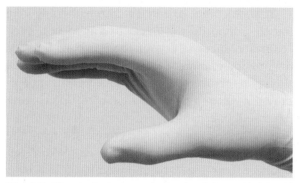

Fig. 4.5 Gloves that are made for the right and left hand are neutral without thumb pull back.

is supported only by the small column of the neck.) Dental personnel should never lean on the table supported by their forearms or bend the wrist from a straight position. A bar rest for the feet provides inadequate support for the lower back; resting the feet on the floor with too great an angle between the hips and knees also puts pressure on the lower back and impairs circulation to the lower leg and feet. The working motion while hand scaling should be a pull stroke that rolls the entire forearm, bending the wrist as little as possible.

Preventive Procedures

Repetitive stress injuries can be prevented in a variety of ways. The types of instruments used can make a significant difference. The use of ultrasonic scalers and hand instruments with the correct types of handles helps. Patient positioning is also relevant. Selecting the correct glove size and regularly performing hand-strengthening exercises are also important preventive measures.

Fitted gloves versus ambidextrous gloves. The use of ambidextrous gloves can cause fatigue. The thumb may be pulled back to a nonneutral position, which exerts excessive force on the thumb as it moves forward (Fig. 4.4). Left and right gloves keep the thumb in a neutral position (Fig. 4.5).

Mechanical dentistry. The use of mechanical-powered dental instruments in place of manual hand instruments reduces the risk of injury. Therefore, mechanical-powered dental instruments should be used whenever possible. Ultrasonic scalers are an excellent choice for the removal of heavy deposits and subgingival root cleaning; these instruments eliminate the need for all but the most cursory scaling.

Instrument handles. Because instruments with "fat" handles are easier to hold, they reduce the fatigue caused by pressing the handles with sufficient force to remove deposits (Fig. 4.6).

Patient positioning. Sandbags are used to position the patient for easy access and visibility, which also improves the operator's positioning. Use of a dental operating light, rather than a surgical light, affords greater flexibility in illuminating the deeper parts of the mouth so that the operator does not need to lean excessively to see the back teeth. Technicians should remember that during the course of a procedure they can change their own position or the position of the patient to reduce the risk of injury. Some teeth are more easily reached from over the head, some from the front of the mouth, and some from the patient's mandible side.

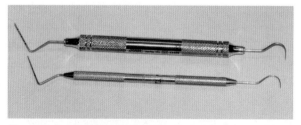

Fig. 4.6 Fat handles are easier to hold on to and less fatiguing than thin handles.

Strengthening exercises. Strengthening the muscles opposite the ones used in dental procedures reduces stress on the working muscles by providing more overall support. Employees should remember to stretch during long procedures or whenever they feel fatigued. Alternating hand and mechanical procedures during treatment also helps rest muscle groups. To relax the shoulders in a standing position, employees can interlace their fingers behind their backs and raise them up as high as possible while leaning forward slightly. This position should be held for 30 seconds (Fig. 4.7).

Another simple way to relax the shoulders while working is to sit up straight, with the hands parallel against the sides. Then, the thumbs should be turned outward as far back as possible while the stomach muscles are tightened. This position should be held for 30 seconds (Fig. 4.8).

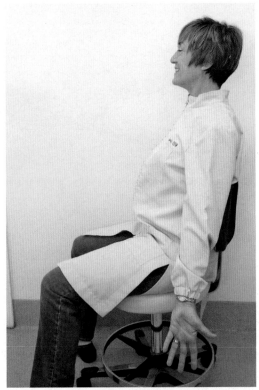

Fig. 4.8 Side shoulder stretch.

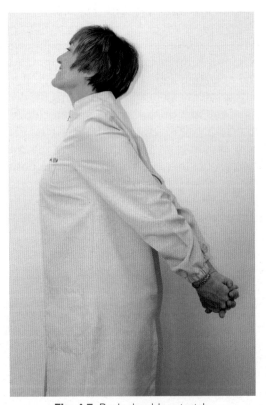

Fig. 4.7 Back shoulder stretch.

To relax the back, the employee should interlace the fingers overhead, with the palms toward the ceiling. With the feet approximately hip width apart and the arms at ear level, the employee should then lean first to the right for 30 seconds and then to the left for another 30 seconds (Fig. 4.9).

To stretch the forearm muscles, employees should raise one arm almost straight forward and then pull their index, middle, and ring fingers back until they feel resistance, taking care not to lock the elbow. This position should be held for 30 seconds (Fig. 4.10).

To stretch the opposite muscles, employees should bend the hand downward, gently push against the fingers, and hold for 30 seconds (Fig. 4.11). Performing these last two exercises several times a day is recommended, particularly when the technician is especially fatigued (e.g., after scaling the teeth of a patient with an unusual amount of calculus).

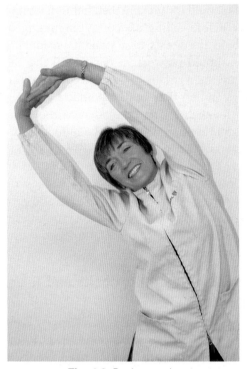

Fig. 4.9 Back stretch.

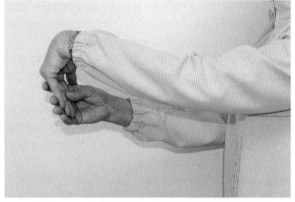

Fig. 4.11 Forearm stretch opposite muscles.

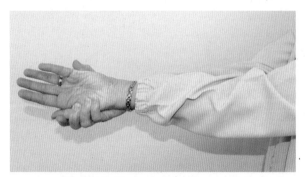

Fig. 4.12 Alternate forearm stretch.

Stretching the muscles that go from the outside of your elbow to the wrist is difficult; the best way to accomplish it is to straighten your elbow and rotate your thumb down and out toward the outside while pulling gently on the outside of the palm and pushing on the thumb area toward the rotation at the same time. Spreading your fingers while holding this helps to stretch the entire forearm (Fig. 4.12).

Lifestyle Ergonomics

Attention to muscle groups used in dentistry must also extend into life outside the workplace. Employees should give their bodies a chance to heal and rest between workdays. Regular exercise that does not repeat the same motions frequently performed at work is a good way to maintain health and general well-being. Employees should make an effort

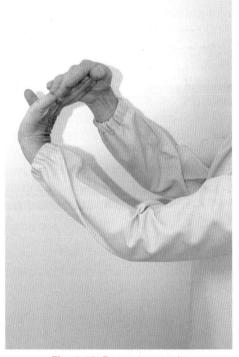

Fig. 4.10 Forearm stretch.

to work opposing muscle groups and acquire balanced muscle development as well as working out regularly to relieve the stresses of the day.

Power walking is one of the better ways to maintain overall body toning and relieve stress without overusing injury-prone areas. Using light hand weights (1 pound) while power walking also helps develop upper body strength without stressing the neck or wrist areas. Heavy Hands handles without weights on them allow carrying weight without the need to hold onto them (no "squeeze factor"). Wrist weights also work as long as they are not tight or moving up and down on the wrist. They should always be carried with the arms bent at a 90-degree angle; straight arms exert pressure on the elbow tendons.

Preventing Injury Away From the Workplace

Performing small-motor activities, such as needlework, prevents the muscles and tendons from relaxing sufficiently after work. Over time, muscles may become sore or irritated. Certain forms of exercise, such as bike riding, put pressure on the wrist, lower back, and neck in much the same way that dental procedures do. Consequently, the body does not have the opportunity to recover from the stresses of the workplace. Carrying heavy items, such as shopping bags, luggage, and large purses, stresses the elbow and wrist tendons excessively and can also cause neck and shoulder pain. Using suitcases with wheels, making frequent trips to deposit shopping bags in the car, and carrying a small purse with only the necessities–all help relieve these problems.

Sleeping with the hands curled into the pillow irritates the wrist tendons. People who habitually do this should try tucking their hands flat under the pillow before falling asleep or purchasing braces that hold the wrists in a straight position. These braces should be worn at night until the habit of bending the wrists is broken. Sleeping on the side or back (rather than on the stomach) is also much better for the neck and shoulders. Although sleeping habits are hard to break, the reduction in neck pain makes the attempt worthwhile. Neck-support pillows (the kind that have a depression in the middle) keep the neck in a good position during sleep. Any measures to reduce stress and promote proper alignment in injury-prone areas lengthen the employee's professional life and reduce the pain caused by repetitive motions.

Ergonomic Operatory Chairs and Tables

Dental Chairs

One of the problems faced in veterinary dentistry is that we need to be able to adjust the chair to both the height of the table and the height of the operator choice of cylinder height. If the table is high (and not adjustable) the standard cylinder with a height adjustment of 18¼ inches to 23¼ inches is best. If the table and operator are short, a short cylinder height range is 16¾ inches to 20¼ inches. The ideal dental chair has a lumbar support that adjusts up-down and front-back. The seat tilt should be adjustable (Fig. 4.13). Chairs with arm rests help ease back problems (see Fig. 4.13C).

Ergonomic Tables

Ergonomic tables have adjustable heights that allow one to position the table in addition to the chair so that the practitioner can obtain a neutral position (Fig. 4.14).

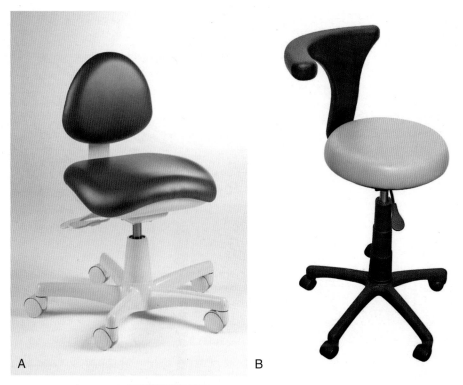

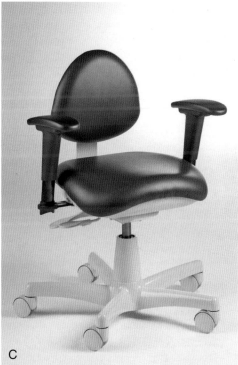

Fig. 4.13 (A) Midmark dental chair. (B) iM3 dental chair. (C) Midmark dental chair with arm rests. (A and C, Courtesy Midmark, Versailles, OH. B, Courtesy iM3, Vancouver, WA.)

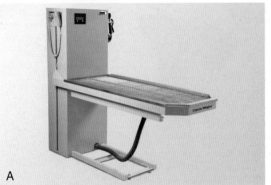

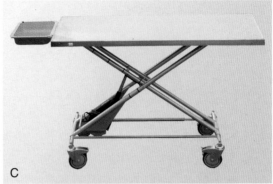

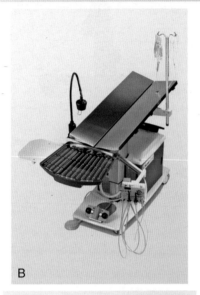

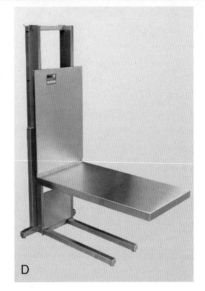

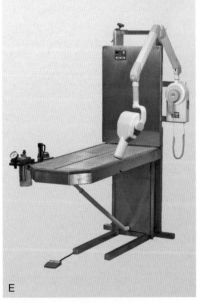

Fig. 4.14 (A) Canis major wet dental treatment lift table. (B) Surgiden theramax DX. (C) Electric transport table with dental tray. (D) Elsam III peninsula table. (E) Elsam IV with equipment. (A, Courtesy Midmark, Versailles, OH. B, Courtesy Surgiden, Towson, MD. C and D, Courtesy Technidyne, Toms River, NJ. E, Courtesy Herb Clay.)

CHAPTER 4 WORKSHEET (ANSWERS ARE ON PAGE 294)

1. Employers are required by _____ to provide employees with preventive safety equipment and require them to wear it during dental procedures.

2. Employees must always be careful to take responsibility for _____ _____ _____.

3. Hazards are classified as follows: _____, _____, _____, and _____.

4. Scaling can also send _____-laden calculus into the dental technician's eyes or mouth.

5. Proper _____ is important for disease control.

6. Employees should be careful to rinse their hands in _____ water.

7. A type I allergic reaction takes place _____ after exposure.

8. Chemical manufacturers and importers must convey hazard information to employers by means of labels on containers and _____ _____ _____ _____.

9. The ultrasonic solutions are not _____ and contain bacteria that can enter the hands through small cuts and openings.

10. Attention to muscle groups used in dentistry must also extend into _____ outside the workplace.

Local Anesthesia

LEARNING OBJECTIVES

When you have completed this chapter, you will be able to:

- List the possible reactions to local anesthetics used in veterinary dentistry.
- Describe the use of bupivacaine in veterinary dentistry and list time of onset of activity and duration of action for this drug.
- State maximal volumes of local anesthetics that should be administered to dogs and cats.
- Describe the purpose and procedure for performing a regional anesthetic block.
- List the four anatomic areas where regional anesthesia is performed before veterinary dental procedures.

KEY TERMS

Bupivacaine
Inferior alveolar nerve block
Infiltration blocks
Infraorbital nerve block

MAC
Major palatine nerve block
Maxillary block
Middle mental nerve block

Regional nerve block
Superior alveolar nerve block

This chapter is devoted to local anesthesia, which is used in veterinary dentistry to reduce the dependence on gas anesthesia during surgery and to control pain during and after the procedure. Reducing the dependence on gas anesthesia can decrease complications of general anesthesia such as hypoventilation, hypotension, and bradycardia.

This chapter focuses on the administration of local anesthetics, benefits, and complications. Local anesthetics are only a part of multimodal anesthesia and analgesia. The veterinary team should utilize all available resources when developing an anesthetic plan for a patient.

Laws regarding the legality of the technician performing these procedures will vary from state to state. In addition, it is up to the supervising veterinarian to prescribe and determine the appropriateness of the technician performing the procedure. While local anesthetics are beneficial, there are potentials for serious complications. The operator should have a strong knowledge of the local anatomy before attempting these nerve blocks.

MECHANISM OF LOCAL ANESTHETICS

Nerve cells work by sending small electrical currents through adjacent nerve cells. Simplified, the currents are caused by the exchange of sodium and potassium ions. Local anesthetics work by blocking the channels the sodium ions use to get into the nerve cell. This cuts off any current and therefore any message of pain. This effect wears off as the anesthetic diffuses throughout the body.

Several local anesthetics are available to the veterinary practitioner. *Bupivacaine* is the most used for dental procedures in dogs and cats. It is most used at a 0.5% solution or 5 mg/mL. The onset of action is typically less than 10 minutes, and the duration of action is 6 to 10 hours. Bupivacaine may be used with or without epinephrine. It is typically recommended to avoid using epinephrine in patients with hypertrophic cardiomyopathy, arrythmias, and history of pheochromocytoma. This is not an exhaustive list and best clinical judgment is recommended.

Lidocaine has been used as well. It does have a shorter time to onset and shorter duration of action. Some have proposed mixing of lidocaine and bupivacaine with the idea of a synergistic effect resulting in a shorter time to onset but a longer duration. The mixing appears not to be synergistic with no change in onset to effect and may decrease the duration of effect.

With challenges in the medical supply chain, bupivacaine has been scarce at times. When not available, ropivacaine is a good alternative due to similar properties. Typically, it does not have a preservative and the bottle needs to be disposed of after 24 hours.

Possible, but rare, reactions to local anesthetics include toxicity to skeletal muscle, anaphylactic reactions, and permanent nerve damage. A simple rule of thumb to avoid toxicity is to never exceed 2.0 mg/kg of bupivacaine in cats and dogs. Exercise care, especially in smaller patients and cats so that these maximal doses are not exceeded. The total volume used depends on the size of the patient and the number of sites that require analgesia. For example, if regional anesthesia is being performed and all four quadrants were blocked in a 10 lb (4.6 kg) cat at 0.1 mL of 0.5% of bupivacaine per site, the cat would receive 0.4 mL or 2.0 mg, well below the maximal dose of 9.2 mg.

BENEFITS OF NERVE BLOCKS

During general anesthesia, the patient can still perceive pain. Analgesics such as opiates and anti-inflammatories do help decrease pain, but unless the transmission of pain signals to the brain is blocked, pain is still detected. To maintain the depth of anesthesia needed to complete surgery, gas anesthetics need to be increased or other analgesics added. All anesthetic medications have the potential to cause harmful side effects, but gas anesthetics have the highest potential, especially when treating compromised patients.

Nerve blocks can help prevent painful stimulus from reaching the brain during the effective period. In this way, the amount of gas anesthetic needed is reduced. This is measured by the minimal alveolar concentration or *MAC*. Reducing the MAC of a gas anesthetic can reduce potentially dangerous side effects and reduce costs as less expensive inhalant is required.

Equally important, the patient perceives less pain, recovers with less pain, and may have less overall pain during the course of surgical recovery. Box 5.1 enlists indications of nerve blocks.

TYPES OF BLOCKS

The two types of local anesthesia are infiltration blocks and regional nerve blocks.

INFILTRATION BLOCKS

Infiltration blocks are not placed over a nerve but into the surgical area in hope that the anesthetic will infiltrate into the associated nervous tissue. It is generally accepted that these are less effective (or not effective) compared to regional blocks in dogs and cats.

REGIONAL NERVE BLOCKS

Regional nerve blocks are performed by placing the local anesthetic directly on the nerve providing sensory innervation to the operated area. The advantage of regional anesthesia is the ability to directly block the nerve that provides sensory function in the area being operated. The disadvantages of regional nerve blocks include transient loss of sensation and function of the area blocked and the possibility of postoperative self-inflicted injury to soft tissues as a sequel to anesthesia. Additionally, local injury can occur to the regional tissues including the eyes, vascular tissue, and target nerve.

Equipment

None of the regional nerve blocks for oral surgery in dogs and cats need any special equipment. Simple 1- or 3-mL syringes and 1 1/4" 25- or 27-gauge needles can be used to deliver the regional anesthetic.

General Technique

The needle is advanced slowly to the desired location. The syringe plunger is drawn back to perform aspiration. The needle is rotated 90 degrees until a full 360-degree rotation has been accomplished. A small amount of the drug is injected, and the aspiration is repeated to ensure that the needle is not in a vessel. If there is no blood drawn back, the agent is slowly injected. If there is blood, digital pressure should be put on the site, a new syringe and needle should be obtained, and the procedure should be repeated.

The regional nerve blocks are similar for the dog and the cat (Fig. 5.1A and B). The author recommends utilizing the inferior alveolar nerve block (sometimes called mandibular nerve block) for painful procedures of the lower jaws and a combination of the infraorbital, superior alveolar, maxillary, and major palatine for painful procedures of the upper jaws.

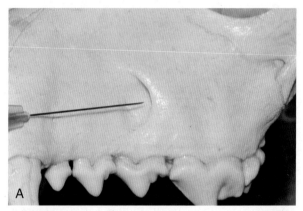

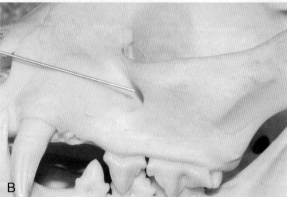

Fig. 5.1 (A) Needle placed on the infraorbital foramen in a dog. (B) Needle placed on the infraorbital foramen in a cat.

The *middle mental nerve block* utilizes the middle mental foramen to access the inferior alveolar nerve. There had been debate about which teeth were affected by the nerve block. Evidence suggests this nerve block is ineffective.

After administration of the block(s), the patient should be evaluated for the effectiveness of the block. If respiration rate, heart rate, and blood pressure increase with surgical manipulation, the block either has not had time for onset or was not correctly placed. If the block is not effective and enough time has elapsed, the block may be repeated as long as the maximal total dose is not exceeded. In cases where local anesthesia cannot be obtained, it is necessary to evaluate the other analgesics used to ensure the patient receives pain control.

Keep in mind that the nervous tissue from the contralateral side may extend to the target area if the incisors are being treated and bilateral blocks may need to be considered.

Technique
Infraorbital and Superior Alveolar Nerve Blocks

The maxillary nerve enters the infraorbital canal to become the superior alveolar nerve and ultimately the infraorbital nerve. The infraorbital exits the infraorbital canal via the infraorbital foramen, just apical or dorsal to the distal root of the maxillary third premolar. Anesthetizing this nerve will likely anesthetize the canine and incisor teeth on that side.

To perform the *infraorbital nerve block*, retract the superior lip dorsally and palpate just dorsal to the distal root of the maxillary third premolar (Fig. 5.2). The infraorbital neurovascular bundle beneath the vestibular mucosa is palpated as a large cylindric band that exits the infraorbital canal. This bundle is retracted dorsally with a digit of the hand that is not holding the syringe. The needle is advanced close to the maxillary bone ventral to the retracted bundle in a rostral to caudal direction to just inside the canal (Fig. 5.3). The needle should pass without hitting the bone around the

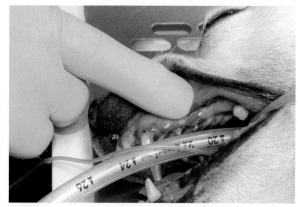

Fig. 5.2 The infraorbital foramen is palpated dorsal to the distal root of the maxillary third premolar.

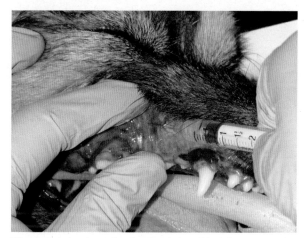

Fig. 5.3 Injection site in the infraorbital foramen of a dog.

infraorbital canal. If a bone is encountered, the needle is withdrawn slightly and redirected. Proper insertion can be confirmed by gentle movement of the syringe as the needle hits the infraorbital canal wall. This will likely anesthetize from the third premolar to the first incisor.

To anesthetize the premolars and molars, the superior alveolar branches need to be in contact with the local anesthetic. The *superior alveolar nerve block* is performed by advancing the needle (as inserted for the infraorbital nerve block) caudally and ventral to the retracted bundle in a rostral to the level of the lateral canthus of the eye. If bone

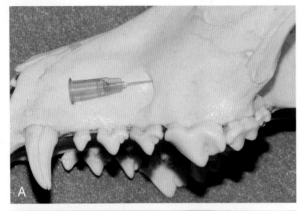

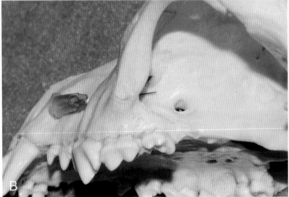

Fig. 5.4 (A) Needle advanced for superior alveolar nerve block in a dog skull. (B) Caudal view in a dog.

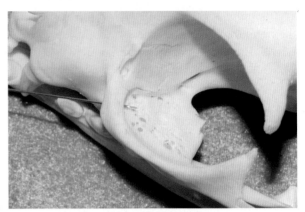

Fig. 5.5 Short infraorbital canal of the cat.

is encountered, the needle is withdrawn slightly and redirected. Proper insertion can be confirmed inability to palpate the needle lateral to the bone as it should be entirely within the infraorbital canal (Fig. 5.4A and B). The infraorbital canal of cats and brachycephalic dogs is very short, and therefore, it is important to keep the syringe and needle parallel to the dental arch line of the maxilla and not extend the needle to the level of the orbital tissues (Fig. 5.5).

Maxillary Nerve Block

Debate exists if the second molar of the dog can be anesthetized via the infraorbital canal. Additionally, the infraorbital canal of all patients cannot be accessed due to anatomic variation and presence of pathology. In these cases, the *maxillary nerve block* is utilized. There are several approaches to this nerve block. The author uses an intraoral approach, inserting the needle at the distolateral line angle of the second molar, advancing just past the alveolar bone of the second molar, and depositing the local anesthetic on the maxillary nerve before it enters the infraorbital canal. The author feels this nerve block presents more risk for iatrogenic trauma to the patient and uses it sparingly.

Major Palatine Nerve Block

The *major palatine block* is used when performing surgery of the hard palate and may provide analgesia to the palatal aspect of the periodontium of the maxillary teeth. The major palatine nerve exits the palatal process of the hard palate via the major palatine foramen located at the level of the mesial edge of the maxillary first molar between the dental arch and midline of the hard palate. The nerve branches at the level of the maxillary canine tooth and part travels through the diastema between the canine and third incisor with the remainder traveling through the palatine fissure. This nerve block is performed by sliding the needle through the mucosa to reach just rostral to the location of the major palatine foramen and injecting the local anesthetic in this region (not into the foramen).

Inferior Alveolar Nerve Block

The mandibular nerve enters the mandibular foramen, located on the lingual (medial) side of the

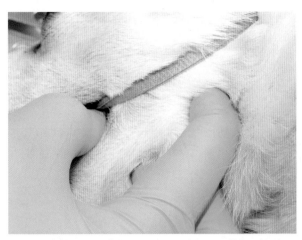

Fig. 5.6 Palpation of the notch caudal mandible of a dog.

mandible at the midpoint of the line that connects the angular process of the mandible and the last molar. When properly performed, the entire mandibular arch should be anesthetized.

The *inferior alveolar block* is performed by extraorally palpating the notch just dorsal to the angle of the mandible and ventral to the condylar process (Fig. 5.6).

The needle is advanced intraorally along the lingual side mandible from just caudal to the third molar in the dog (Fig. 5.7A) or first molar in the cat (Fig. 5.7B). Because the inferior mandibular nerve is located outside of the mandibular canal in this region, it is important that the needle tip is located just caudal to the foramen and rostral to the angular process of the mandible (Fig. 5.8A). Because the mandibular first molar is missing in the cat in Fig. 5.8B, the mandibular notch is palpated, the position of the first molar is approximated, and the needle is directed to the injection site, midway between where the tooth was and the notch.

An alternative method is to use the lateral canthus of the eye as the landmark. An imaginary line is drawn from the lateral canthus of the eye directly to the ventral mandible. The index finger is used to palpate the foramen on the inside of the ramus. Depending on the size of the patient, a 25-g ⅝- or 1½-inch needle is advanced up from the ventral mandible, aiming the point of the needle toward the

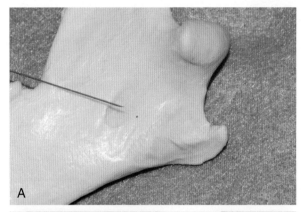

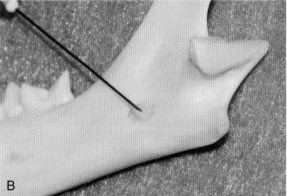

Fig. 5.7 (A) Intraoral mandibular needle placement in the dog skull for inferior alveolar nerve block. (B) Intraoral needle placement for inferior alveolar nerve block in a cat.

index finger, which is in position over the foramen. The needle is advanced along the lingual surface of the ramus. When the needle is felt by the index finger, without advancing through the mucosa, the plunger is pulled back to make sure a blood vessel is not hit and that the local anesthetic is injected. The bleb of local anesthetic should be felt developing under the index finger as the local anesthetic is injected to confirm proper needle placement. This should be about one to one-third of the distance from the ventral to the dorsal mandible.

Increasing the Duration of Local Anesthesia

Opioids inhibit the pain signal at multiple steps along the pain pathway. There are opioid receptors

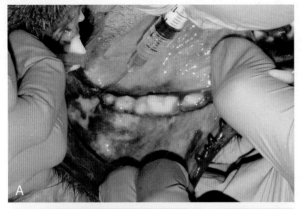

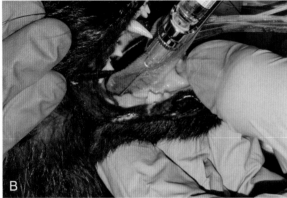

Fig. 5.8 (A) Intraoral mandibular needle placement in a dog. (B) Intraoral mandibular needle placement in a cat.

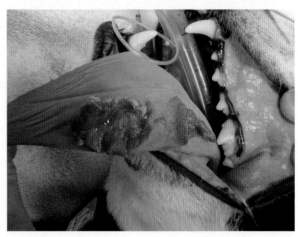

Fig. 5.9 Injured tongue by local anesthesia. This patient awoke and could not feel its tongue and, as a result, chewed its tongue.

If the inferior alveolar nerve block is placed too far caudally or lingually, there is risk of anesthetizing the lingual nerve and causing the tongue to become numb. In turn, this may lead to the patient biting into the tongue (Fig. 5.9). Treatment ranges from the distraction of the patient to sedation and general anesthesia until the regional anesthesia wears off or the dysphoria stops.

in the peripheral nervous system. Because of these receptors, buprenorphine has been shown to effectively double the analgesic duration when combined with bupivacaine. To mix, 0.05 mL of 300 µg/mL buprenorphine is added to 1 mL bupivacaine with the following doses administered as previously described in this chapter.

Complications of Local Anesthesia

The first potential complication of local anesthesia is that the local anesthetic is ineffective. This may be due to improper placement of the anesthetic or other patient and local factors. It is known that genetics play a factor efficacy of local anesthetics in humans, making the regional blocks ineffective or less effective. Regional changes in pH may also affect uptake of the anesthetic by the nerve cell.

BOX 5.2 Potential Complications of Nerve Blocks

Infraorbital and Superior Alveolar Nerve Block
- Retrobulbar hemorrhage
- Direct eye trauma (cats and small dogs)

Maxillary Nerve Block
- Direct eye trauma

Inferior Alveolar Nerve Block
- Anesthesia of the lingual nerve leading to self-trauma

All Nerve Blocks
- Systemic toxicity
- Inadequate analgesia
- Paresthesia

When performing the infraorbital nerve block in a cat or brachycephalic dog, there is a risk of injecting the local anesthetic into the eye if the needle is directed dorsally. There is risk of globe penetration when performing the maxillary nerve block in any animal. If this occurs, there is a high risk that the eye will need to be enucleated.

As the nerve targets for regional nerve blocks are associated with blood vessels, there is a risk of penetrating these vessels with the needle. The obvious risk is insertion of the local anesthetic intravascularly, hence necessitating the need to aspirate before injecting. Injection of the local aesthetic into a vessel may increase the risk of toxicity. Damage to the surrounding vessels may also induce hemorrhage. If hemorrhage is suborbital or retroorbital, there is potential to cause temporary exophthalmos. Potential complications of nerve blocks are enumerated in Box 5.2.

CHAPTER 5 WORKSHEET (ANSWERS ARE ON PAGE 295)

1. It is up to the _____ to prescribe and determine the appropriateness of the technician performing the procedure assuming state law allows for it.
2. Bupivacaine is the most used local anesthetic at a _____% solution or _____ mg/mL.
3. The total dose of bupivacaine should never exceed _____ mg/kg in dogs and cats.
4. The site for the infraorbital foramen is just dorsal to the _____ root of the maxillary _____ premolar.
5. To perform the superior alveolar nerve block, the needle is advanced more _____ via the _____ canal.
6. The inferior alveolar nerve block is performed by injecting the local anesthetic over the _____ on the _____ side of the mandible.
7. To perform inferior alveolar block, the needle is advanced intraorally along the mandible from just caudal to the _____ molar in the dog or _____ molar in the cat.
8. Always _____ prior to injecting.
9. If the _____ nerve is anesthetized while trying to perform the _____nerve block, the tongue may be anesthetized, leading to trauma.
10. _____ or _____ may be added to the local anesthetic to increase the duration of anesthesia.
11. Previously used to anesthetize the rostral mandibles, the _____ nerve block is not recommended as it is thought not to be effective.
12. Local anesthetics work by blocking _____ channels, preventing the nerve from firing.
13. If bupivacaine is not available, _____ is an alternative that has similar properties.
14. _____ blocks are not placed over the nerve and are thought to be less effective than regional nerve blocks.
15. _____ gauge needles are typically recommended for performing regional nerve blocks.

FURTHER READING

Krug W, Losey J. Area of desensitization following mental nerve block in dogs. *J Vet Dent.* 2011 Fall;28(3):146–150. doi:10.1177/089875641102800301.

Lawal FM, Adetunji A. A comparison of epidural anaesthesia with lignocaine, bupivacaine and a lignocaine-bupivacaine mixture in cats. *J S Afr Vet Assoc.* 2009;80(4):243–246.

Snyder LBC, Snyder CJ, Hetzel S. Effects of buprenorphine added to bupivacaine infraorbital nerve blocks on isoflurane minimum alveolar concentration using a model for acute dental/oral surgical pain in dogs. *J Vet Dent.* 2016;33(2):90–96. doi:10.1177/0898756416657232.

Pathogenesis of Periodontal Disease

CHAPTER OUTLINE

LEARNING OBJECTIVES

When you have completed this chapter, you will be able to:

- List the factors that contribute to the development of periodontal disease in dogs and cats.
- Define periodontal disease and describe the appearance of the gingival and other supporting tissues when periodontal disease is present.
- Discuss the etiology of periodontal disease and define the terms "plaque" and "calculus."
- Become familiar with the hypotheses of why periodontal disease develops.
- Learn the typical indices for recording periodontal disease.
- Describe the staging of periodontal disease using the American Veterinary Dental College (AVDC) classification system.

KEY TERMS

Anaerobic bacteria
Biofilm
Calculus
Crestal bone loss
Epithelial attachment
Furcation

Gingivitis
Halitosis
Pellicle
Perio to endo lesion
Periodontal disease
Periodontitis

Plaque
Pocket
Tartar
Thiols

Periodontal disease (PD) is one of the most diagnosed diseases in dogs and cats and the most treated disease in the veterinary dental practice. Having a good working knowledge of the pathogenesis, consequences, and treatment strategies is important for the whole team.

Many factors determine the reason why one patient develops PD and another does not. These factors include age, species, breed, genetics, chewing behavior, diet, grooming habits (that can cause impaction of hair around the tooth and in the gingival sulcus), orthodontic occlusion, health status, home care, frequency of professional dental care, and bacterial flora of the oral cavity (Box 6.1). As our understanding of PD improves, other factors are coming to light.

PERIODONTAL DISEASE

Periodontal disease is an inflammation and infection of the periodontal tissues (Fig. 6.1). The resultant inflammation of the periodontium is known as *periodontitis*. With ongoing periodontitis, the periodontal tissues may be progressively lost. Locally, this leads to root exposure, tooth mobility, and

potential inflammation and infection of the pulp. Several local and systemic consequences can occur as well.

Etiology and Pathogenesis
Plaque
The saliva provides substrates such as glycoproteins to form a layer on the tooth called the *pellicle*. The pellicle forms on the enamel nearly immediately after dental cleaning or brushing. It allows for bacterial attachment to the surface of the tooth soon after formation. This bacterial layer is known as *plaque*. With continued plaque maturation, the overall bacterial population switches from predominantly gram-positive aerobic bacteria to predominantly gram-negative anaerobic bacteria, which are generally considered more harmful to the periodontal tissues. The now-established community of bacterial colonies protected by a polysaccharide complex, known as *biofilm*, is protected within the glycoproteins and other products present, greatly reducing the efficacy of antiseptics and antibiotics on plaque bacteria. Therefore, the disruption of this biofilm is the key factor in the control of PD and not antimicrobial therapy.

Plaque is found in several areas around the tooth. Plaque can be supragingival and attached to the tooth or gingiva, or it can be subgingival free-floating in the pocket or sulcus. As the soft

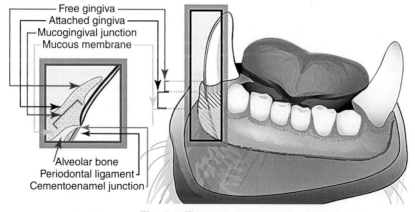

Fig. 6.1 The periodontium.

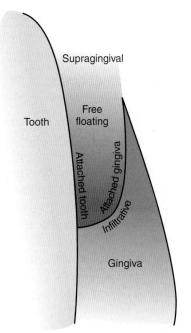

Fig. 6.2 Types of plaque: supragingival, free-floating subgingival, attached to tooth or gingiva, and invasive into gingiva.

tissues become compromised, bacteria from plaque can infiltrate into the periodontal and connective tissues (Fig. 6.2).

Calculus

When minerals from saliva (and other minor sources) interact with plaque, precipitation of mineral crystals occurs within the plaque, which propagates to form *calculus*. The mineral composition is mainly calcium carbonate and calcium phosphate. In common vernacular, calculus is called *tartar*.

Theories of Periodontitis

There are five theories explaining why some patients develop periodontitis while others are minimally affected. These are the nonspecific plaque hypothesis, the specific plaque hypothesis, the ecologic plaque hypothesis, the keystone pathogen hypothesis, and the polymicrobial synergy and dysbiosis hypothesis. The nonspecific plaque hypothesis is a model where periodontitis

is caused by a simple overpopulation of all plaque bacterial species. The specific plaque hypothesis is like the previous hypothesis that the bacterial population changes from gram-positive aerobic bacteria to gram-negative anaerobic bacteria. The ecologic plaque hypothesis suggests that local environmental factors such as pH and oxygen concentration are the inciting factors, allowing plaque bacteria to flourish. The keystone pathogen theory describes the presence of a specific bacteria species leading to periodontitis directly and indirectly. Polymicrobial synergy and dysbiosis hypothesis describes interactions between different bacterial species that create "cooperation" between the species and increase virulence. It may be obvious that there are similarities between the models and there is no consensus regarding whether one model is more likely. There are likely parts of each model that work, and no one model can explain periodontitis entirely.

Local Effects of Plaque and Calculus

Healthy periodontal tissues are coral pink and do not bleed during probing. The exception to coral pink tissue is healthy pigmented tissue, which is dark purple to black in color. Plaque and calculus contribute to the inflammation of the periodontal tissues. Plaque contributes directly to inflammation through bacteria-induced inflammation and the patient's own inflammatory response. Calculus causes minor inflammation directly as an irritant to the soft tissues. More importantly, it serves as a surface for increased plaque accumulation.

Initially, the inflammation begins as an inflammation of the gingiva only, *gingivitis*.

If inflammation is allowed to continue, the gingival attachment to the tooth is compromised. As a result, the gingiva separates from the tooth, past the original level of the gingival sulcus. This space is known as a *pocket*. Without the gingival *epithelial attachment*, which is the epithelium attaching the gingiva to the tooth, the gingiva may begin to recede in an apical direction.

Other periodontal tissues become inflamed and are lost as well, typically beginning with crestal bone loss. *Crestal bone loss* is the resorption of the peaks of bone mesial and distal to teeth or within the interdental space. This can be observed radiographically and is an early indicator of periodontitis. If the patient is not treated and the disease is allowed to progress, deeper pockets form. With increased bone loss, root exposure, infrabony pockets, and loss of furcation, exposure occurs. In multirooted teeth, the *furcation,* which is the area at which the roots join the crown, and loss of bone in this area creates exposure of this portion of the tooth. This creates more regions for plaque to attach and thus cause more inflammation. As attachment loss progresses apically, the apical delta or lateral canals to the pulp may be compromised. This can lead to infection and inflammation of the pulp and is known as a *perio-to-endo lesion.*

Finally, if the loss of attachment is sufficient, the tooth may fall out.

Depending on the location and severity of periodontal attachment loss, several serious local complications can occur. If the maxillary incisors, canines, or premolars are severely affected, an oronasal fistula may occur, leading to possible rhinitis. Disease of the maxillary fourth premolar or molars may lead to infection of the suborbital tissues. Bone loss of the mandibular incisors can lead to loss of the bony attachment of the mandibular symphysis, resulting in laxity of this joint. And bone loss of the mandibular third incisor region to the first molar region can compromise the mandibular body, resulting in a pathologic fracture.

Systemic Effects of Periodontal Disease

The systemic effects of PD are well documented in humans. Diseases such as atherosclerosis, stroke, and diabetes mellitus appear to have a correlation with periodontitis. Periodontitis may contribute to these diseases through the direct effects of periodontal bacteria, indirectly via the effect of associated inflammatory mediators, or a combination of both. Research in veterinary medicine is still ongoing. While it is difficult to make a direct causative link from PD to other systemic diseases, it appears likely that PD affects many body systems in dogs and cats.

Presenting Complaints and Initial Signs

Most commonly, clients report *halitosis,* or bad breath, as the patient's PD progresses. This is often mistakenly called "doggy breath." This condition, however, is not normal. It is caused by *thiols,* which are sulfur-containing byproducts of plaque bacteria metabolism. Clients may report that their pets are not eating well. Occasionally, patients drool and blood may be noted in the saliva. Clients may also observe the patient pawing at its mouth.

Often, pet owners are not aware of a problem as veterinary patients are expert at hiding pain and discomfort. Therefore, it is up to the veterinary team to be the advocate for the pet. On oral examination, red, inflamed gingiva may be noted. The gingiva may bleed easily during the examination. Fragile capillaries in the inflamed tissue cause this bleeding. An accumulation of plaque and calculus is evident. However, it is important to note that the amount of plaque and calculus does not always correspond to the degree of PD present. It is not uncommon to find patients with mild to moderate changes noted on the conscious examination have severe periodontal bone loss noted during the anesthetized examination.

Patients with PD may also have visible root exposure, mobile teeth, or missing teeth. PD is not the only disease to cause bad breath, mobile teeth, and lack of appetite. Renal and gastrointestinal diseases can cause both bad breath and lack of appetite. As stated before, there are several causes of mobile teeth. It is important that the patient be assessed before recommending general anesthesia.

Assessing and Recording Periodontal Disease

Periodontal disease examination findings should be recorded. Some findings such as calculus accumulation and degree of gingival inflammation are easily recorded in the standard examination.

Others including tooth mobility and periodontal pocket depths require a dental chart, which is described in detail ahead in the text.

Tracking these findings will allow the team to monitor progression of disease and success of treatment. Standardized descriptions have been established for findings that are not simply objective (as periodontal pocket depth is). These include the indices for plaque, calculus, gingivitis, and mobility as well as the stage of furcation exposure. These indices have been summarized in Box 6.2.

Keep in mind that not all tooth mobility is secondary to PD. Teeth may also be mobile due to root fracture, bone fracture, tooth resorption, metabolic disease, or neoplasia; therefore, full evaluation including imaging is necessary (Fig. 6.3).

Most PD findings are based on visual examination and periodontal probing. In addition to a thorough anesthetized examination, dental radiography is necessary to fully assess PD. Early periodontitis, marked by crestal bone loss, cannot be detected by examination alone and treatment options cannot be fully evaluated without radiographs. Dental imaging is discussed in more detail later in the text. Regardless, dental radiograph is necessary for the full evaluation.

Other diagnostic tools are readily available. OraStrip is used to test for thiols. The presence of thiols indicates the presence of PD. The OraStrip is first removed from its protective pouch, taking care not to touch the small pad on the top of the strip. Next, the patient's upper lip is lifted while supporting the pad end of the test strip with the index finger on the nonpad side. The pad is gently glided against the upper gum line. Salivary fluid is drawn into the pad, taking no longer than 5 to 10 seconds. Care should be taken not to cause bleeding because this may interfere with the results. Once the sample has been collected, remove the strip from the patient's mouth and wait 10 seconds before reading the result. The strip is held near the colors shown on the comparator card color chart, and the number of the color closest to the color on the pad is noted. The color should be based on the

---

BOX 6.2   Plaque Index (Silness and Loe)

Grade 0: None
Grade 1: Thin layer at gingival margin only detectable by scraping with probe
Grade 2: Moderate layer visible to naked eye
Grade 3: Abundant with interdental spaces filled

Calculus Index
Grade 0: None
Grade 1: Thin band of calculus at free gingival margin only
Grade 2: 1/3 to 2/3 of the crown is covered
Grade 3: >2/3 of the crown is covered or bridging calculus is present

Gingival Index (Loe and Silness)
Grade 0: None
Grade 1: Slight erythema with no bleeding
Grade 2: Moderate erythema, bleeding on probing
Grade 3: Severe erythema, spontaneous bleeding, possible ulceration

Furcation Involvement Index
Stage 1 Furcation (FI): Probe extends less than half the distance under the crown
Stage 2 Furcation (F2): Probe extends greater than half the distance under the crown but not fully through
Stage 3 Furcation (F3): Probe able to pass completely through furcation

Tooth Mobility Index
Stage 0 (M0): Physiologic mobility up to 0.2 mm.
Stage 1 (M1): The mobility is increased in any direction other than axial over a distance of more than 0.2 mm and up to 0.5 mm.
Stage 2 (M2): The mobility is increased in any direction other than axial over a distance of more than 0.5 mm and up to 1.0 mm.
Stage 3 (M3): The mobility is increased in any direction other than axial over a distance exceeding 1.0 mm or any axial movement.

---

most intense color seen on the pad. A numerical result of 1 or above is associated with active PD. A score of 0 is not associated with active periodontal

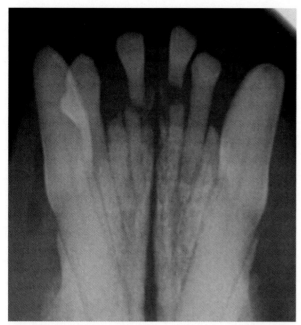

Fig. 6.3 Fractured roots will cause tooth mobility, but not due to periodontal disease.

infection. For dogs with a history of PD, a score of 0 reflects favorable ongoing management of existing disease.

Plaque-disclosing solutions can be used to make plaque more visible. These come in many forms. The liquid form can be gently dabbed on teeth, which stains plaque a visible pink, blue, or green color. This aids in quantifying plaque accumulation. It also aids the operator in ensuring all plaque is removed from the teeth. Plaque-disclosing solutions can also stain the patient and clothing.

PERIODONTAL DISEASE CLASSIFICATION

The American Veterinary Dental College (AVDC) has created a classification system for PD. It differs from the system presented in the previous edition of this text. This system is a radiographic system and not a clinical grading system. To use this system, you must have radiographs to evaluate the state of periodontal health with the AVDC's system. Staging is performed only after the radiographs have been taken. The degree of severity of PD relates to a single tooth; a patient may have teeth that have different stages of PD described ahead:

Normal (PD 0): Clinically normal: No gingival inflammation or periodontitis clinically evident (Fig. 6.4).

Stage 1 (PD 1): Gingivitis only without attachment loss. The height and architecture of the alveolar margin are normal (Fig. 6.5A and B).

Stage 2 (PD 2): Early periodontitis: Less than 25% of attachment loss or, at most, there is a stage 1 furcation involvement in multirooted teeth. There are early radiologic signs of periodontitis. The loss of periodontal attachment is less than 25%, as measured either by probing of the clinical attachment level or by radiographic determination of the distance of the alveolar margin from the cementoenamel junction relative to the length of the root (Fig. 6.6A and B).

Stage 3 (PD 3): Moderate periodontitis: 25% to 50% of attachment loss, as measured either by probing of the clinical attachment level or by radiographic determination of the distance of the alveolar margin from the cementoenamel junction relative to the length of the root, or there is a stage 2 furcation involvement in multirooted teeth (Fig. 6.7A and B).

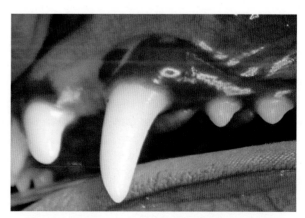

Fig. 6.4 Teeth and gingiva of a normal young dog.

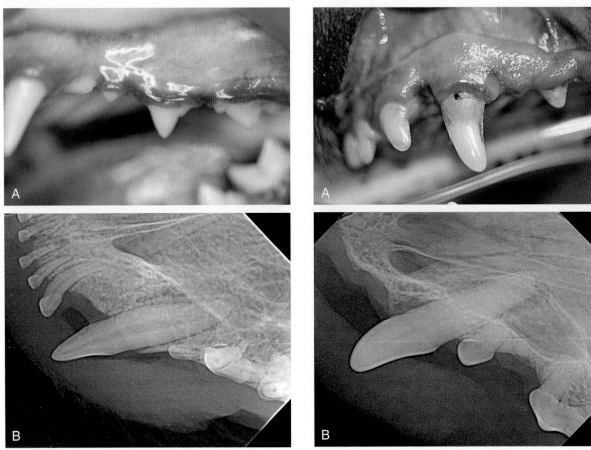

Fig. 6.5 (A) Periodontal disease stage 1 (PD 1) in a cat. (B) PD 1 radiograph of a cat.

Fig. 6.6 (A) Periodontal disease stage 2 (PD 2) in a dog. (B) PD 2 radiograph of a dog with a missing left maxillary second premolar.

Stage 4 (PD 4): Advanced periodontitis: More than 50% of attachment loss, as measured either by probing of the clinical attachment level or by radiographic determination of the distance of the alveolar margin from the cementoenamel junction relative to the length of the root, or there is a stage 3 furcation involvement in multirooted teeth (Fig. 6.8).

Patients may have teeth with mixed stages of PD (Fig. 6.9A and B). In Fig. 6.9, the premolars are stage 4 and the canine is stage 2. Taking the worst tooth's grade, this would be considered stage 4 (PD 4).

Chapters regarding the prevention and treatment of PD follow. Of note, although clients do not always perceive an obvious problem when their pet has PD, they typically appreciate that their pet is more active and seems "happier" after the treatment of PD.

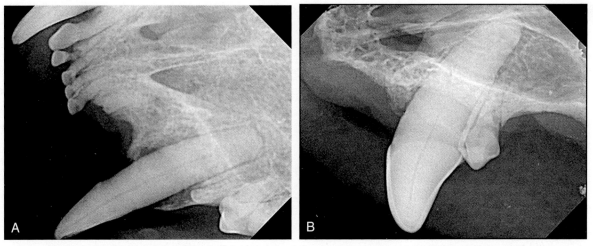

Fig. 6.7 (A) Stage 3 periodontal disease of the left maxillary canine tooth in a cat. Note retained third incisor root. (B) Radiograph of periodontal disease stage 3 (PD 3): left maxillary canine tooth and first premolar.

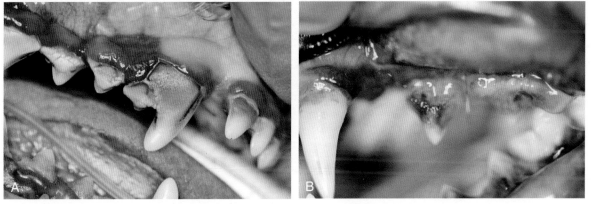

Fig. 6.8 (A) Periodontal disease stage 4 (PD 4) in a dog. (B) PD 4 in a cat.

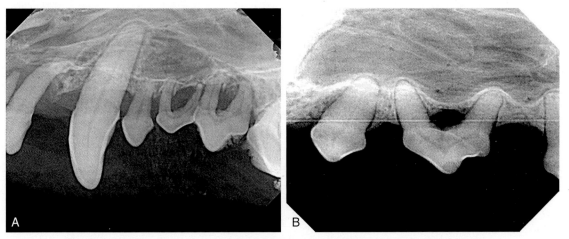

Fig. 6.9 Mixed stages of periodontal disease are graded by the worst tooth present.

CHAPTER 6 WORKSHEET (ANSWERS ARE ON PAGE 295)

1. Periodontal disease is an _____ and _____ of the tissues surrounding the tooth. It is characterized by movement of the gingiva toward the apex and migration of the junctional epithelium, with associated loss of the periodontal ligament and bone surrounding the tooth.
2. A glycoprotein component of saliva, known as the _____, attaches to the tooth surface allowing for bacterial attachment.
3. Healthy periodontal tissues are _____ and have no _____ during probing.
4. Stage _____ periodontal disease is gingivitis only without attachment loss.
5. Periodontal disease has _____ stages, including stage 0.
6. Loss of bone at the furcation that allows the probe to pass fully through the furcation indicates stage _____ furcation involvement.
7. While it is difficult make a direct _____ from periodontal disease to systemic disease, it is likely that periodontal disease affects other body systems.
8. The clinical term for bad breath is _____.
9. The sulfur containing compounds that cause bad breath are _____.
10. _____ can be due to periodontal disease, neoplasia, root fracture, or metabolic disease.
11. Other causes of inappetence (besides periodontal disease) include _____.
12. The presence of _____ protects bacteria from antiseptics and antibiotics.
13. There are _____ theories regarding why some patients develop periodontitis.
14. The established hypothesis that gram-negative anaerobic bacteria overpopulate the plaque flora during periodontitis is called _____.
15. Mineral from _____ interacts with plaque to create _____.

CHAPTER OUTLINE

LEARNING OBJECTIVES

When you have completed this chapter, you will be able to:

- List the instruments and equipment needed to perform a professional dental cleaning and periodontal therapy.
- List the steps in performing a professional dental cleaning.
- Explain the rationale for performing endotracheal intubation prior to anesthetizing a patient for a dental prophy.
- Describe circumstances under which the veterinarian may prescribe antibiotics for dental patients.

- Describe the proper use of a mouth gag during the dental prophy.
- Explain the purpose of the water flow through the ultrasonic dental scaler.
- Describe the general technique used for scaling teeth with an ultrasonic scaler.
- Describe the instrument used and general technique for evaluating depth of the sulcus.
- Describe the modified pen grasp for holding dental instruments.
- Describe the general technique used for polishing teeth.

KEY TERMS

Closed position

Disclosing solution

Four-handed charting

Modified pen grasp

Open position

Periodontal therapy

Professional dental cleaning

Prophylaxis

Pull stroke

Veterinarians and technicians often speak of performing a "dental prophylaxis," "prophy," or "dental." This usage is incorrect and may often mislead the client regarding the patient's true condition. The word *prophylaxis*, which means prevention of or protective treatment for disease would indicate a procedure to prevent disease, and not treat disease. Typically, the veterinary patient has some state of periodontal disease or other dental pathology that is being treated. Uncommonly is the patient receiving purely preventative treatment (that would be ideal). This important distinction must be kept in mind when discussing treatment plans with the client.

Once the patient has periodontal disease, far more extensive treatment is required. In this case the clinician should discuss with the client the necessary steps and options (that may include extractions) to treat the condition.

Several acronyms (COHAT, COAPT, etc.) have been proposed to describe the various procedures performed in professional prevention and treatment of periodontal disease. While these acronyms do serve a purpose, the absence of a universally accepted acronym leads to confusion. Currently, the AVDC describes dental and scaling under general anesthesia as a *professional dental cleaning* (PRO) and treatment of diseased periodontal tissues as *periodontal therapy*. These procedures require several important instruments and pieces of equipment (Box 7.1).

As a note, many texts (including the previous editions of this text) use the term "Complete Prophy" to describe all the steps in PRO. This term has been omitted from this text not as a criticism of its use, but to reflect current AVDC nomenclature. One will note that different texts describe this

---

> **BOX 7.1   Instruments and Equipment Needed for Professional Dental Cleaning**
>
> Universal and area-specific hand scaler
> Universal and area-specific hand curette
> Calculus-removing forceps
> Periodontal probe/explorer with appropriate marking for patient
> Ultrasonic scaler
> Low-speed handpiece
> Prophylaxis angle
> Prophylaxis cup
> Prophylaxis paste
> Disclosing solution
> Chlorhexidine rinse
> PPE (eye protection, mask, gloves)

procedure differently, but the essential pieces are the same.

PREPARATION FOR THE PROCEDURE

Before performing PRO, the veterinarian should discuss the procedure with the client and provide a written estimate of its cost and potential complications. After obtaining the client's consent, the veterinarian should develop a contingency plan in case additional problems are discovered under anesthesia and the client must be contacted. The client should provide instructions so that the veterinary team knows how to proceed in case the client is unavailable during the procedure. Options may include the following:

1. Proceed with recommended procedures.
2. Attempt to call first; if the client cannot be reached, proceed with recommended procedures.
3. Do nothing if the client cannot be contacted.

If the client cannot be reached, and a newly recommended procedure has significant complications, the veterinarian should use discretion before proceeding without permission as they will be liable for any operative complications not discussed.

Along with the discussion of the procedure itself, the client should also be educated about their pet's anesthesia, including how anesthesia will be performed and monitored and the patient's anesthetic risk assessment. Consideration should be given to preoperative blood profiles, intravenous fluids, preoperative antibiotics (if indicated), and anesthetic protocol (including preoperative agents, induction, anesthesia, and patient monitoring). Inhalation anesthesia with an endotracheal tube is necessary to prevent the aspiration of fluids, dental calculus, and other debris.

STEPS TO THE PROFESSIONAL DENTAL CLEANING

Professional dental cleaning entails several steps (Box 7.2). According to the general sequence, the oral cavity is evaluated, large pieces of calculus are removed and supragingival scaling is performed. Then teeth are examined for the presence of subgingival calculus and the subgingival calculus is removed, and the teeth are evaluated to ensure that they and the entire periodontal area are completely clean. Then the teeth are polished, and the oral

---

BOX 7.2 Steps of the Professional Dental Cleaning

1. Preliminary examination and evaluation
2. Supragingival gross calculus removal
3. Periodontal probing (and periodontal charting)
4. Subgingival calculus removal
5. Detection of missed plaque and calculus
6. Polishing
7. Sulcus irrigation and fluoride treatment
8. Application of a sealer
9. Imaging
10. Final charting
11. Home care

---

cavity is cleansed including irrigation of the sulcus. Full dental charting is performed and further diagnostic tests, including full-mouth dental radiographs, are performed. Home-care instruction should be given to the client after the procedure.

Treatment beyond cleaning has been omitted from this summary as it is not part of PRO, but part of periodontal therapy and oral surgery. These steps are typically performed after dental charting and diagnostics.

When to Use Antibiotics

Ultimately, the decision to administer antibiotics is the veterinarian's. The veterinarian evaluates the patient and prescribes antibiotics, if indicated. Generally, antibiotics are not necessary for healthy patients with periodontal disease. Antibiotics may be indicated for patients who are potentially immunocompromised or have evidence of periodontal infection away from the periodontal tissues. This may include patients with draining sinus tracts, lymph node enlargement, or evidence of cellulitis.

Patient Care

Once anesthetized, the patient may be positioned in lateral or dorsal recumbency. Neither position is better than the other and both have advantages and disadvantages. Lateral recumbency reduces pooling of fluids in the oropharynx, which may be aspirated or introduced to the nasopharynx. However, visualization of the teeth is compromised, and the patient must be rotated to the opposite lateral side to complete the procedure. Doral recumbency gives superior visualization but oral fluids must be contended with. This may include use of suction, neck extending pads or prudent use of pharyngeal packs. It is vitally important if pharyngeal packs are used, that the operator assures it is removed before extubating. Failure to do so can be deadly to the patient. Regardless of the positioning of the patient, the patient is kept on a grate over a table sink or on a specially designed dental table that allows the fluids used in the dental procedure to drain. If the patient is kept on a grate, a padded structure should

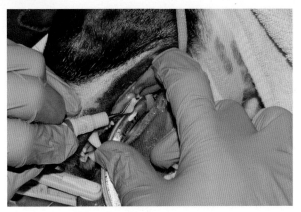

Fig. 7.1 Holding mouth open.

be under the body to decrease pressure on the soft tissues caused by the wires on the grate.

Oral speculums or mouth gags should not be used or used very sparingly. When they are used, care should be taken not to overextend the TMJs. The spring-loaded oral speculum can begin to slip over time, leading to stretching and tearing of the ligaments and muscles of the jaw. In cats, spring-loaded speculums have been associated with cortical blindness and death due to compression of the maxillary artery between muscles of mastication. Thus, spring-loaded oral speculums should not be used in cats. Typically, the mouth should be propped open with the nonworking hand (Fig. 7.1) and spring-loaded speculums only be used, when necessary, in dogs. If the need for a speculum arises when working with feline patients, a 1-cc syringe, cut to size, can be used to open the mouth no more than 50% of full extension.

Step 1: Preliminary Examination and Evaluation

Ideally, the patient has allowed the practitioner to perform a preliminary examination of the oral cavity before induction of anesthesia. However, some patients may not allow this examination at all or, at best, only for a brief time. Therefore, the first step in a prophy is a more complete evaluation of the necessary diagnostic and treatment measures.

Step 2: Supragingival Gross Calculus Removal

The next step of the procedure is to remove supragingival gross calculus. Many types of instruments may be used to perform this step.

Hand Scalers

Hand scalers are used for supragingival removal of calculus. They should not be inserted below the gumline. Scalers are particularly effective in removing calculus from the developmental groove of the fourth premolar. A *pull stroke* (a stroke pulling the calculus toward the coronal aspect) is used to remove calculus.

Hand Instrument Technique

Modified pen grasp. The modified pen grasp is the preferred method for holding hand scalers and curettes. To obtain the *modified pen grasp*, the thumb and index finger are placed at the junction of the handle and the shank of the instrument (Fig. 7.2A). The pad of the middle finger is placed on the shank. The ring finger is held straight and placed on the surface closest to the tooth being worked on as a rest and fulcrum (Fig. 7.2B). The position of the fingers creates a "triangle of forces" that provides stability and control when the wrist-rocking motion is initiated. The closer the fulcrum is to the tooth being scaled, the more effective the working stroke, because of its greater power. This grip can be practiced by holding a pencil and drawing a small circle by rotating only on the fulcrum (ring finger) and moving the wrist. The fingers should not flex at all during this motion.

Calculus Removal Forceps

The use of calculus removal forceps is a quick method for removing supragingival calculus. The longer tip is placed over the crown, the shorter under the calculus. The calculus is cleaved off when the tips are brought together (Fig. 7.3). When using calculus removal forceps, the operator should be extremely careful not to damage the gingiva or create an iatrogenic dental fracture.

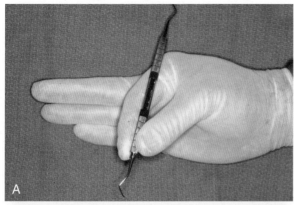

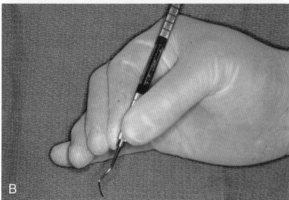

Fig. 7.2 (A) First grab pen grasp. (B) Modified pen grasp.

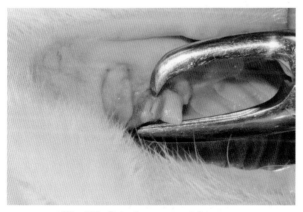

Fig. 7.3 Calculus removal forceps.

Ultrasonic or Sonic Scalers

Ultrasonic or sonic scalers are used to quickly remove the smaller deposits of supragingival calculus. Ultrasonic scalers vibrate in the range of 18,000 to 45,000 cycles per second. When properly applied, this vibration breaks up or pulverizes calculus on the surface of teeth. Because ultrasonic instruments can damage teeth by mechanical etching or thermal heating, they should be used with caution (Fig. 7.4). For supragingival scaling, use of the side of a beavertail tip is preferable rather than the end of the tip. This section of the chapter discusses supragingival scaling, but the same principles apply to the use of ultrasonic or sonic scalers in subgingival scaling.

Power instrument grasp. The ultrasonic instrument should be grasped lightly, not tightly. It should feel balanced in the hand, with minimal pull from the handpiece cord. The handpiece, not the hands, must be allowed to do the work (Fig. 7.5A). The handpiece is balanced on the index or middle finger. A modified pen grasp is not as important in holding the ultrasonic or sonic scaler as it is with hand instruments (Fig. 7.5B). To decrease stress on the hand from the pull on the handpiece cord, the cord may be looped over the little finger (Fig. 7.5C). As opposed to hand instruments, in which a fulcrum is used to provide leverage for the pulling stroke, ultrasonic scalers do not require a fulcrum. The hand is used as a guide for the ultrasonic handpiece.

Water flow. Water flow is required to prevent overheating of the teeth and damage to the pulp. With the broad-based, beaver-type inserts,

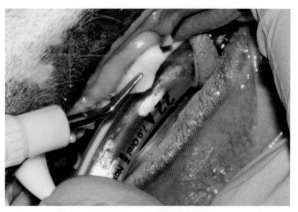

Fig. 7.4 Supragingival scaling.

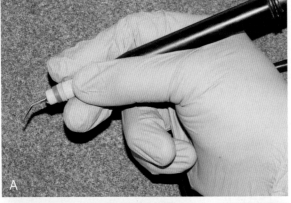

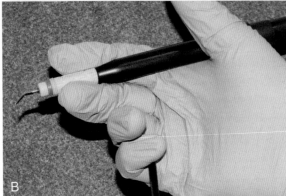

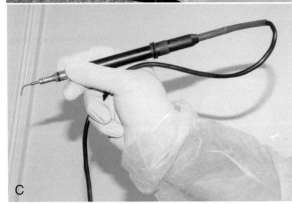

Fig. 7.5 (A) Holding ultrasonic. (B) Balanced ultrasonic. (C) Loop.

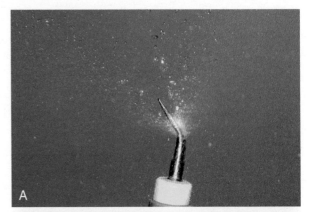

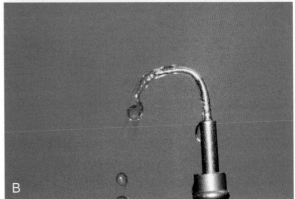

Fig. 7.6 (A) Large flow. (B) Drip.

an ample supply of water is necessary for irrigation (Fig. 7.6A). Less water is required to cool the smaller tips. The water flow can be adjusted to a smaller halo, almost a drip, just enough to cool the tip (Fig. 7.6B). Figure 7.6 demonstrates both ample water flow and reduced water flow.

Pressure. The operator should use a light touch, keeping the tip moving while traveling around the circumference of the tooth and not stopping in any area.

Adaptation. Unlike hand instruments, ultrasonic and sonic instruments do not need cutting edges. However, the tip motion of the instrument must be understood to take advantage of the maximal cleaning stroke. The side of the tip should be held parallel to the tooth surface. The tip of the ultrasonic instrument should not be pointed at the tooth surface or held at a 90-degree angle to the tooth. Doing so could damage the tooth surface by heating up the pulp; it also provides less cleaning surface and therefore is less effective. The instrument tip is kept parallel with the long axis of the tooth. The instrument should only be kept in contact with the tooth for less than 10 seconds at a time.

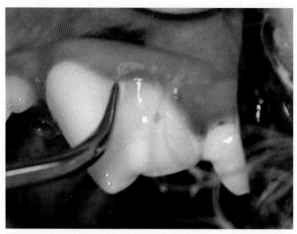

Fig. 7.7 The side of the scaler should be held gently against the tooth and moved in an apical to coronal direction with broad overlapping strokes.

Ultrasonic technique. The ultrasonic technique includes the following steps:

- Scale one quadrant at a time, making sure to not engage any one tooth for more than 10 seconds at a time.
- Use broad, overlapping strokes from an apical to coronal direction (7).
- Clean each surface (vestibular, mesial, distal, palatal/lingual, occlusal) before moving to the next quadrant.

Power settings—dial-type units. Higher power settings should be used for the broad-based, bea-vertail-type tips. The power should be decreased to lower settings when thin subgingival tips are used. Failure to decrease the power may cause fracturing of the tip or render it ineffective because tips are manufactured to operate in optimal frequency ranges. Often the dial will note optimal settings for different procedures (subgingival scaling, supragingival scaling, etc.). If not, refer to the manufacturer's instructions of what power setting is used for each procedure.

Rotary Scalers

Since its introduction to veterinary medicine, the rotary scaler has been very controversial. Its acceptance in human dentistry has been limited because the rotary scaler can easily damage teeth and requires a great deal of training and practice for safe use. Rather than scaling the teeth, this bur frequently ends up burnishing the calculus. Ineffective removal or burnishing of calculus can lead to a periodontal abscess. The use of rotary scalers in dogs and cats is generally unaccepted except for trimming composites.

Step 3: Periodontal Probing (and Periodontal Charting)
Probing Technique

A periodontal probe should be used to measure the depth of the sulcus or pocket. Caution is necessary when applying the periodontal probe. A healthy sulcus will bleed if more than 20 gm of pressure is applied to the probe. If too much pressure is applied, the probe can puncture the junctional epithelium. The probe should be held parallel to the long axis of the tooth for an accurate reading (Fig. 7.8A). Holding the probe at an angle will result in an inaccurate measurement (Fig 7.8B). The measured depth must be carefully evaluated when using a periodontal probe. The measurement of sulcular or pocket depth is not necessarily the same as that of attachment loss. If the gingival margin is at the normal cementoenamel junction, the probed depth will correspond to attachment loss. If the gingival margin is coronal to the cementoenamel junction, an increase in probing depth may indicate some form of gingival enlargement (edema, gingival hyperplasia, neoplasia, etc.) If a previous recession of gingiva has occurred and the gingival margin has moved apically, the pocket depth will be less than the actual loss of attached gingiva.

Charting

Record keeping is an important part of the dental procedure. Dental charts are used for dental charting and record keeping. Because periodontal disease is progressive, charting is an important aid for follow-up visits. Accurate records establish a baseline: Subsequent measurements of the pockets,

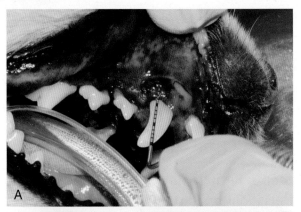

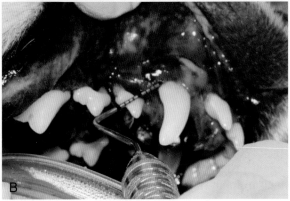

Fig. 7.8 (A) Probe correct. (B) Probe incorrect.

furcation exposure, and mobility are compared at each appointment, which is useful in evaluating treatment and client compliance.

The method used to chart teeth should be consistent to ensure that all pathology is accurately recorded. Dental abnormalities, such as missing or fractured teeth, are noted. Points on each side should be measured while charting the sulcular/pocket depth. The distal, midsection, and mesial portions of the tooth are measured. An effective way to record pathology on the dental chart is using four-handed charting. *Four-handed charting* entails one individual probing and examining each tooth while verbally noting all abnormalities, allowing a second person to record the pathology in the chart. Two hands are performing the examination and two are recording, thus the term four-handed.

Step 4: Subgingival Calculus Removal

A curette or select ultrasonic scaler should be used to remove the calculus below the gumline. Ultrasonic scalers with subgingival tips can be used to scale and remove calculus below the gumline. Several companies make specialized inserts that can be used subgingivally. Removal of subgingival calculus is an extremely important part of the procedure. Turning on the handpiece before insertion provides a water supply and thereby eases the insertion of the tip in the sulcus should subgingival scaling be performed at the same time as supragingival scaling.

If subgingival calculus remains, the patient will not receive long-term benefits from treatment and bacterial plaque will continue destroying the periodontium, leading first to bone deterioration and eventually to tooth loss.

Regardless of the technique used, if a periodontal pocket greater than 6mm deep is present, subgingival calculus cannot be adequately removed without surgical techniques (Chapter 9).

Adapting to the Tooth

The curette is adapted to the tooth root surface (Fig. 7.9A). If the instrument does not fit the curvature of the tooth, the opposite end of the instrument is adapted (Fig. 7.9B).

As the curette is inserted into the pocket, the face of the instrument should face the root surface. This is called the *closed position*. The instrument is moved over the calculus and then repositioned so that the cutting surface is under the calculus ledge. This is called the *open position*. With a rocking pull or oblique stroke, calculus is cleaved from the root surface.

Step 5: Detection of Missed Plaque and Calculus

An explorer is used to evaluate the tooth surface while checking for subgingival calculus. The tooth is inspected for missed plaque and calculus by the application of a disclosing solution or by gently air-drying the tooth.

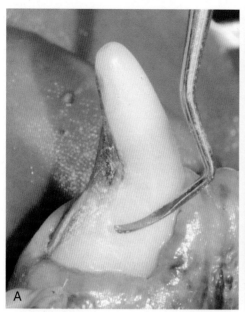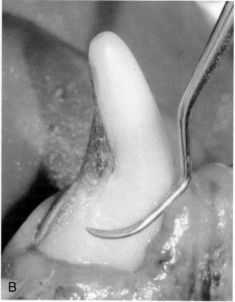

Fig. 7.9 (A) Nonadapting. (B) Adapting.

Application of Disclosing Solution

Disclosing solution can be used to maintain quality control of the teeth-cleaning procedure. A *disclosing* solution is a dye that adheres to plaque and calculus. Painting a small amount of disclosing solution on the teeth with a cotton-tipped applicator allows the detection of plaque and calculus that were missed while scaling (Fig. 7.10A). After being rinsed with water, areas where plaque remains assume a red, blue, or green pigment, depending on the brand of the disclosing solution (Fig. 7.10B). Clean teeth do not retain the stain. Care should be exercised when using the disclosing solution because it can stain hair and clothing.

Air-drying

Another technique to detect plaque and calculus is to dry the tooth with compressed air. Plaque and calculus appear chalky white when dry (Fig. 7.11). This technique should not be used if the integrity of the periodontium is in question because air could be blown into tissues, resulting in air being trapped in the subcutaneous tissues or possibly entering the bloodstream.

Step 6: Polishing
Mechanical Polishing

Mechanical polishing is the use of a prophy angle and abrasive paste. Polishing with an electric- or air-powered polisher removes any plaque that may have been missed and smooths the tooth surface. Because polishing generates considerable heat, a liberal amount of prophy paste or pumice slurry should be used and only a brief period should be spent on each tooth (Fig. 7.12). Paste is placed on each tooth in a quadrant before turning on the unit. The teeth are polished with a low-speed handpiece and prophylaxis angle and cup at approximately 3000 to 8000 rpm. If a pumice slurry is used, the prophy cup should be filled with the slurry consistently during use. The prophy cup must be kept moving and should never linger over one area. A slight flare of the prophylaxis cup is used to polish teeth subgingivally. Disposable prophylaxis angles that oscillate instead of spin are recommended (Fig. 7.13) as the oscillating motion reduces the risk of hair becoming wrapped in the spinning cup.

Some researchers have expressed concern that excessive polishing could cause enamel loss. The

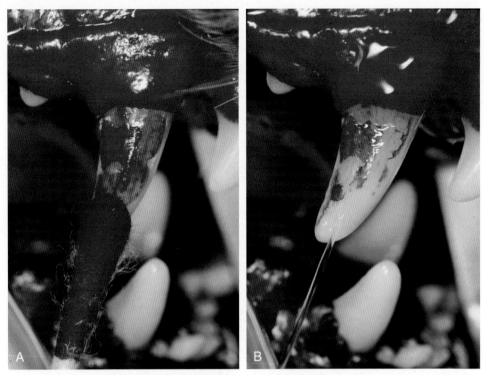

Fig. 7.10 (A) Apply disclosing solution. (B) Rinse disclosing solution.

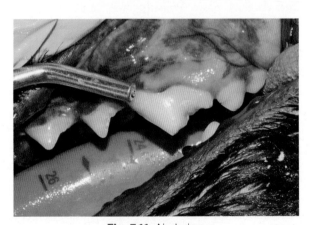

Fig. 7.11 Air-drying.

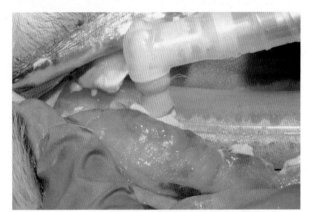

Fig. 7.12 Polishing.

risk of enamel loss may be a factor with humans, whose teeth may be polished 3 or 4 times a year for many years; however, veterinary patients will not have their teeth cleaned as often as humans.

Many different brands of fine commercial prophy pastes are available, in many different flavors.

Most contain fluoride and oils that may interfere with restorations. These pastes may be stored in a large bulk jar or individual containers. If used from a large bulk jar, a tongue depressor or other instrument should be used to remove some paste from the jar to prevent cross-contamination.

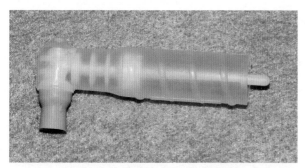

Fig. 7.13 Oscillating prophy angle.

The pumice, which is commercially available, is a highly silicious material of volcanic origin. When performing restorations, pumice should be used in place of paste. It should be mixed with oil-free (filtered) water until it reaches the consistency of a thick paste.

Pastes and pumice are available in fine and coarse textures. The fine paste is used to smooth down the tooth surface. The coarse paste is used to remove stains and should be followed up with fine prophy paste.

Air Polishing

Air polishing uses an air, water, and powder projection method on the dental surface with a specialized handpiece (Fig. 7.14). This should not be confused with air abrasion that is used for cavity preparation. Its advantages are that it is faster

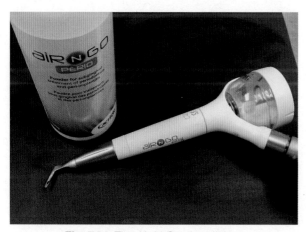

Fig. 7.14 The Air N Go air polisher.

and less demanding, reducing the operator's hand fatigue; it is less abrasive than abrasive pastes; there is no production of heat; and it gives better access to the teeth and no direct contact with the dental surface treated. The disadvantage is that it is more expensive than a mechanical polisher and without the judicious use of suction, it can be messier.

Step 7: Sulcus Irrigation and Fluoride Treatment

Gentle irrigation of the sulcus flushes out trapped debris and oxygenates the intrasulcular fluids. A saline, or diluted chlorhexidine (typically ~0.12%) solution may be used. A blunted 23-gauge irrigation needle with a syringe is effective for this. The full-strength disinfectant chlorhexidine that is commonly found in veterinary hospitals should never be used as a disinfectant without proper dilution as it can cause severe mucosal injury. Given the availability of commercially available chlorhexidine rinses, it is difficult to justify the use of other chlorhexidine solutions. Alternatively, a fluoride gel may be applied to slow the reattachment of plaque after the dental cleaning; it is then wiped (not rinsed) from the tooth surface.

Step 8: Application of a Sealer

Periodontal sealers are available that may decrease the accumulation of plaque. Sanos is a self-hardening liquid designed to work on the gingiva; it should be applied as thick as possible into the gingival sulcus to inhibit plaque contact with the gingiva. The brush is dipped into the single-use vial after every one or two tooth circumferences (Fig. 7.15). Sanos should not be used in combination with fluoride or subgingival antibiotics. If there is sulcular bleeding, the area should be gently wiped, pressure lightly applied, and a waiting period for sulcular bleeding to subside. OraVet is a waxlike product that is applied to the clean tooth surface with a sponge applicator or gloved fingers (Fig. 7.16). It reduces plaque and tartar formation by repelling water and preventing bacteria from attaching to the teeth. This is followed by a weekly application at home.

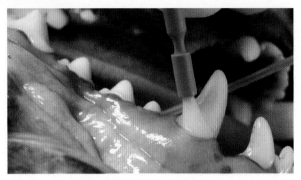

Fig. 7.15 Sanos application.

Step 9: Imaging

Diagnostics should always include periodontal probing full mouth dental radiographs or cone beam CT. Radiographs and cone beam CT evaluate the dental and bony structures for periodontal bone loss, endodontic disease, and other conditions. The patient in Fig. 7.17A has healthy-appearing gingiva and teeth; however, the dental radiographs in Fig. 7.17B show severe subgingival tooth resorption.

All probing, examination findings and imaging findings should be recorded.

Step 10: Final Charting

Final charting involves a review of the previously performed diagnostic and periodontal charting. This final review should include any additional treatment performed.

Step 11: Home Care

The last step to complete dental cleaning is home-care instruction. This subject is discussed in detail in Chapter 8.

NONPROFESSIONAL DENTAL SCALING (NPDS)

Unfortunately, many clients have been misled into thinking they can have their pet's teeth cleaned without anesthesia. It is impossible to do a thorough job in this situation, and disease is missed. This procedure is sometimes carried out in grooming facilities and pet stores. In this case, the

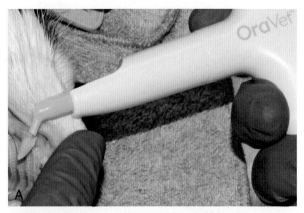

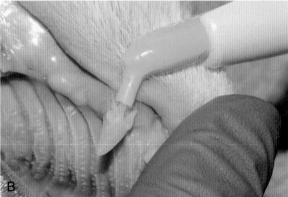

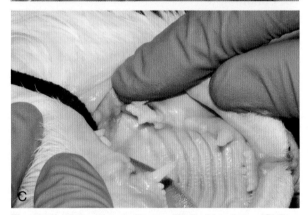

Fig. 7.16 (A) OraVet applicator. (B) OraVet close. (C) OraVet (Merial Inc., GA, USA) being applied with fingers.

practice is illegal in most states because it constitutes the practice of veterinary medicine without a license. Unfortunately, several companies have been formed to also come into veterinary offices and persuade the veterinarian to allow this service.

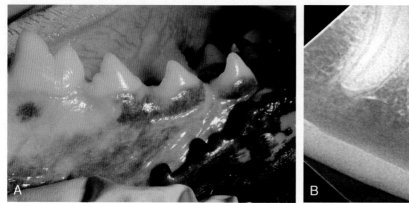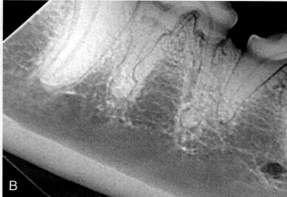

Fig. 7.17 (A) Healthy-appearing gingiva and teeth. (B) Radiograph of severe subgingival tooth resorption.

In this case the practice is legal; however, without intraoral radiographs, dental probing, and charting, it is below the standard of practice and the veterinarian may be held guilty of neglect.

The AVDC has a website that can help explain the risks of NPDS to pet owners. This is https://afd.avdc.org/.

CHAPTER 7 WORKSHEET (ANSWERS ARE ON PAGE 295)

1. The use of _____ is a fairly quick method of removing supragingival calculus.
2. _____ is required to prevent the overheating of the teeth and damage to the pulp.
3. The operator should use a _____ touch, keeping the tip moving while traveling around the circumference of the tooth and not stopping in any area.
4. The _____ pen grasp is the method of holding dental instruments.
5. Gentle irrigation of the sulcus flushes out trapped debris and _____ the intrasulcular fluids.
6. The two sealants that can be placed after a professional dental cleaning are _____ and _____.
7. A _____ prophylaxis angle and cup may prevent hair entanglement.
8. A _____ can stain plaque and calculus, making visualization easier.
9. When the face of the scaler or curette is against the tooth, the instrument is in _____ position.
10. The use of _____ is associated with cortical blindness when used in cats.

FURTHER READING

Martin-Flores M, Scrivani PV, Loew E, Gleed CA, Ludders JW. Maximal and submaximal mouth opening with mouth gags in cats: implications for maxillary artery blood flow. *Vet J.* 2014;200(1):60–64. doi:10.1016/j.tvjl.2014.02.001.

Homecare Instruction and Products

LEARNING OBJECTIVES

When you have completed this chapter, you will be able to:

- Discuss issues related to client education for dental care of their pets.
- Discuss methods used to acclimate patients to tooth brushing.
- Describe the advantages and disadvantages of the various brushing devices available for use with dogs and cats.
- List and describe homecare products used for promoting oral health in dogs and cats.
- Explain the general rules for choosing toys and chews for dogs and cats.
- Describe the action of chlorhexidine and list products that contain chlorhexidine.
- Describe the use of fluoride-containing products in the dental care of dogs and cats.

KEY TERMS

Chemical plaque control
Chlorhexidine
Coronal direction
Glucose oxidase

Lactoperoxidase
Mechanical plaque control
Monofluorophosphate fluoride
Periodontal disease

Stannous fluoride
Veterinary Oral Health Council
Xylitol
Zinc ascorbate

Effective periodontal home care is necessary for the successful treatment of periodontal disease. The veterinary team can provide excellent professional care, but if plaque cannot be reduced daily, periodontitis will return, and periodontal disease will progress. Therefore, much of the success lies in the pet owner's ability and willingness to be a part of their pet's care. Client education should begin before the procedure is performed. The decision to save a tooth or extract depends on the client's desire and ability to comply with homecare instructions.

CLIENT EDUCATION

Home dental care entails daily plaque removal and methods to reduce calculus formation. The gold standard for plaque reduction is daily toothbrushing. Daily to every other day toothbrushing has been shown to reduce plaque and gingivitis in dogs, whereas less frequent appears to be minimally effective.

Team members should review brushing and homecare techniques with clients. If possible, a "demonstrator" dog (or cat) can be used (Fig. 8.1). Otherwise, plastic dental models can be used to show brushing techniques (Fig. 8.2). Some of these models show pathologic as well as healthy conditions. Skulls may be bothersome and distracting to clients and their use for brushing demonstrations is discouraged. When demonstrating, a circular or oval motion with emphasis on the coronal direction, away from the gumline, is recommended (Fig. 8.3). Clients should be encouraged to return for further instruction as often as necessary.

There are instances in which toothbrushing is not possible due to patient demeanor or client abilities. Other products are available that can aid in decreasing plaque and calculus. These are discussed

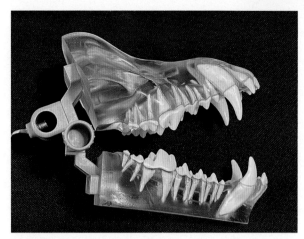

Fig. 8.2 Canine dental models are great for demonstrating brushing techniques. Skulls should be avoided as they are distracting to clients.

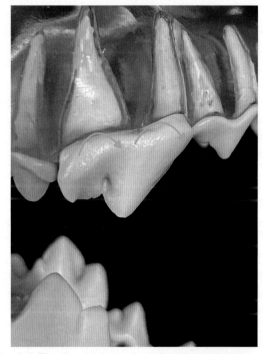

Fig. 8.3 The brushing motion should be circular with emphasis on the coronal direction. The motion is outlined in *green.*

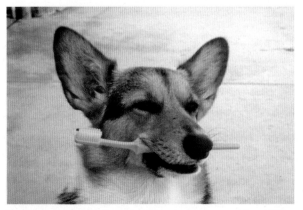

Fig. 8.1 A demonstrator dog can be a useful addition to the staff.

in the section regarding the Veterinary Oral Health Council (VOHC). None of these products replace toothbrushing.

Every member of the veterinary team can contribute to client education. While demonstration of brushing techniques may fall to the medical team, the client service team can still help direct clients to effective plaque and calculus control products.

Visual Aids

Visual aids and client handouts are beneficial in reinforcing the need for brushing and homecare. Many manufacturers offer professionally designed displays and handouts. Some commercial handouts leave spaces for the inclusion of the practice's name and phone number. The veterinary team should evaluate each display or handout before using in their practice to make sure it fits within the practice philosophy and the information is accurate.

The practice can also customize a handout specifically for the practice. Photographs of the dental area and equipment may increase client awareness of veterinary dentistry procedures performed in the hospital or clinic.

Many social media materials are available. If the practice decides to incorporate these into their practice, the information should be closely evaluated as not all self-proclaimed experts produce accurate content. If statements seem contrary to typical belief and cannot be backed by data, the information may not be accurate.

PLAQUE CONTROL AND HOMECARE

Toothbrushing

Pet owners frequently ask how often they should brush their pets' teeth. Because of how plaque and calculus form, daily brushing is best. Plaque forms 6 to 8 hours after brushing and calculus within 3 to 5 days. Thus, daily brushing is recommended. Even if pet owners are less compliant and brush every other day, it is still effective. Recall less than every other day is not effective.

Starting pets early in these routines improves patient acceptance. Gently manipulating the lips and rubbing the teeth before the pet is fully grown can acclimate them to toothbrushing in the future.

This is like manipulating a puppy's feet early to acclimate them to nail trims.

Brushing Devices

Ideally, a medium-bristled toothbrush is used. Electric toothbrushes are also great. There often is a conditioning period for the patient to get used to the vibration and noise, but it can be done. The smaller head of some electric toothbrushes can make brushing the caudal aspect of the mouth easier in smaller dogs.

Due to the size of some patient's mouths and the reduced ability of clients to brush due to physical limitations, other brushing devices are available. Rubber finger brushes are available and are easier for the client to adapt to their pet's teeth (Fig. 8.4). However, they may not be as effective as other toothbrushes and canine and feline toothbrushes (Figs. 8.5 and 8.6). Smaller brushes useful for brushing the interproximal and furcation areas are available at human pharmacies (Fig. 8.7). Wipes are also available that help introduce the concept of oral hygiene. These may not be effective for removing subgingival plaque.

Brushing Agents

The mechanical action of brushing or wiping is an important factor in plaque control, not the agent

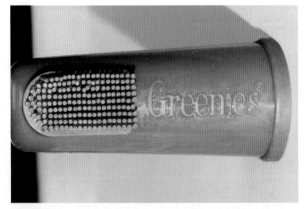

Fig. 8.4 A rubber fingerbrush may be used as a starter brush, but clients should be encouraged to use a child's preschool-sized toothbrush.

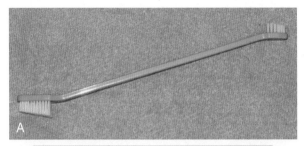

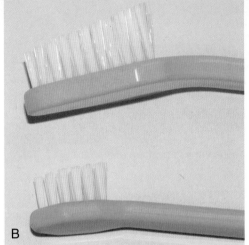

Fig. 8.5 (A and B) Canine toothbrush.

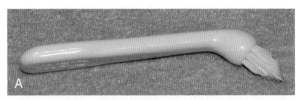

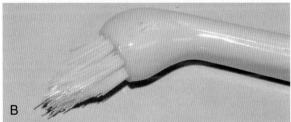

Fig. 8.6 (A and B) Feline toothbrush.

itself. Brushing with plain water and a toothbrush can still remove plaque. This may be necessary for patients with food allergies and other dietary restrictions.

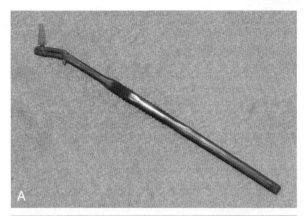

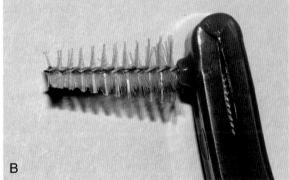

Fig. 8.7 (A and B) Proxabrush.

If no restrictions are present, pet-formulated toothpastes are recommended. These are formulated for pets in the fact they may be swallowed with little risk to the patient and are often flavored to encourage the pet to be compliant. In addition to abrasive materials, some toothpastes contain glucose oxidase and lactoperoxidase that combine to produce the hypothiocyanite ion, which is the same ion produced naturally in saliva to help inhibit bacterial growth. A number of toothpastes, wipes, and gels have been approved by the VOHC.

Other materials such as chlorhexidine rinse have been used. The advantage of chlorhexidine is its substantivity or its ability to adhere to oral tissues and release its agents slowly and its ability to break open the cell wall of bacteria. It can stain the teeth and may have a bitter taste.

Tips for difficult cases. For patients who resist attempts to brush, flavored material or toothpaste can be placed on the toothbrush. The patient is allowed to lick the brush, with no effort made to brush the teeth or restrain the patient in any way. Once the patient begins to become comfortable with the process, the client can begin to swipe at the teeth. Eventually, full brushing can take place. Cats may respond positively to liquid drained out of water-packed tuna. It is advised to encourage the patients with positive rewards during brushing. This can be a small food treat. Although food can contribute to caries, which are rare in dogs, food does not significantly contribute to periodontal disease.

Advanced techniques. The occlusion of the dog and cat do not allow the mandibular molars to be brushed when the mouth is closed (Fig. 8.8). Once the patient is accustomed to having its teeth brushed, a chew, or other prop may be placed in the mouth (Fig. 8.9). The mouth is gently held closed, and the teeth are brushed. This exposes the mandibular molars.

The pet owner should be advised that all chews have a potential for causing choking or a gastrointestinal foreign body. The size appropriate for the patient should be fed, and they should not be fed unattended as there is always the possibility of choking or other complications if the patient swallows the product whole.

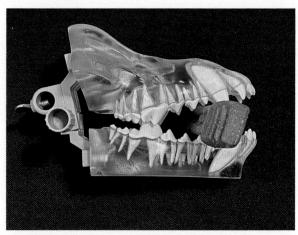

Fig. 8.9 A treat such as a Greenie can be used to prop the mouth open and gain access to the mandibular fourth premolar and molars. As a bonus, the pet gets a dental treat after brushing, which is beneficial to periodontal health and positive reinforcement.

Homecare Products

The three methods of controlling plaque are the following: mechanical, chemical, and the combination of mechanical/chemical. The number of dental homecare products is increasing steadily, and all claim to be effective. Unfortunately, pet owners may be overwhelmed and confused by the number of products with claims of promoting dental health. The VOHC is an organization established to evaluate products with claims of plaque or calculus prevention. If product testing is approved and deemed effective, the product is awarded the VOHC seal of acceptance (see Fig. 8.10). VOHC-accepted products for dogs and cats are listed in Tables 8.1 and 8.2, respectively. The product may receive acceptance as a plaque or calculus preventative or both.

As these products are constantly updated, the reader is recommended to periodically check the VOHC website at www.vohc.org. There are requirements showing the product is safe and that no consumer complaints regarding safety have been submitted. Despite the VOHC acceptance of products, caution must be exercised in recommending all chew products. The VOHC is not responsible for conducting safety studies, and it

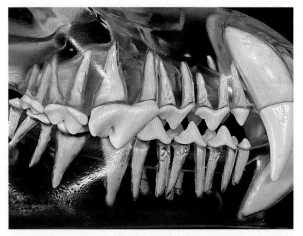

Fig. 8.8 When the mouth is closed, the maxillary fourth premolar and molars block access to the mandibular fourth premolar and molars.

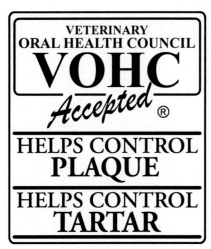

Fig. 8.10 Veterinary oral health council seal of approval.

is the responsibility of the manufacturer to assure that the product is safe.

Dental Diets

Dental diets are formulated either to remove plaque by mechanical means or prevent plaque and/or calculus by chemical means. Some such as Hill's t/d are larger kibble that requires the patient to chew the food (as opposed to simply swallowing the food)

and has a texture that helps abrade plaque from the teeth. Others, such as the Eukanuba diets with the Dental Defense System, have polyphosphates that sequester minerals in saliva and help reduce calculus. These are not the only dental diets or the only means of plaque and calculus control within diets.

Some veterinary professionals incorrectly believe that feeding these diets as a snack gives the same benefit as feeding it as a complete diet. It is important to realize that the data showing that these diets are effective is based on feeding as a complete diet, and it does not necessarily translate to feeding as a snack or treat only.

Dental Treats

Many treats are available that can help reduce plaque and/or calculus. As with dental diets, some dental treats work by mechanical means and some by chemical. These have been tested as a daily treat, given along with a complete diet. As with all treats, caloric intake should be monitored as adding calories may cause weight gain.

As many of these treats are "high value" to the pet, using these as a reward after brushing gives additional benefits.

Product	Type	Plaque	Tartar
TABLE 8.1 VOHC-Accepted Products for Dogs (Updated March 2024)			
Hill's T/D (Original and Small Bites)	Diet	X	X
Hill's Science Diet Oral Care (Including Small and Mini Formulas)	Diet	X	X
Eukanuba Adult Maintenance	Diet		X
Purina Prol Plan DH (Including Small Bites)	Diet		X
Royal Canin Dental (Including Small Dog)	Diet		X
Canagan Dental	Diet	X	X
Purina Busy HeartyHide Chew	Rawhide		X
Purina Pro Plan Dental Chewz	Rawhide		X
Tartar Shield Soft Rawhide Chews	Edible Treat		X
Greenies (Multiple Sizes and Types)	Edible Treat	X	X
Checkups Chews	Edible Treat	X	X
Milk-Bone Brushing Chews	Edible Treat		X
OraVet Dental Hygiene Chews	Edible Treat		X

(Continued)

TABLE 8.1   VOHC-Accepted Products for Dogs (Updated March 2024)—cont'd

Product	Type	Plaque	Tartar
Purina DentaLife Daily Oral Care Dog Treats	Edible Treat		X
Hill's Science Diet Canine Oral Care Chews	Edible Treat	X	X
ProDen PlaqueOff Dental Bites and Dental Care Bones	Edible Treat	X	X
Member's Mark Dental Treats	Edible Treat	X	X
HealthyMouth Chew Treat	Edible Treat	X	X
Pedigree Dentastix	Edible Treat	X	X
Whimzees Brushzees and Toothbrush Dog Treats	Edible Treat	X	X
CET Veggiedent Fr3shchews, Zen Chews and Flex Chews	Edible Treat	X	X
Clenz-A-Dent Dental Sticks	Edible Treat	X	X
Purina DentaLife ActivFresh Daily Oral Care	Edible Treat		X
Yummy Combs Treats	Edible Treat		X
WholeHearted Smart Smiles	Edible Treat		X
HealthyMouth Water Additive	Water/Food Additive, Gel, Spray, or Toothpaste	X	
HealthyMouth Topical Gel	Water/Food Additive, Gel, Spray, or Toothpaste	X	
HealthyMouth Spray	Water/Food Additive, Gel, Spray, or Toothpaste	X	
Petsmile Toothpaste	Water/Food Additive, Gel, Spray, or Toothpaste	X	
Pettura Oral Care Gel	Water/Food Additive, Gel, Spray, or Toothpaste		X
ProDen PlaqueOff Powder	Water/Food Additive, Gel, Spray, or Toothpaste	X	X
TropiClean and Nautrel Promise Solutions	Water/Food Additive, Gel, Spray, or Toothpaste	X	
Bluestem Water Additive	Water/Food Additive, Gel, Spray, or Toothpaste		X
Vetradent Water Additive	Water/Food Additive, Gel, Spray, or Toothpaste		X
Plaqtive+ Water Additive	Water/Food Additive, Gel, Spray, or Toothpaste		X
Skout's Honor Water Additive	Water/Food Additive, Gel, Spray, or Toothpaste		X
HealthyMouth Toothpaste/Brush Kit	Toothbrushes and Wipes		X
HealthyMouth Anti-Plaque Wipes	Toothbrushes and Wipes		X
Sanos	Professional Sealant	X	X

TABLE 8.2 VOHC-Accepted Products for Cats (Updated March 2024)

Product	Type	Plaque	Tartar
Hill's T/D	Diet	X	X
Hill's Science Diet Oral Care	Diet	X	X
Purina Pro Plan DH	Diet	X	X
Royal Canin Feline Dental Diet	Diet	X	
Feline Greenies	Edible Treat		X
Whiskas Dentabites	Edible Treat		X
Purina DentaLife Daily Oral Care Cat Treats	Edible Treat		X
Purina Pro Plan Crunchy Bites	Edible Treat	X	X
ProDen PlaqueOff Powder	Water/Food Additive, Gel, Spray, or Toothpaste	X	X
HealthyMouth Water Additive	Water/Food Additive, Gel, Spray, or Toothpaste	X	
HealthyMouth Topical Gel	Water/Food Additive, Gel, Spray, or Toothpaste	X	
HealthyMouth Topical Spray	Water/Food Additive, Gel, Spray, or Toothpaste	X	
HealthyMouth Toothpaste/Brush Kit	Toothbrushes and Wipes	X	
HealthyMouth Anti-Plaque Wipes	Toothbrushes and Wipes	X	

Water and Food Additives

Several water and food additives are accepted by the VOHC. Although not as effective as brushing, they are helpful as an adjunct to brushing and are useful for those patients who do not accept brushing.

Zinc. Zinc ascorbate reduces plaque and stimulates gingival healing. MaxiGuard Gel contains vitamin C and zinc sulfate, which are reported to clean the mouth and help decrease inflammation. MaxiGuard may be used before or after surgery (Fig. 8.11). For routine brushing, the manufacturer recommends the use of MaxiGuard OraZn. Both of these products are applied by brushing, spraying, or wiping.

Fluoride gels. Several types of fluoride gels are available. Stannous fluoride, the most bactericidal agent, is stable at a pH of 6.5. The 0.4% strength should be used. Fluoride has been shown to aid in plaque prevention when deposited on the surface of the enamel. Although it is unlikely to cause toxicity at this strength, the client should be cautioned to use the product sparingly. Any food in the stomach at the time of ingestion will likely neutralize the fluoride.

Selecting the Appropriate Homecare Regimen

The type of dental product recommended depends on the severity of the pathologic condition. The only way to thoroughly judge oral health is by periodontal probing and intraoral radiographs. The need for oral hygiene can be prescribed only after knowing the pathologic condition using these parameters.

Ideally, homecare would begin soon after the permanent teeth have erupted and before periodontal disease has been established.

When the disease is established, the regimen should be tailored to the patient's needs. Patients

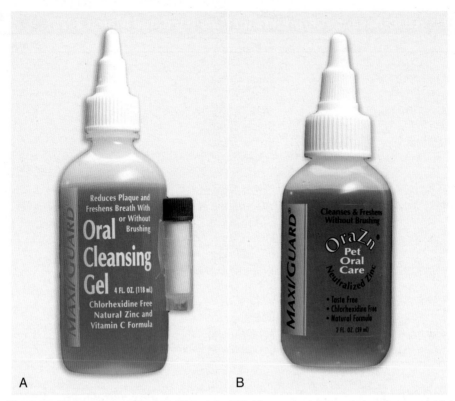

Fig. 8.11 (A) MaxiGuard. (B) MaxiGuard OraZN. (Courtesy Addison Labs, Fayette, MO.)

with gingival inflammation may benefit from products that may reduce gingival inflammation such as zinc ascorbate. If calculus accumulation is a concern, polyphosphates can be helpful. In these patients, brushing should be delayed until after treatment to prevent the pet from associating brushing with oral pain.

When considering performing more involved periodontal surgery such as guided tissue regeneration, homecare is extremely important. If there is doubt about whether daily tooth brushing can be performed, more advanced periodontal procedures may not be in the best interest of any involved parties.

Plaque-Removing Chew Toys

Clients frequently ask veterinary staff to recommend chew toys. Objects such as antlers, hooves, bones, and other animal parts are simply too hard and will fracture teeth.

The following three rules should be explained to the client in choosing toys and chews:
1. The item must bend or break easily when flexed.
2. If the item is hit on your kneecap and it hurts, it should not be fed.
3. If you think the item is too hard to chew yourself, your pet should not chew it.

It is unclear if toys actually help decrease plaque and calculus. However, they are enriching for pets. As with all chews, they should be used with supervision.

CHAPTER 8 WORKSHEET (ANSWERS ARE ON PAGE 295)

1. Client education should begin _____ the procedure is performed.
2. If possible, a "_____" dog (or cat) should be used to demonstrate tooth brushing to the client.
3. How often should brushing be recommended?
4. _____ breaks open the bacterial cell wall and can be used as a brushing agent.
5. The Veterinary Oral Health Council evaluates claims of _____ and _____ control in veterinary products.
6. _____ sequester mineral in saliva to reduce calculus formation.
7. The client must be reminded that all toys should be used under _____ supervision
8. Plaque forms _____ hours after brushing.
9. State "True" or "false": t/d is just as effective if given as a treat compared to given as a complete diet?
10. _____ aids in reducing plaque and stimulating healing of gingiva.

FURTHER READING

Harvey C, Serfilippi L, Barnvos D. Effect of frequency of brushing teeth on plaque and calculus accumulation, and gingivitis in dogs. *J Vet Dent.* 2015;32(1):16–21. doi:10.1177/089875641503200102.

9

Nonsurgical Periodontal Therapy

LEARNING OBJECTIVES

When you have completed this chapter, you will be able to:

- Describe the difference between root scaling and root planing.
- Describe the purpose and procedure for performing root planing.

- Explain the purpose and result of periodontal debridement.
- Describe the use of ultrasonic scalers in periodontal therapy.
- Discuss the use of local antibiotic therapy with veterinary dental patients.

KEY TERMS

Local antibiotic therapy
Periodontal debridement
Root planing
Root scaling

Once periodontal disease beyond stage 1 is established, periodontal therapy is necessary. This is beyond preventative care and the difference between the two is important. As discussed in Chapter 7, a prophylaxis is performed to prevent periodontal disease and when stage 1 periodontal disease is present, only a dental cleaning is required. When a patient has stage 2 or higher periodontal disease, periodontal therapy is appropriate. This chapter focuses on nonsurgical periodontal therapy. This entails the treatment of suprabony and minor infrabony periodontal pockets. This entrails the treatment of pockets of 5 mm or less. Larger infrabony pockets and areas of gingival dehiscence require more advanced treatment, which is covered later. The following treatments are performed along with typical dental scaling and polishing.

ROOT SCALING

Scaling is the mechanical removal of plaque, calculus, and stains from the crown and root surfaces.

The act of scaling does not necessarily treat periodontal disease. It only removes the surface irritants. The technique for scaling of the crown is discussed in Chapter 7. Calculus can also be scaled from the tooth root when present. Although this is known as *root scaling*, the procedure is performed with a curette, not a scaler.

The curette is inserted into the pocket in closed position. The handle of the curette is tipped to engage the blade of the curette against the root in open position. Calculus is removed with a pull stroke and the pocket irrigated.

ROOT PLANING

The objective of *root planing* is the removal of calculus and diseased cementum from the root surface and the creation of a clean, smooth root surface.

Root Planing: Technique

A routine, systematic approach should be used on each quadrant and each tooth. The working end of the curette is positioned against the root surface in closed position. The instrument is manipulated into open position, engaging the blade against the root. The curette is pulled with overlapping strokes in horizontal, vertical, and oblique directions (Fig. 9.1), removing debris from the pocket with each stroke. This crosshatch pattern of planing creates a smooth surface and maintains root anatomy.

BALANCE BETWEEN ROOT SCALING AND ROOT PLANING

A healthy cementum is necessary for the complete attachment of periodontal tissues to the tooth. When possible, cementum should be spared. Newer research has shown that bacterial plaque is loosely bound to, and molecular growth factors are contained within the cementum, aiding in the reattachment of the periodontal ligament to the root surface. Now, only the removal of plaque and calculus is mandatory.

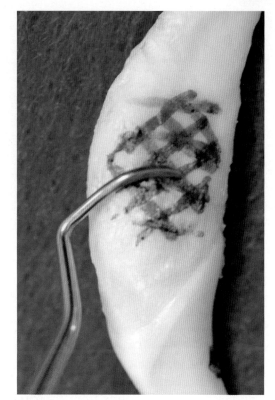

Fig. 9.1 Crosshatch directions for scaling strokes.

It is up to the clinician to decide when to remove cementum via root planing and when to simply perform root scaling. If calculus is embedded within cementum, root planing in that area may be necessary. In cases of gingival recession that will be managed as an area of root exposure, root planing may be warranted.

Ultrasonic Periodontal Therapy

With the increased availability of ultrasonic scalers and thinner periodontal tips, ultrasonic root scaling and periodontal debridement is sometimes used in lieu of using hand instrumentation. Unlike the wider tips used in ultrasonic scaling for gross calculus removal, the tips for ultrasonic root scaling and periodontal debridement are thinner and can enter the periodontal pocket with less distention of the gingiva and less risk of harm to the tissues, which sometimes occurs with curettes

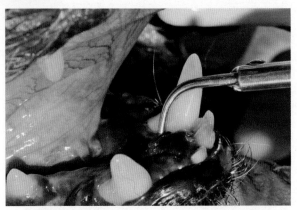

Fig. 9.2 Using an ultrasonic scaler for subgingival scaling.

(Fig. 9.2). When choosing an ultrasonic tip, the practitioners should look for tips compatible with their equipment.

When properly used, ultrasonic scalers remove less cementum as compared to hand instruments. In addition, the ultrasonic scalers provide water lavage that allows better visualization of the tissues and flushes or removes debris from the pocket. Because they irrigate the tissues, ultrasonic scalers also improve cleanliness and wound healing.

Ultrasonic scalers can clean the root surface more efficiently than hand instruments. The result is less time for treatment and less time when the patient is under anesthesia. Moreover, ultrasonic energy can produce a cavitation effect, disrupting the bacterial cell wall. The combination of removing debris from the pocket, removal of inflammatory mediators, and the cavitation effect of ultrasonic instruments is known as *periodontal debridement*.

No instrument is 100% effective in removing irritants from the root and granulation tissue from the periodontal pocket. Typically, a combination of ultrasonic and hand instrumentation is required.

LOCAL ANTIBIOTIC THERAPY

Antibiotics may be applied directly into periodontal pockets after root planing and root scaling as *local antibiotic therapy*. This was once coined as a "perioceutic" in veterinary medicine. This term is a proprietary term and not an accepted medical term. These are only designed to be placed in periodontal pockets and are not meant to fill the alveolus after extraction. The application of local antibiotic therapy is a treatment beyond cleaning and should only be prescribed and performed by the veterinarian.

Doxirobe

Antibiotic therapy can be used with periodontal debridement techniques. One product is Zoetis's Doxirobe gel (doxycycline hyclate), which delivers doxycycline directly to the periodontal pockets of 4 mm or greater depth. The medication provides local delivery of an antibiotic to afford local control of the microorganisms responsible for periodontal disease. According to the manufacturer, the gel reduces periodontal pocket depth, increases attachment levels, and reduces gingival inflammation by inhibiting collagenase produced by inflammatory cells. The two-syringe system necessitates mixing before use. Syringe A contains the polymer delivery system, and syringe B contains the active ingredient (doxycycline) (Fig. 9.3A and B). A blunted cannula is used for delivery (Fig. 9.3C).

The A and B syringes should be connected to each other (Fig. 9.4A). The material is transferred back and forth 100 times (Fig. 9.4B). The material is transferred into the "A" syringe for the final mix, placed on the edge, and allowed to sit for a few minutes to allow the material to settle so that air can be expressed (Fig. 9.4C). The material is inserted into a pocket with the provided cannula (Fig. 9.5A). The gel solidifies to a wax-like consistency when exposed to water. The solidified material is gently packed into the pocket with a plastic working instrument (Fig. 9.5B). The pocket should not be overfilled so as to distend the soft tissues.

Arestin

Arestin (minocycline hydrochloride) is a sustained-release, locally applied antibiotic. Like

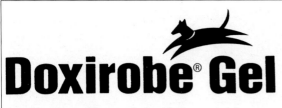

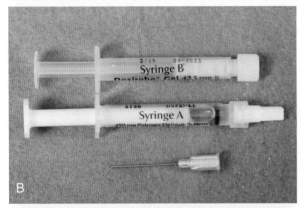

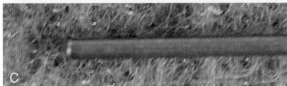

Fig. 9.3 (A) Doxirobe label. (B) Doxirobe contents. (C) Close-up of tip of a Doxirobe needle.

Doxirobe, Arestin is indicated along with periodontal debridement. Unlike Doxirobe, Arestin is a powder that is applied with a special applicator.

Clindoral

Clindoral (Clindoral, AL, USA) is a sol-to-gel liquid of clindamycin hydrochloride that is slowly released from the sol-to-gel matrix over 7 to 10 days to fight periodontal pathogens by inhibiting protein synthesis in the bacterial cell. It is applied in a similar fashion to Doxirobe, except it does not solidify in water and does not need to be manipulated thereafter.

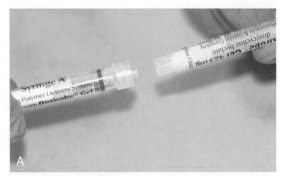

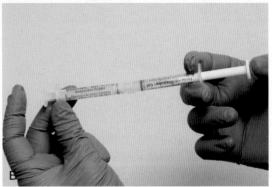

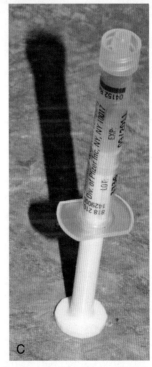

Fig. 9.4 (A) Connecting Doxirobe. (B) Mixing Doxirobe. (C) Settling Doxirobe. (Zoetis, NJ, USA).

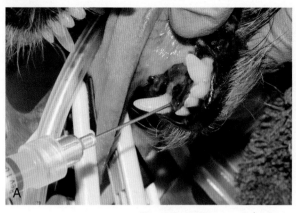 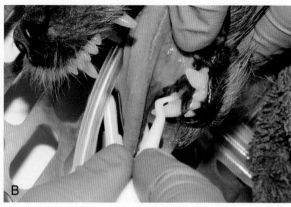

Fig. 9.5 (A) Placing Doxirobe. (B) Plastic working instrument.

Efficacy of Local Antibiotics

Research conducted by the manufacturers suggests that Doxirobe gel and Clindoral will reduce the depth of periodontal pockets when used for root scaling and planing. A study comparing root planing alone to root planing with either Doxirobe gel or Clindoral did not demonstrate a significant change in pocket depth but did show an improvement in gingivitis in the groups receiving local antibiotic treatment.

OTHER PERIODONTAL THERAPY

Surgical procedures are available to treat deeper periodontal pockets, regenerate bone, and mediate gingival recession. These are discussed in the advanced dental procedure chapter.

CHAPTER 9 WORKSHEET (ANSWERS ARE ON PAGE 295)

1. The objective of _____ is to create a clean, smooth, glasslike root surface.
2. The energy produced by ultrasonic scalers has a cavitation effect, _____ the bacterial cell wall.
3. Doxirobe gel should be mixed _____ times before use.
4. Compared to hand instruments, ultrasonic scalers remove less _____ from the root.
5. Doxirobe gel, Arestin, and Clindoral are examples of _____ used after root planing or root scaling.
6. Arestin is a minocycline powder that is applied with _____.
7. State whether "True" or "False": The use of local antibiotics is always shown to result in the reduction of periodontal pockets.
8. A _____ pattern of root planing provides a smooth surface.
9. If a patient has stage _____ or less periodontal disease, only a simple dental cleaning is required.
10. State whether "True" or "False": Special periodontal tips are required for subgingival ultrasonic scaling.

FURTHER READING

Martel DP, Fox PR, Lamb KE, Carmichael DT. Comparison of closed root planing with versus without concurrent doxycycline hyclate or clindamycin hydrochloride gel application for the treatment of periodontal disease in dogs. *J Am Vet Med Assoc.* 2019;254(3):373–379. doi:10.2460/javma.254.3.373.

Feline Dentistry

CHAPTER OUTLINE

LEARNING OBJECTIVES

When you have completed this chapter, you will be able to:

- Differentiate between feline stomatitis, gingivitis, and periodontitis.
- List the diagnostic testing used for the evaluation of patients with suspected feline stomatitis.
- Describe the management of patients with feline stomatitis.

- Describe the classification scheme used to stage tooth resorption.
- List the possible causes of feline orofacial pain syndrome.
- Describe alveolar bone expansion.
- Know the types of medications associated with medication-related osteonecrosis of the jaws.
- Know the sites affected by patellar fracture and dental anomaly syndrome.

KEY TERMS

Caudal stomatitis
Feline stomatitis
Feline orofacial pain syndrome

Medication-related
osteonecrosis of the jaws
Stomatitis

Tooth resorption

Cats are affected by the same diseases previously discussed in the other chapters. However, some conditions of the oral cavity are more common in cats than they are in other species. This chapter focuses on these conditions but does not intend to minimize the importance of other diseases previously discussed with regard to all species.

FELINE STOMATITIS

Stomatitis is defined as "inflammation of the mucous lining of any of the structures in the mouth." In itself, it is not a diagnosis or disease. Domestic cats are affected by a painful form of stomatitis known as *feline stomatitis* (FST) that can be debilitating due to pain and inflammation. It has been previously called stomatitis, faucitis, feline chronic ulcerative gingivostomatis, plasma cell stomatitis-pharyngitis, and lymphocytic-plasmacytic gingivitis-stomatitis, and feline chronic gingivitis and stomatitis.

Clinically, cats present with inflammation of the caudal oral mucosa (Fig. 10.1), where the upper and lower jaws meet, just lateral to the palatoglossal folds. This is known as *caudal stomatitis*. While other oral soft tissues are typically inflamed, inflammation of the caudal oral mucosa is necessary for a diagnosis of FST. Most cats have gingivitis and typically periodontitis. Often enlargement of the submandibular lymph nodes is present. Blood profiles commonly demonstrate elevated blood protein (hyperproteinemia) due to elevated globulin (hyperglobulinemia).

These patients suffer from various degrees of oral pain that can lead to decreased appetite, complete anorexia, weight loss, and lack of grooming. Drooling and dehydration is not uncommonly seen.

Factors that can complicate management owing to their contribution to overall inflammation and/or immunomodulation are feline immunodeficiency virus (FIV) and feline leukemia virus (FeLV). Since the onset, the client should be advised that initial treatment is extensive and long term, therapies have potentially dangerous side effects, and some drugs used have not been approved for use in cats.

Cause and Diagnosis

Some evidence suggests that this disease is a disease of immune dysfunction. There is a known change in subsets of the T lymphocyte population. Data also points to calicivirus being involved in the immune dysfunction. This appears to make affected cats much more susceptible to periodontal infection, resulting in severe inflammation of the oral cavity. It does not appear that antiviral medication is effective in treatment, as it does not treat the immune dysfunction.

Diagnosis begins with a history and a complete physical examination of the mouth, which may require chemical restraint. Diagnostics should go beyond a brief physical examination; however, clinical appearance and clinical signs may be enough for a diagnosis. This should include testing for calicivirus, FeLV, and FIV and also include a blood biochemistry profile and a complete blood count (CBC), considering future treatment options involving the use of anesthesia and pain relief.

Full-mouth examination under general anesthesia must include intraoral dental radiographs and periodontal charting. The examination should include observation of the buccal mucosa, tongue, gingiva, teeth, pharynx, tonsillar region, and the hard and soft palates. All surfaces should be examined for color, shape, size, consistency, surface texture, ease of bleeding, and response to pain. Gingival bleeding is one of the earliest signs that may be noted. Inflamed gingiva and mucosa may appear swollen, cobblestone-textured, bright red, or raspberry-like, which is often symptomatic of stomatitis.

A biopsy of unusual-appearing or unilateral different-appearing tissue will rule out conditions such as eosinophilic granuloma or squamous cell carcinoma.

Treatment

Currently, treatment of FST focuses on elimination of plaque. This is accomplished by

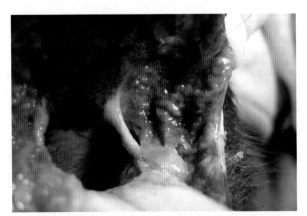

Fig. 10.1 Caudal stomatitis affecting a cat with feline stomatitis.

extraction of teeth with periodontitis and often all the teeth. Even with full-mouth extraction 30% of cases will require continued medical management, and some may not respond to any treatment.

For those cats that still do not respond, long-term antibiotic and steroid therapy is used to control the patient's condition. This treatment will need to be continuous and adapted to each patient.

Additional therapies that have worked on individual—but not all—patients include diet modification, azithromycin, pentoxifylline, cyclosporine, bovine lactoferrin, mesenchymal stem cells, and vitamin supplementation.

EARLY ONSET GINGIVITIS AND PERIODONTITIS

Juvenile cats can develop marked gingivitis and periodontitis soon after the eruption of the permanent dentition (Fig. 10.2). This manifests as generalized gingivitis, sometimes with edema or enlargement of the gingiva and often periodontitis is present in the form of horizontal bone loss. It is not clear if this is an early form of FST or an unrelated disease. Where FST is often associated with calicivirus, one study showed only four of seven cats with early onset of gingivitis (EOG). In this same study, 2 of 27 cases later developed caudal mucositis.

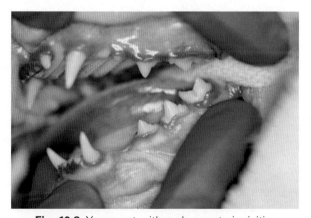

Fig. 10.2 Young cat with early onset gingivitis.

Treatment may include selective extractions and periodontal therapy or full-mouth extraction.

TOOTH RESORPTION

Another condition common in cats is *tooth resorption* (TR), which is a progressive resorption of dental hard tissues by odontoclasts, leading to pain and tooth loss. Odontoclasts are a multinucleated giant cell similar to osteoclasts. As these cells migrate through the tooth, they destroy the hard tissue, weakening the tooth.

TR has had a number of names: feline odontoclastic resorptive lesion (FORL), neck lesions, cervical line lesions, and cat cavities. FORL was removed from the vernacular as TR affects other species than cats (although it most commonly affects cats) and odontoclastic infers a histologic diagnosis was made, which is not typical. Both terms, "neck lesion" and "cervical line lesion," are no longer used as these indicate the lesion only affects the region where the crown and root meet (neck of the tooth). Cavities, or carious lesions, have a completely different pathogenesis from TR, and the existence of cavities in feline patients is controversial. The classification of TR has been provided in Box 10.1.

The incidence of TR varies according to the study, but most research suggests that a little less than one-half of the cat population is clinically affected. Intraoral radiographs may increase this number to 75%. The effects of TR include resorption of the tooth and proliferation of the gingiva or pulp to cover the resulting lesion. The signs of TR are essentially those of pain. Because all patients react to pain differently, the signs may be difficult to interpret. The patient's behavior might change; some cats become aggressive or start hiding. Appetite decreases, and the animal may drop food or even hiss at it. Additionally, missing teeth in cats are often due to previous TR.

Cause and Diagnosis

At the current time, there is not a consensus on what causes TR.

BOX 10.1   Classification of Tooth Resorption

Types: Based on the Radiographic Appearance of Roots

Type 1: Focal or multifocal lucency of tooth with otherwise normal radiopacity of roots with normal periodontal ligament space

Type 2: Loss of periodontal ligament space and decreased radiopacity of roots

Type 3: Features of type 1 and 2 associated with the same tooth

Stages: Based on the Amount of Tooth Missing

Stage 1 TR1: Mild cementum and/or enamel loss

Stage 2 TR2: Cementum and/or enamel loss with dentin loss but no exposure of pulp

Stage 3 TR3: Hard tissue loss extends into pulp with majority of hard tissue intact

Stage 4 TR4: Extensive hard tissue loss with majority of tooth missing
- TR4a: Crown and root are equally affected
- TR4b: Crown more severely affected
- TR4c: Roots more severely affected

Stage 5 TR5: Crown missing with gingiva intact

AVDC Stages and Types

The American Veterinary Dental College (AVDC) has created a system of classifying TR by stages.

Stage 1 (TR 1): Mild dental hard tissue loss (cementum or cementum and enamel) (Fig. 10.3).

Stage 2 (TR 2): Moderate dental hard tissue loss (cementum or cementum and enamel with loss of dentin that does not extend to the pulp cavity) (Fig. 10.4).

Stage 3 (TR 3): Deep dental hard tissue loss (cementum or cementum and enamel with loss of dentin that extends to the pulp cavity); most of the tooth retains its integrity (Fig. 10.5).

Stage 4 (TR 4): Extensive dental hard tissue loss (cementum or cementum and enamel with loss of dentin that extends to the pulp cavity); most of the tooth has lost its integrity. In Fig. 10.6, the crown and root are equally affected. Fig. 10.7 shows the crown more severely affected than the root. In Fig. 10.8, the root is more severely affected than the crown.

The clinical sign of inflamed gums may initially lead the clinician to suspect that TR lesions are present. Some lesions are immediately apparent, and others are covered by hyperplastic gingiva. In most cases, the extent of the lesion is impossible to determine by visual clinical examination alone and an anesthetized dental examination with radiographs is necessary. Visually, a portion of the tooth may be missing. In some cases, only small defects are present that cannot be seen but can be detected with a dental explorer. As previously mentioned, TR is a common cause for missing teeth in the cat. This may be clinically evident by absence of the mandibular third premolar that is affected in 93.4% of cats with TR.

Dental radiographs may detect resorption that is not visible or palpable. Radiographs also aid in the examination of the tooth roots. The roots may be unaffected, may be missing hard tissue, or may be resorbed by alveolar bone.

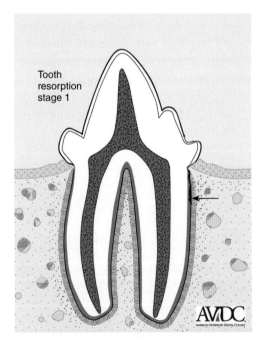

Fig. 10.3 Tooth resorption, stage 1: Enamel or cementum loss (*arrow*). (With permission from the American Veterinary Dental College.)

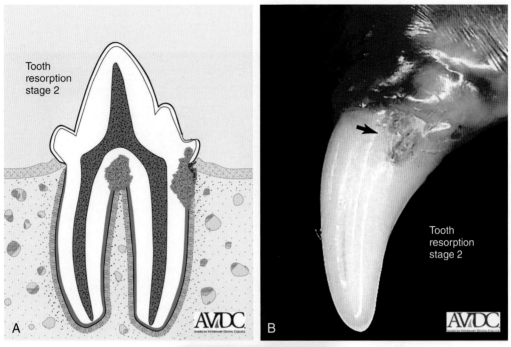

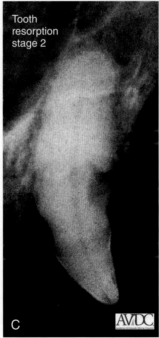

Fig. 10.4 (A–C) Tooth resorption, stage 2: Deeper than stage 1 but not into pulp. (With permission from the American Veterinary Dental College.)

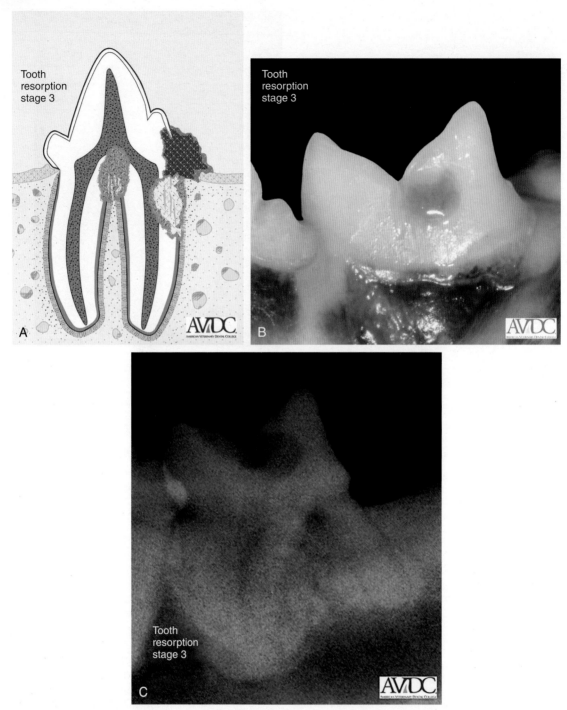

Fig. 10.5 (A–C) Tooth resorption, stage 3: Into pulp but tooth maintains integrity. (With permission from the American Veterinary Dental College.)

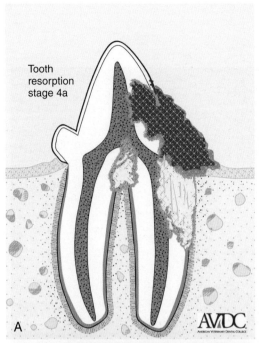

Tooth resorption stage 4a

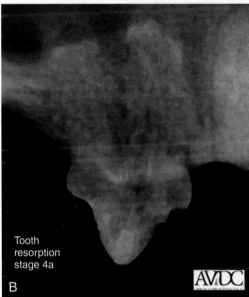

Tooth resorption stage 4a

Fig. 10.6 (A and B) Tooth resorption, stage 4a: Extensive tooth destruction of crown and root. (With permission from the American Veterinary Dental College.)

Stage 5 (TR 5): Remnants of dental hard tissue are visible only as irregular radiopacities, and the gingival covering is complete (Fig. 10.9).

The three types of TR (I, II, and III) describe if the root is being replaced by alveolar bone (bone replacement resorption). In type I, each root of the affected tooth is intact, and the bone has not replaced the root. This does not simply mean the periodontal ligament space is not visible, as it may be too thin to evaluate on radiographs. If the root can be visualized, one should assume type I resorption is present.

Type II resorption occurs when the alveolar bone replaces each root of the affected tooth. This is noted by the inability to differentiate between the root and the bone and the irregular appearance of the root.

Type III resorption occurs when a multirooted tooth demonstrates both type I and type II resorption of different roots.

Treatment of Tooth Resorption

After radiographic evaluation, TR is treated by extracting the remaining dental tissue. This means roots with type I resorption are extracted in their entirety and roots with type II resorption have the obvious dental tissue removed. There is no need to remove the new bone produced during bone replacement resorption. In the cases of stage 5 resorption, unless there is evidence of inflammation, the remaining root does not necessarily need to be extracted.

Prevention of Tooth Resorption

At this point, little is known about the prevention of TR. A 2005 study demonstrated that cats with TR had a significant increase in serum vitamin D levels compared to unaffected cats. In a study examining 64 healthy cats, no correlation was found between serum vitamin D levels and the incidence of resorption. Two studies suggest that cats that are affected by TR respond differently to vitamin D and in turn produce more osteoclasts in response to higher vitamin D levels. Although it is not known for sure, the reduction of vitamin D in the diet may have some benefits.

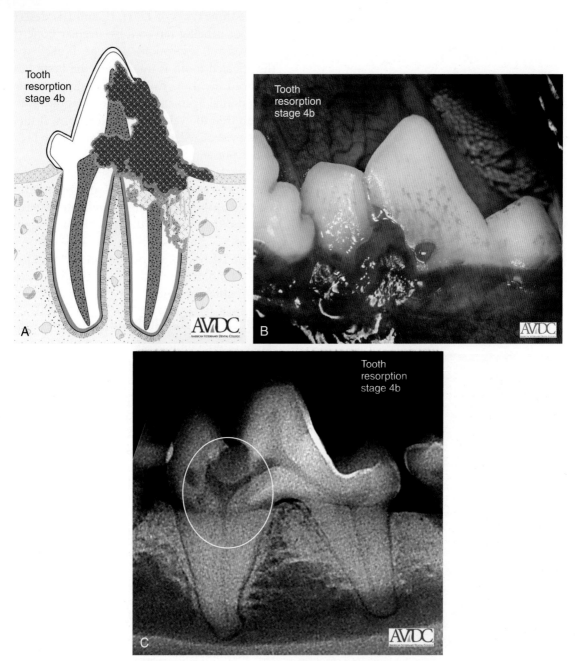

Fig. 10.7 (A–C) Tooth resorption, stage 4b: Extensive tooth destruction, crown worse. (With permission from the American Veterinary Dental College.)

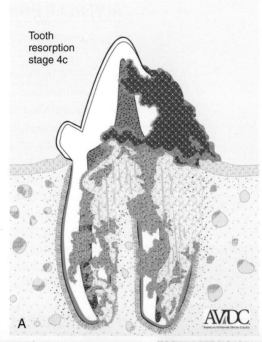

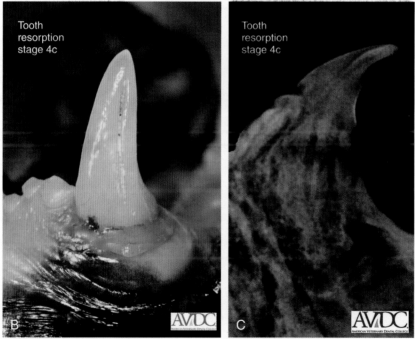

Fig. 10.8 (A–C) Tooth resorption, stage 4c: Extensive tooth destruction, root worse. (With permission from the American Veterinary Dental College.)

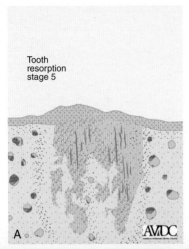

Tooth resorption stage 5

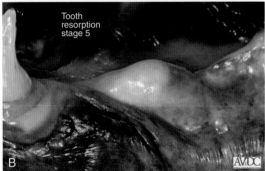

Tooth resorption stage 5

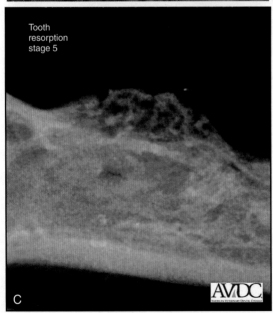

Tooth resorption stage 5

Fig. 10.9 (A–C) Tooth resorption, stage 5: End stage. (With permission from the American Veterinary Dental College.)

ALVEOLAR BONE EXPANSION

The cat often expresses periodontal disease of the canine teeth by a process called alveolar bone expansion (ABE). This is an enlargement of the alveolar bone of the canine teeth, resulting in the loss of the normal anatomy and the relationship between the tooth and alveolar bone and vertical bone loss. It is commonly associated with advanced periodontal disease. Early cases can be treated by periodontal debridement, possible resective osseous surgery, and ongoing periodontal preventative care. Advanced cases need extraction (Fig. 10.10A and B). In some cases, the tooth may luxate, resulting in the inability of the patient to close the mouth due to the luxated tooth presenting a mechanical blockage. Not uncommonly, this luxation is misdiagnosed as a temporomandibular joint luxation.

FELINE OROFACIAL PAIN SYNDROME

Feline orofacial pain syndrome (FOPS) is a likely neuropathic disorder of cats that manifests as severe oral and facial pain. It occurs mainly in Burmese cats. FOPS is thought to be caused by dysfunction to nerves of the peripheral nervous system, possibly involving central and/or ganglion processing of sensory trigeminal information. The predominance within the Burmese cat breed suggests that it is an inherited disorder. Patients will have sporadic one-sided discomfort, followed by pain-free intervals. Mouth movements appear to trigger discomfort. The disease is often recurrent and, with time, may become constant. It can be resistant to traditional pain medication but responds to anticonvulsants. Clients should establish diaries regarding dates and times, the activity before the attack, and a description of the attack. Video recording is also very useful, and video taken by a cell phone can be sufficient to make the diagnosis.

There is no known way to definitively diagnose FOPS and in turn it is a diagnosis of exclusion. Other causes of oral pain and tooth grinding (TR, retained tooth roots, and gastrointestinal or renal pain) need to be ruled out before FOPS can be diagnosed.

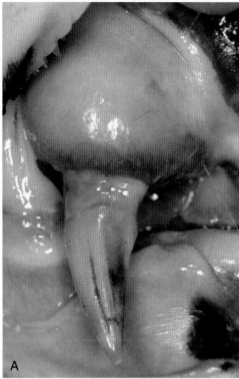

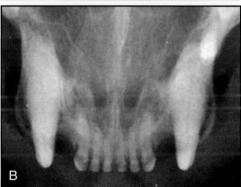

Fig. 10.10 (A) Alveolar osteitis: clinical. (B) Alveolar osteitis: radiograph. This patient has alveolar osteitis caused by periodontal disease and tooth resorption. The radiograph shows a deep pocket between the tooth root and bone. (Courtesy Dr. Jan Bellows.)

MEDICATION-RELATED OSTEONECROSIS OF THE JAWS

Increased use of bisphosphonates to treat idiopathic hypercalcemia in cats has brought to light a serious condition called bisphosphonate-related osteonecrosis of the jaws (BRONJ) or medication-related osteonecrosis of the jaws (MRONJ).

Medication-related osteonecrosis of the jaws is a condition in which the administration of bisphosphonates leads to necrosis of the jaw bones and long bones. In the jaw, this may manifest after jaw trauma such as TR or extractions (Fig. 10.11). When present in the jaws, the bone is exposed and enlarged. This may require involved surgical debridement of the bone or conservative management. In long bones, this can lead to pathologic fracture. Case reports and data unpublished at the time of writing demonstrate that this is not a rare side effect. The practitioner must seriously consider the value of prescribing bisphosphonates in cats considering potential side effects. As the

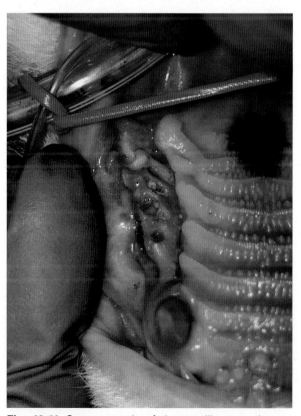

Fig. 10.11 Osteonecrosis of the maxilla secondary to bisphosphonate administration.

half-life of bisphosphonates in bone may be years, management is lifelong for these patients.

PADS

Patellar fracture and dental anomaly syndrome (PADS) is a congenital disease of cats that manifests as bone fractures (most commonly the patella), osteomyelitis of the jaws, persistent deciduous teeth, and impacted permanent teeth. Currently, treatment consists of extraction of unerupted permanent teeth and persistent deciduous teeth and judicious debridement of necrotic bone. Clients should understand that this will require lifelong management.

CHAPTER 10 WORKSHEET (ANSWERS ARE ON PAGE 295)

1. _____ is defined as an inflammation of the oral mucosa, including the buccal and labial mucosa, palate, tongue, floor of the mouth, and gingiva.
2. Approximately _____% of cats undergoing full-mouth extraction still require medical treatment.
3. A process in which the alveolar bone of the canine teeth becomes inflamed and enlarged is _____.
4. _____ is a pain disorder of cats with behavioral signs of oral discomfort and tongue mutilation.
5. Stage _____ TR lesions involve the cementum or enamel only.
6. The most common treatment for TR is _____.
7. MRONJ or BRONJ is caused by _____.
8. A congenital disease in which there is a risk of long bone fracture, impacted permanent teeth, and osteomyelitis of the jaws is _____.
9. Which breed is most associated with FOPS?
10. Type _____ TR is characterized by completely intact roots without bone replacement resorption.

FURTHER READING

Bell CM, Edstrom E, Shope B, et al. Characterization of oral pathology in cats affected by patellar fracture and dental anomaly syndrome (PADS). *J Vet Dent*. 2023;40(4):284–297. doi:10.1177/08987564231175594.

Booij-Vrieling E, de Vries TJ, Schoenmaker T, et al. Osteoclast progenitors from cats with and without tooth resorption respond differently to 1,25-dihydroxyvitamin D and interleukin-6. *Res Vet Sci*. 2012;92(2):311–316.

Booij-Vrieling HE, Tryfonidou MA, Riemers FM, Penning LC, Hazewinkel HAW. Inflammatory cytokines and the nuclear vitamin D receptor are implicated in the pathophysiology of dental resorptive lesions in cats. *Vet Immunol Immunopathol*. 2009;132(2–4):160–166.

Girard N, Servet E, Hennet P, Biourge V. Tooth resorption and vitamin D3 status in cats fed premium dry diets. *J Vet Dent*. 2010;27(3):142–147. doi:10.1177/089875641002700301.

Heaton M, Wilkinson J, Gorrel C, Butterwick R. A rapid screening technique for feline odontoclastic resorptive lesions. *J Small Anim Pract*. 2004;45(12):598–601. doi:10.1111/j.1748-5827.2004.tb00181.x.

Reiter AM, Lyon KF, Nachreiner RF, Shofer FS. Evaluation of calciotropic hormones in cats with odontoclastic resorptive lesions. *Am J Vet Res*. 2005;66(8):1446–1452. doi:10.2460/ajvr.2005.66.1446.

Soltero-Rivera M, Vapniarsky N, Rivas IL, Arzi B. Clinical, radiographic and histopathologic features of early-onset gingivitis and periodontitis in cats (1997–2022). *J Feline Med Surg*. 2023;25(1). doi:10.1177/1098612X221148577.

Intraoral Imaging

LEARNING OBJECTIVES

When you have completed this chapter, you will be able to:

- List and describe the indications and contraindications for performing intraoral radiography.
- List and describe the components of digital veterinary dental radiology systems.

- Differentiate between parallel and bisecting-angle dental radiographic techniques and describe when each would be used.
- List and describe the views needed for a complete intraoral radiographic study.
- Describe common complications in dental radiology related to improper exposure, positioning, and digital artifacts.

- Describe normal radiographic anatomy of dogs and cats and common abnormalities that may be seen with radiographic evaluation.

- Understand the fundamentals of cone beam computed tomography (CBCT)

KEY TERMS

Bisecting-angle technique
Computerized radiology
Cone beam tomography
Digital radiology

Lamina dura
Multiplanar reconstruction
Parallel technique

Periapical lucency
phosphor plate
SLOB rule

The value of dental radiography is widely recognized in small animal practice. At one time it was thought of as a "luxury" or "fancy" diagnostic tool; it is now accepted as a necessity to provide dental care. Yet making full-mouth radiographs in a reasonable time and interpretation of the images is still regarded as a challenge for many. After reading this chapter and with practice, the team can become more capable of producing great dental radiographs.

INDICATIONS FOR DENTAL RADIOGRAPHY

Dental radiographs are necessary for the complete diagnosis of dental pathology and are used to document and study the progression of disease and success of treatment. Dental radiographs are also valuable in assessing oral neoplasia, certain metabolic diseases, and oral trauma. However, other imaging modalities (computed tomography, standard radiographs, ultrasound) are also needed for assessing neoplasia and many trauma cases.

In canine patients, full-mouth dental radiographs demonstrated clinically important findings in 27.8% of dogs without clinical lesions, additional information in 50% of dogs with clinical lesions, and essential information in 22.6% of dogs with clinical lesions. In feline patients, full-mouth dental radiographs demonstrated clinically important findings in 41.7% of cats without clinical lesions, additional information in 53.9% of cats with

clinical lesions, and essential information in 32.2% of cats with clinical lesions.

As dental radiographs are required to discover essential information in 1/4 to 1/3 of patients, the need to assess full-mouth radiographs on every dental patient is obvious. The only contraindication for dental radiology is in the case of a patient who cannot undergo general anesthesia.

GOALS OF DENTAL RADIOGRAPH ACQUISITION

When making dental radiographs, the images should capture every tooth in its entirety, including at least 2 mm of tissue around the apex of each tooth. Ideally, the ventral cortex of the mandible is fully imaged to assess for pathology and preplanning for treatment. There should be minimal overlap of adjacent teeth and other structures. The images should approximate the normal shape of the tooth (no foreshortening or elongation). The images should be reproducible when repeated at future visits.

PROTECTIVE MEASURES

Personnel should protect themselves by wearing lead safety aprons or using screens. They should also maintain a safe distance from the beam of radiation emitted by the radiographic unit. The safe distance is a minimum of 6 feet from the tube and in a radius that is 90 to 135 degrees from the primary beam trajectory.

All team members who may be exposed to X-rays should wear a dosimetry badge near his or her thyroid gland. If a team member is pregnant, she should follow regulations provided by the local authority. This may include limited to no exposure or wearing an additional badge for the developing child.

A variety of devices may be used to hold the film in place. Placing the film in holders, resting the film against the endotracheal tube, and securing the film with gauze sponges are a few common methods.

The patient and dental X-ray generator should always be positioned in such a way that radiation is never aimed directly at team members. Shields and protective devices should always be used if there is any chance of exposure.

DENTAL RADIOGRAPHIC EQUIPMENT

Dental Radiograph Generators

The dental radiograph generator is the equipment that produces the X-ray radiation necessary to make a radiograph. Of note, an X-ray is not a diagnostic image. It is a form of radiation. The radiograph is the image we evaluate. The advantage of the dental radiographic unit is its articulating radiographic head and jointed extension arm (excluding hand-held units). The unit can be moved into position and angled easily, which minimizes the need for patient repositioning. This also allows the patient to remain on the operatory table without moving for diagnostic images.

Dental radiographs can be made using standard medical radiographic units. However, these require considerable effort in positioning the patient. With the stationary radiographic unit, the patient must be moved several times to reorient the head. This often leads to prolonged anesthesia and less than diagnostic radiographs.

The radiographic tube has a cylindrical position indicating device (PID) from which radiation is emitted. The PID is already collimated to the appropriate size. As there is no light projected from the PID, the boundary of the cylinder indicates where the radiation will project.

There are two types of current that can be input into dental X-ray machine heads: Alternating current (AC) and direct current (DC). In most dental machines, the amount of voltage applied to the tube determines the power of the X-ray. An AC unit (that produces a sine wave) produces impulses of X-rays. In the United States, the rate is 60 pulses every second; in some parts of the world, the rate is 50 pulses per second. The amount is measured at its kilovoltage peak (kVp). DC units are more like very high-frequency AC units—they produce a wave in the 70,000 cycles per second range. Thus, the high pulse is not perceived and is expressed as kilovolt (kV), and the power is more consistent. Therefore a DC unit is used with less kV than an AC unit's kVp. Milliamperage (mA) is often fixed in AC dental X-ray units—most typically at 7 mA, but it can be 6 or 8 mA; mA is usually variable in DC X-ray units—typically in a range of 4 to 8 mA.

The kVp in most dental radiographic units is fixed between 60 and 90 kVp, with 70 being the most common. Likewise, the mA is fixed for most units. Time, however, is a variable that may require adjustment according to the thickness of the area to be studied. Some units measure time in portions of a second and others set time in pulses—one impulse equals one-sixtieth of a second; thus, 30 pulses would equal 0.5 second.

Many units have preselected settings that change based on patient size, the tooth being imaged, and if film, digital radiography (DR) or Computerized radiology (CR) is being used.

Choosing a Dental Radiograph Generator

There are two important criteria in choosing an X-ray unit. First, the stability of the arm is important, especially if there is a long reach between where the X-ray unit is mounted and the patient. Good arms do not wobble after they are positioned. The second criterion is the focal spot size inside the tube head—the smaller the spot, the sharper the image; a 0.4-mm spot will be much sharper than a 0.7-mm spot.

Dental X-ray units may be mounted on the wall (Fig. 11.1A), on stands (Fig. 11.1B and C), or hand-held (Fig. 11.1D). The advantage of a wall-mounted unit is that it has a smaller footprint than stand-mounted units. However, wall-mounted units cannot be moved from room to room. Stand-mounted units take space in the dental operatory but can be moved around to different rooms or tables. Hand-held units tend to be less powerful than stand-mounted (floor-mounted) units.

Image Capture

There are three ways in which X-rays can be captured to produce a radiograph: standard film, DR, and CR. Each modality has advantages and disadvantages. The practitioner should consider all of these before deciding on which modality to use.

Intraoral Film

Intraoral radiographic film is inexpensive, small, and flexible. It fits neatly into the oral cavity and conforms to the area in which it is placed. An intraoral film is a nonscreen film that provides greater detail than the screen films used in standard radiographs. An intraoral film can be processed by a chairside developer using hand or through automatic developers.

Most intraoral film packets are composed of a series of layers. A plastic coating covers the external portion. Between the plastic coating and the radiographic film is a layer of paper. The next layer is the radiographic film, sandwiched by another layer of paper. Finally, a layer of lead is followed by another layer of paper that can be peeled from the plastic coating (Fig. 11.2). As intraoral film is infrequently used, less time is given to this modality in the current text.

Digital Radiology

Digital radiology uses a sensor (Fig. 11.3) to capture X-rays, which are then translated into radiographs.

This is typically via a charge-coupled device (CCD) or a complementary metal oxide superconductor (CMOS). These systems are directly wired into a computer (some wireless models exist). They produce a radiographic image directly to the provided software within seconds.

The sensors are typically a standard size 2, although variations exist. The housing is wider than the portion that collects radiation and also makes the unit thicker than the alternatives (film, CR).

If the sensor is cared for properly, it should generate 200,000 images. A computer is used to process the image, which is then displayed on the monitor. At least, the minimal system requirements recommended by the sensor manufacturer should be met, and the monitor must be high quality and capable of image reproduction. The computer, which is used in image production, will need to have the appropriate driver software installed. If viewing software is installed and the computer has access to the file database, remote-viewing stations can be used as well.

The equipment should be protected because it is very fragile and subject to damage from being dropped or bitten or from water getting inside. Protective covers should be placed on the unit and secured. Another way to be safer is to use Velcro to attach a wire from the sensor to the X-ray arm. Some units come with the sensor attached to the radiographic machine arm.

The protective cover will not protect the sensor from animal bites. The patient must be completely anesthetized. Even the slightest flexing may damage a sensor (Fig. 11.4).

Computerized Radiography

Another digital system has a phosphor plate (Fig. 11.5A) and a processing unit (Fig. 11.5B); this system is known as indirect or CR. The phosphor plates are of standard dental radiograph sizes: 0, 2, 3, and 4 with some manufacturers making proprietary sizes. Size 2 is often known as periapical film size. In veterinary dentistry, this type of film is suitable for small patients. Size 4, also called occlusal

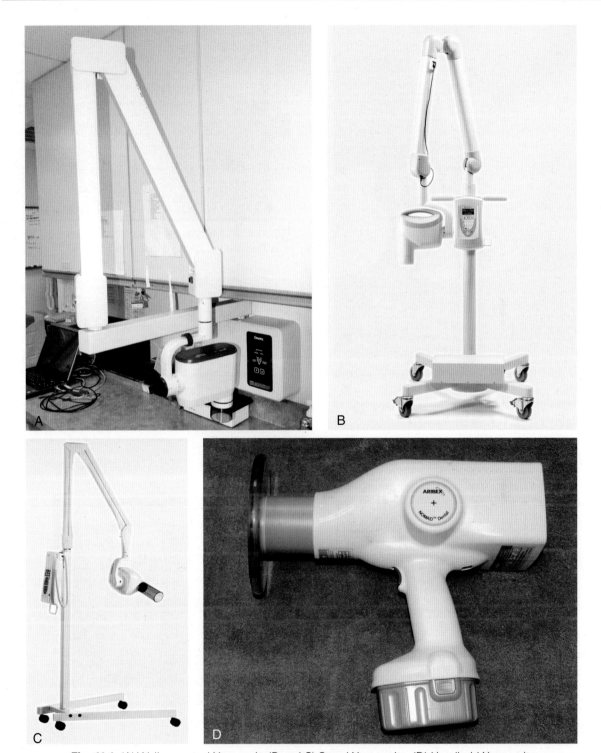

Fig. 11.1 (A) Wall-mounted X-ray unit. (B and C) Stand X-ray units. (D) Handheld X-ray unit.

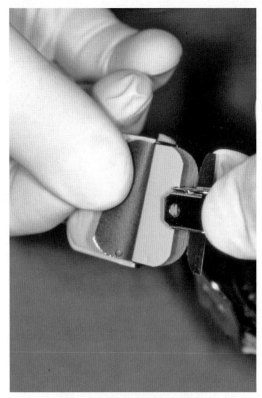

Fig. 11.2 Inside intraoral film.

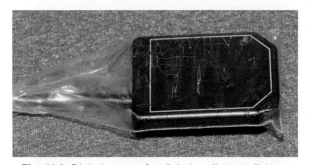

Fig. 11.3 Digital sensor for digital or direct radiology.

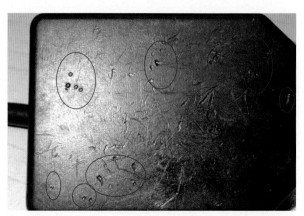

Fig. 11.4 This sensor damage on the outside (*red circles*) may destroy the electronics inside.

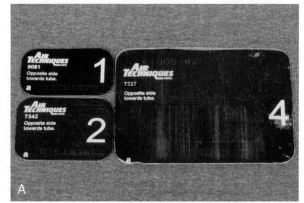

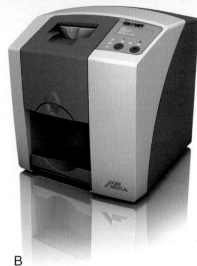

Fig. 11.5 Plates (A) and processing unit (B) for computerized radiography.

film size, is appropriate for larger patients. For cats, size 0 may be useful for radiographic evaluation of the mandibular premolars and molars. Each plate is thin and flexible. The bulk of the plate is made of polyester with a phosphor coating on one side, which captures X-rays. The plate is placed in the mouth with the phosphor facing the generator. After exposure, the plate is placed into the scanner, and a laser aids in releasing the stored energy of the X-rays, producing visible light. This light is then translated into a radiograph. As the plate moves through the scanner, the previous image is erased.

The plates are placed in a protective envelope that protects them not only from visible light but also from scratching. The plate should always be kept in the envelope except during scanning or should be kept in its protective case. The envelopes are disposable. It may seem frugal to reuse envelopes, but this increases the risk of damage to the plate or worse, the scanner. The plates can be cleaned, and the user is directed to the manufacturer's instructions so as not to void any warranties. The plates do have a finite life span. They should be replaced if the edges are roughened or if damage to the phosphor is noted.

The scanner itself should be periodically cleaned. Some scanners are designed to be opened by the user for cleaning. Others use special cleaning sheets that pull out dust and debris. Regardless, periodic professional cleaning may be necessary and as with the plates, the user is referred to the manufacturer's recommendations.

The computer requirements of CR are like that of DR.

Comparison of DR and CR

The resolution (measured in line pairs) of all modern DR and CR systems is better than what the human eye can detect. The detector latitude of DR is like a film but that of CR is superior. This produces more "shades of gray" in an image and makes soft tissue structure more visible. DR systems produce a single image directly to the computer faster than CR as CR requires manual scanning. When processing multiple images at a time, some CR systems may be faster depending on the operator. CR does require more maintenance due to cleaning and more dispensable materials (envelopes) are required. However, replacing a CR plate is orders of magnitude less expensive than replacing a DR sensor if damaged. DR sensors may be more difficult to position due to the size of the sensor compared to the smaller CR plate and the presence of a wire. Both are capable systems, and the choice is based on preference. The three main image capture modalities are compared in Table 11.1.

TABLE 11.1 Comparison of Dental Radiograph Image Capture Options			
	Film	Direct Digital (DR)	Indirect Digital or Scanner (CR)
Time	Slowest	Fastest	
Resolution (note, all produce resolution better than unmagnified vision)	Best	Near to film	Least
Image Latitude or Shades of Gray	Similar to DR	Similar to film	Best
Shortcomings	• Difficult to archive • Chemical handling and clean-up required	• Limited sensor sizes available • Housing of sensor is not flexible	• Additional steps during processing (compared to DR) • Additional materials to purchase (envelopes, cleaners)

Radiographic Technique

In general, the following tips are helpful to obtain the best technique in setting up radiographs.

The patient is positioned appropriately for the radiograph to be taken. The sensor or plate is placed in the proper position. As an aid in positioning the film, a film wedge, or other object can be placed behind the film. The head of the X-ray machine is placed 8 to 12 inches or as close as possible to the structure being evaluated and positioned for the study. The image is exposed and then scanned, if necessary.

The number of images in a complete radiographic study is dependent on patient size and the technology used. Typically, a complete canine study includes an occlusal view of the maxillary incisors a lateral oblique of each maxillary canine a bisecting angle of the first three maxillary premolars, a bisecting angle, and caudal to rostral oblique of the maxillary fourth premolar and molars, an occlusal of the mandibular incisors and canines, a lateral oblique of the mandibular canines, a bisecting angle of the mandibular premolars, and a parallel view of the mandibular molars. The cat is similar except often a bisecting-angle view of the mandibular premolars is not necessary as both can be obtained with a parallel technique.

Patient Positioning

Full-mouth radiographs can be made in sternal/dorsal recumbency or in each lateral recumbency. The position is based on practice workflow. Both should be practiced as intraoperative films may need to be made in the position the patient is in during the procedure.

If using sternal/dorsal recumbency, all maxillary radiographs can be made with the patient in sternal recumbency after intubation; then all mandibular radiographs can be made in dorsal recumbency.

Placing Film

The sensor or plate should be placed in the mouth so that the active side is facing toward the subject and head (position-indicating device) of the radiographic unit. This is the side opposite the wire with DR systems and the phosphor side with CR systems. A maximal amount of root and supporting bone should be included in the film. Placing the radiographic film in such a way that most of the film is not over tooth and bone is ineffective. The edge of the sensor or film should not hang too far past the tooth in a buccal/facial direction.

Parallel Technique

The parallel technique for oral radiographs is indicated to evaluate the mandibular molars of the dog and often the mandibular premolars and molars of the cat. The sensor or plate is placed parallel to the structure to be radiographed and between the tongue and mandible. The PID is pointed directly at the sensor or plate. Fig. 11.6A demonstrates the parallel technique to image the seventh right mandibular first molar. The direction of the X-ray radiation is indicated in green, and the position of the film is indicated in red. Fig. 11.6B demonstrates the obtained radiograph.

Bisecting-Angle Technique

In areas where the parallel technique cannot be used, the *bisecting-angle technique* should be used. The bisecting angle is obtained by visualizing an imaginary line that bisects the angle formed by the sensor/plate, and the structure being radiographed and the PID is aimed perpendicular to this line (Fig. 11.7). If the X-ray beam is aimed at the tooth, the image on the finished film will be distorted by elongation (Fig. 11.8). If the X-ray beam is aimed at the film, the image will still be distorted, this time by foreshortening (Fig. 11.9).

When first learning this technique, some technicians find it helpful to use props, such as sticks (cotton-tipped applicators) to help visualize the bisecting angle.

Positioning for Full-Mouth Dental Radiographs

The following technique works for both sternal/dorsal recumbency and lateral recumbency. As specific angles (in relation to the teeth and film) are

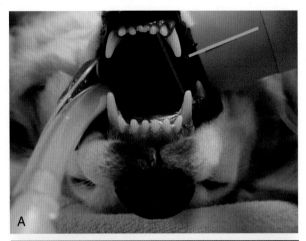

A

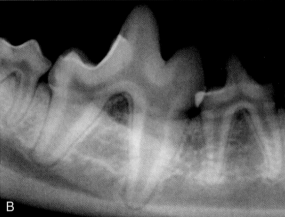

B

Fig. 11.6 (A) Parallel radiographic technique with X-ray radiation direction marked in green and film position marked in red. (B) Radiograph of right mandibular first molar obtained with parallel technique.

not used, only the concepts of parallel technique and bisecting-angle technique need to be used. The illustrations will have the plane of the film annotated in red, the plane of the teeth in white, the bisecting angle in blue, and the direction of the X-ray radiation in green.

Maxillary incisors. In both the dog and the cat, the sensor/plate is placed adjacent to the roof of the mouth with the rostral edge of the film just rostral to the incisor teeth. The PID is aimed perpendicular to the bisecting angle (Fig. 11.10A). Often the bisecting angle is parallel to the alar fold of the nose. The resulting radiograph is shown in Fig. 11.10B.

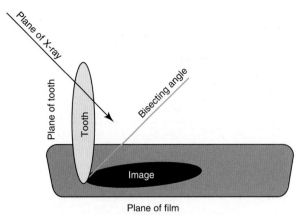

Fig. 11.7 The plane of the tooth is at a 90-degree angle to the film. The bisecting angle is therefore 45 degrees. The radiographic cone is aimed at this imaginary line. As a result, the image is recorded with slight magnification.

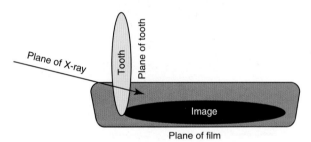

Fig. 11.8 Elongation caused by aiming the radiographic cone at the tooth rather than the bisecting angle.

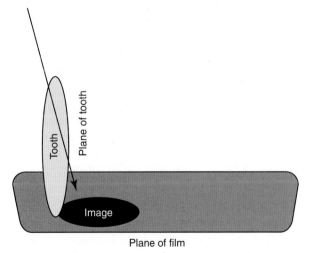

Fig. 11.9 Foreshortening caused by aiming the radiographic cone toward the film.

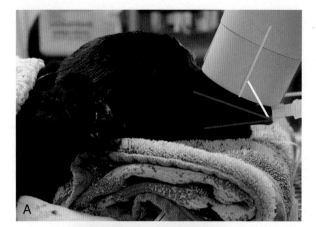

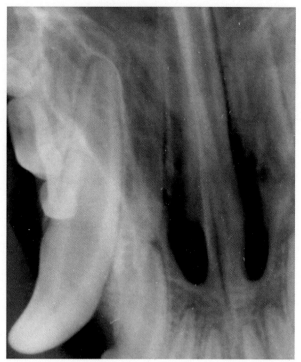

Fig. 11.11 If the maxillary canines are imaged from rostral to caudal, the premolars overlap the canine tooth.

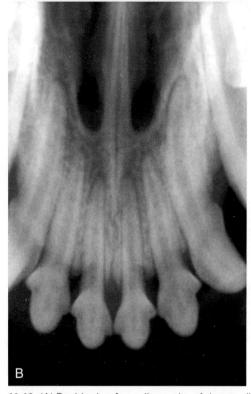

Fig. 11.10 (A) Positioning for radiographs of the maxillary incisors. (B) Radiograph of maxillary incisors of a dog.

Maxillary canine. Due to overlap of the maxillary first and second premolars in the dog, the canine teeth cannot be evaluated on the same image as the incisors (Fig. 11.11). Instead, PID is shifted from a rostral to caudal direction to an angle 45 degrees from the front of the patient and 45 degrees from the side of the patient while maintaining the bisecting angle (Fig. 11.12A–C).

Maxillary first, second, and third premolars. To take a radiograph of the first three maxillary premolars, the film is placed in the mouth parallel to the hard palate. The PID is aimed perpendicular to the bisecting angle (Fig. 11.13A and B). In some patients, the line between the premolars is not parallel with the median line of the patient and the PID may need to be shifted in a slight rostral to caudal direction to compensate.

Maxillary fourth premolar and molars. For the maxillary fourth premolars and molars, the film is simply placed across the maxilla parallel to the hard palate. The long end of the film is parallel to the muzzle. The PID is positioned like imaging for the first three premolars. This provides a lateral view of the three teeth. In this view, the mesial roots of the maxillary fourth premolar are superimposed (Fig. 11.14). To image the mesial

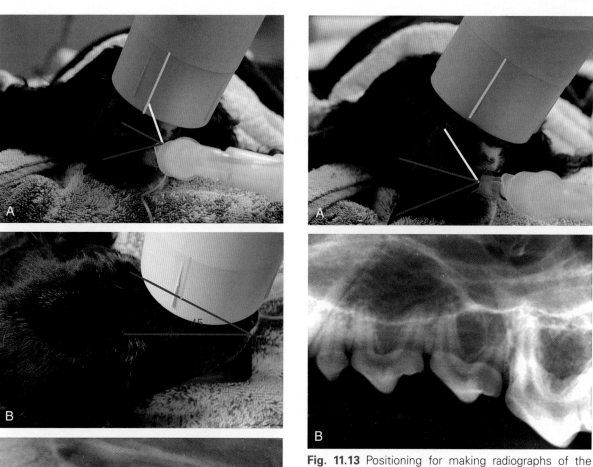

Fig. 11.12 (A) Rostral view of position for making radiographs of the left maxillary canine tooth. (B) The PID is shifted from a rostral to the caudal direction to aim 45 degrees from the midline of the patient. (C) Radiograph of left maxillary canine tooth with minimal overlap.

Fig. 11.13 Positioning for making radiographs of the maxillary premolars and the radigraph achieved.

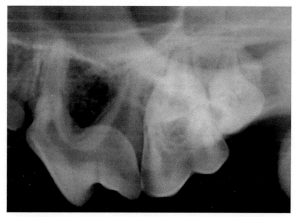

Fig. 11.14 Lateral view of left maxillary fourth premolar and molars.

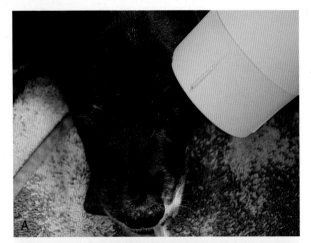

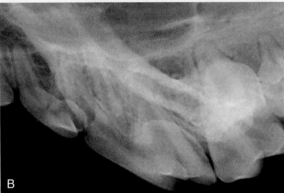

Fig. 11.15 (A) Caudal to cranial oblique to image mesial roots of let maxillary fourth premolar without superimposition. (B) Caudal to rostral oblique radiograph of left maxillary fourth premolar to image the mesial roots. The mesiobuccal root is the most rostral root, the mesiopalatal the middle root and the distal root remains distal.

roots of the maxillary fourth premolar, the PID must be shifted to a caudal-to-rostral oblique angle (Fig. 11.15A). With this view, the root on the image that appears in the middle is the lingual (palatal) root. The buccal root appears more rostral (Fig. 11.15B). This is known as the *Same Lingual, Opposite Buccal (SLOB) rule*. The readers can use their fingers to learn this rule. For the right maxillary fourth premolar use your right hand. Hold up the thumb to represent the distal root, the index finger to represent the mesiobuccal root, and the

middle finger to represent the palatal root. Holding the index and middle fingers so they line up would represent an overlap of the mesiobuccal and palatal roots. If the observer's head is tilted to the left without moving the fingers, the middle finger, representing the palatal (lingual) root, will move in the same direction (right or forward) as the tilting head (Fig. 11.16).

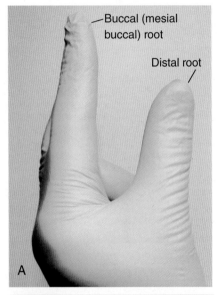

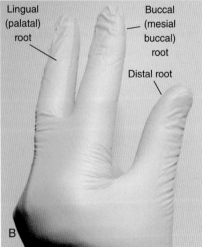

Fig. 11.16 Example of using fingers. (A) Lined-up position. Left maxillary fourth premolar. (B) Moved to left positioning.

Mandibular incisors. To take a radiograph of the mandibular anterior teeth, the film is placed in the mouth parallel to the mandibles with the tongue between the film and the teeth. The PID is aimed perpendicular to the bisecting angle (Fig. 11.17A and B). Due to the table pushing the film, this can be difficult to position in lateral recumbency.

Mandibular premolars. The mandibular premolar radiographs are very similar to the maxillary premolar radiographs (Fig. 11.18A and B). This view is often positioned in a way that makes the image elongated. This should be kept in mind when positioning.

Mandibular molars. The mandibular molar radiograph is simple in concept. The sensor/plate is placed between the tongue and teeth and the PID is aimed perpendicular to the sensor/plate. The challenge is the musculature and angle of the jaw, making it difficult to position the sensor back far enough to reach the mandibular third molar. The solution is to move the machine head further caudal and aim it more rostral.

Feline caudal maxillary teeth. Owing to the shape of the head and zygomatic arch, many times the zygomatic arch will obscure visualization of the roots of the third and fourth premolar. Two techniques are used to overcome this. The extraoral technique places the sensor directly on the tabletop. The patient's head is placed on the sensor, with mouth opened about 1½ inches and mandibular canines tipped about 1 inch off the table. The X-ray beam is directed so that it skylines the palate (Fig. 11.19).

The almost parallel technique places the film on the opposite side of the mouth that is being studied. The radiographic beam is directed so that it skylines the palate (Fig. 11.20).

Overlapping Dental Structures

To determine the identity of three-dimensional structures seen on a two-dimensional plane, particularly in the evaluation of maxillary fourth premolar palatal and mesiobuccal roots, a second film is taken, with the X-ray beam moved either anterior or posterior to the previous position of the radiographic cone head. The structure that is more lingual (the palatal root) will be shadowed on the film in the

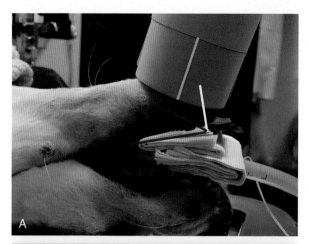
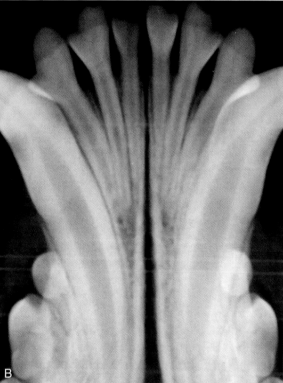

Fig. 11.17 (A) Position for making radiographs of the mandibular incisors. Note the same position is used to make an occlusal view of the canine teeth as long as the film is placed far enough casual to image the apices. (B) Radiograph of the mandibular incisors.

same direction as the X-ray beam. The structure that is more buccal (the mesiobuccal root) will be shadowed in the opposite direction as the X-ray beam.

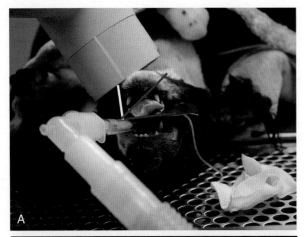

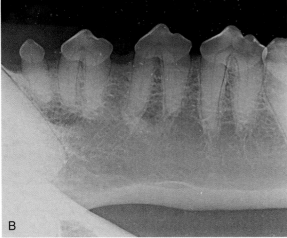

Fig. 11.18 (A) Imaging the left mandibular premolars. (B) Radiograph of the left mandibular premolars.

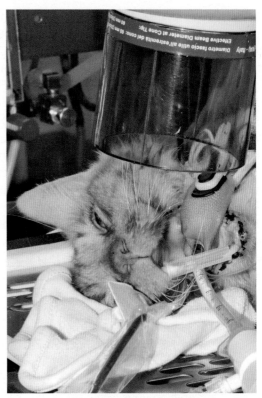

Fig. 11.19 Extraoral technique.

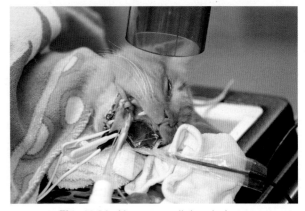

Fig. 11.20 Almost parallel technique.

This phenomenon may be remembered by the SLOB rule. When successive radiographs are taken, the most lingual (palatal) root will move in the same direction on the radiograph as the cone head was repositioned. If the cone is moved forward, the lingual root will be the root that moves forward.

Four Simple Rules for Positioning

- Make sure you are aiming at the subject and sensor/plate.
- Do not take a radiograph of air.
- If the image is elongated, aim at the sensor/plate.
- If the image is foreshortened, aim at the subject.

Mounting Radiographs

Radiographs should be viewed with the crowns of the maxillary teeth pointed down and the crowns of the mandibular teeth pointed up. When viewing the right-side images, the more rostral teeth should be on the right and caudal to the left. The opposite holds true for the left side. This is known as labial imaging. Radiographic software should position the films in this way as a default. However, if a phosphor plate is placed into the mouth with the phosphor opposite the radiograph generator, a mirror image will be produced. If that occurs, the image can be flipped horizontally. In the case of DR, the electronics of the sensor will be imaged.

When film was used, the film had to be marked in such a way that told the viewer as to which side was being imaged. A raised dot on the film aided in knowing which side of the film faced the generator and using anatomic knowledge, the viewer could ascertain which teeth were being imaged. This still required the film to be marked with the patient's information and the date taken.

COMPLICATIONS IN DENTAL RADIOLOGY

Complications in dental radiology occur because of improper exposure, positioning, and developing. Table 11.2 is a troubleshooting guide.

Failure to Position Film Sensor or Plate Properly

There is a tendency to attempt to get as close to the tooth as possible. This may result in the film or sensor's "real estate" being wasted (Fig. 11.21).

Blurred or Double Images

Movement of either the patient or the X-ray machine head causes blurred or double images. If the movement continues throughout the exposure, the image will be blurred. When the film is in one position for part of the exposure and then moved to a second position for the remainder of the exposure, a double image results. Tongue movement in lightly sedated patients may also cause the film to move.

Elongation of Image

If the image appears elongated, the radiographic cone head was probably aimed too directly at the

TABLE 11.2   Troubleshooting Guide for Dental Radiology

Error	Correction
Backside of sensor electronics or no image	Turn over the sensor
Missing tooth	Reposition sensor or machine cone
Elongation	Reposition machine cone to aim more at film
Foreshortening	Reposition machine cone to aim more at the sensor
Blurring	Make sure patient is not moving
	Make sure radiographic unit is not swinging
Underexposure	Increase exposure time or decrease distance
Overexposure	Decrease exposure time or add distance
Cervical burnout	Take multiple exposures at multiple timings
Out of dynamic range	Take multiple exposures
No exposure	Was button held down long enough?
	Are the lights on?
	Make sure the unit is plugged in
	Check fuses
	Check digital sensor (is it backward?)
	Reboot computer

subject as opposed to the bisecting angle between the subject and the film or sensor. Another possibility is that the film was placed incorrectly (Fig. 11.22). To correct, first check film placement and, if this is correct, aim the machine head more toward the film.

Foreshortening of Image

If the image appears foreshortened, the radiographic cone head may have been aimed too directly at the radiographic film or sensor as opposed to the

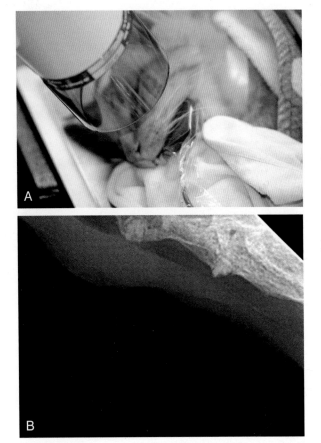

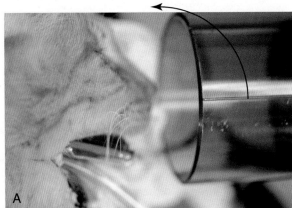

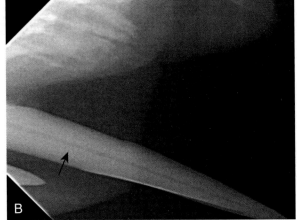

Fig. 11.21 (A) Too much air positioning. (B) Too much air radiograph.

Fig. 11.22 (A) Elongated incorrect positioning. (B) Extremely elongated radiograph of canine tooth (*arrow*).

bisecting angle. Another cause is improper positioning of the film (Fig. 11.23).

Radiographic Errors
Positioning
Aside from correct positioning, the three results from positioning are as follows:

1. The sensor and radiographs can miss the intended subject or not contain enough subject. It is important that the image contains 2 to 3 mm of bone around the apex. Most commonly, the sensor is placed very close to the crown, missing the root and imaging only air. In this case, the sensor and radiograph cone head must be repositioned.
2. The image can be elongated. In this case, the radiographic cone has been aimed too much at

the subject. The correction is to reposition the radiographic machine head so that it is aimed more at the sensor. The next error that can occur is the image is foreshortened. In this case, the radiographic cone has been aimed too much at the sensor. In this case, the cone should be redirected so that it aims more at the tooth.

3. Although the positioning may be correct, other errors may occur. Blurring can be caused by patient motion or machine head motion. The image can be overexposed or underexposed. One weakness of DR is the dynamic range. Dynamic range is the difference between the least and most amount of radiation that can be recorded on the sensor. When the dynamic range is exceeded, one part of the image is overexposed

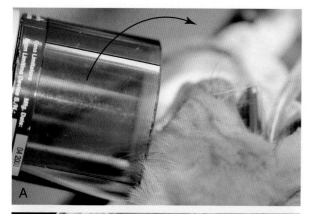

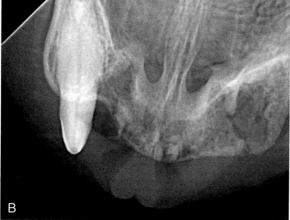

Fig. 11.23 (A) Foreshortened positioning. (B) Foreshortened radiograph.

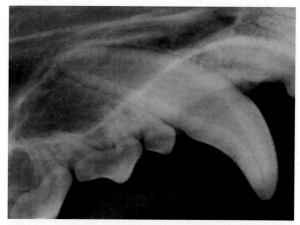

Fig. 11.24 Normal radiographic anatomy of the right maxillary canine tooth. Note the radiodensity of enamel at the periphery of the crown compared to dentin and pulp (*radiolucent*).

Radiographic Anatomy

The important landmarks in reviewing an individual tooth are enamel, dentin, pulp chamber, periodontal ligament space, and alveolar bone. The enamel is the most radiodense structure followed by dentin, cementum, and alveolar bone, then the pulp chamber and periodontal ligament space. Each of these areas should be recognized and evaluated (Fig. 11.24).

Normal Young Patient

In the young patient, the dentinal wall is thin, and the pulp chamber is large. As the tooth develops, odontoblasts that line the pulp chamber produce dentin resulting in a thicker dentinal wall and thinner pulp chamber. The apex may not have formed, depending on the age of the patient. In the young patient, the dense cortical alveolar bone forming the wall of the alveolus appears radiographically as a distinct, opaque, uninterrupted, white line parallel to the tooth root (Fig. 11.25A). This line is known as the *lamina dura*. The radiolucent structure between the lamina dura and tooth is the periodontal ligament space. On the other side of the lamina dura is the trabecular bone, which is less radiodense than the lamina dura.

and another is underexposed. The neck region of the tooth is one area in which this may cause a misdiagnosis. If overexposed, it may appear that there are tooth resorption (TR) lesions, yet this overexposure may be necessary to evaluate the root structure.

RADIOGRAPHIC FINDINGS

Radiographic findings can be recorded in the medical record, dental chart, or radiology notes chart. These should be organized by quadrant and tooth or by grouping within pathology categories such as periodontal disease and endodontic disease findings.

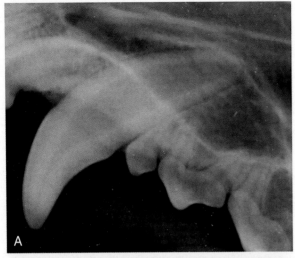

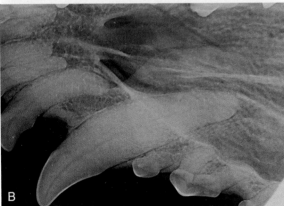

Fig. 11.25 (A) Radiograph of left maxillary canine of an approximately one-year-old dog. Note the width of the root canal. (B) Radiograph of the left maxillary canine of an approximately 7-year-old dog. Note the root canal width is much narrower compared to the patient in Fig. 25A.

Normal Older Patient

The dental radiograph of a healthy adult shows a decreased canal size and increased dentinal wall thickness (Fig. 11.25B). Generally, the periodontal ligament space becomes narrower with age. The lamina dura may become less visible but is typically present in the healthy tooth.

Periodontal Disease

Radiographic evidence of periodontal disease begins with rounding and loss of the crestal bone.

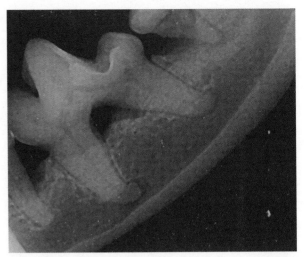

Fig. 11.26 Horizontal bone loss of the left mandibular first molar. Note that there are areas of vertical bone loss.

This is particularly visible in the interproximal space between teeth. Periodontal disease may also be noted as horizontal bone loss (Fig. 11.26). In this pattern of bone loss, the plane of the remaining alveolar bone is relatively parallel to its original position. Loss of interradicular bone within the furcation can be noted. If vertical bone loss has occurred, increased periodontal ligament space will be evident. The plane of bone loss is oblique to its original position, creating a gap between the bone and the root (Fig. 11.27). Periodontal bone loss is typically a mixed pattern of horizontal and vertical.

Endodontic Disease

Signs of endodontic disease include decreased radiodensity around the apex of the tooth root, often called a *periapical lucency*, widening of the periodontal ligament space, relatively wide pulp chamber, resorption of the tooth root internally, or resorption of the tooth root externally (Fig. 11.28). Fractures may be noted above or below the gumline. Apical periodontitis. Apical periodontitis is due to inflammation and infection of the pulp extending through the apical delta into the periapical tissues. This can lead to inflammation and widening of the periodontal ligament and demineralization of the

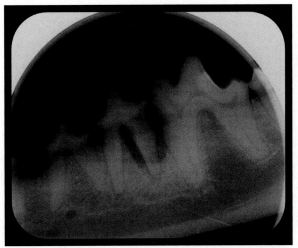

Fig. 11.27 Vertical bone loss of the left mandibular fourth premolar and first molar.

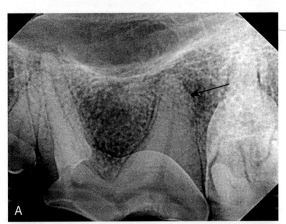

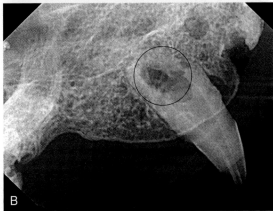

Fig. 11.28 (A) Endodontic root resorption in a dog (*arrow*). (B) Endodontic root resorption in a cat (*circle*).

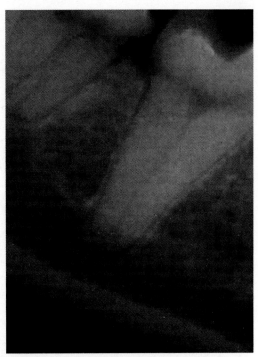

Fig. 11.29 Right mandible. A normal chevron sign in a nondiseased tooth.

periapical bone, creating a lucency or periapical rarefaction.

Distinguishing the chevron sign around the apex from pathology is a very common problem for the practitioner. The chevron sign tends to be distinct with sharp demarcation between the chevron sign, which represents the area where vessels and nerves are entering the apex and bone (Fig. 11.29). It is congruent with the shape of the apex and is typically symmetrical when compared to the opposite side of the patient.

Pathologic apical periodontitis, also called a lesion of endodontic origin, is less distinct. The shape is irregular, and it is not symmetrical. A patient had a chronically complicated fractured right first molar. Radiographs were taken before endodontic therapy was performed, right after endodontic therapy, 6 months postoperative, and 1 year postoperative. Bone has filled in, indicating a successful procedure (Fig. 11.30A and F). Although bone density may never be "normal," there is resolution of the periapical periodontitis.

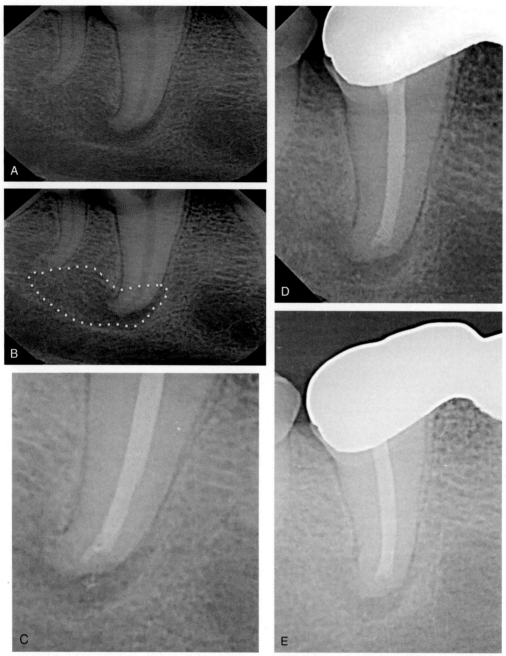

Fig. 11.30 (A) Preoperative periapical periodontitis. Radiograph upon presentation and before treatment. (B) Periapical periodontitis outlined. The area of the lucent bone has been outlined in *yellow*. (C) Postoperative endodontic therapy: Endodontic therapy has been performed on the tooth. Note the slight "puff" of sealer in the periapical region, indicating the filling of the apical delta. (D) Six months resolved apical periodontitis. The bone density is becoming more uniform as the periodontitis resolves. A metal crown has been placed on the tooth and is radiodense. (E) One-year postoperatively resolved apical periodontitis. Bone continues to fill in.

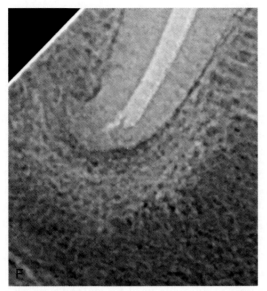

Fig. 11.30, cont'd (F) A 2.5-year pathologic apical (PA) post. Bone has filled in nicely.

Tooth Resorption

Radiographic signs of a TR lesion range from a barely visible coronal lucency to resorption of the entire root and replacement with new alveolar bone (Fig. 11.31A and B). See Chapter 10 for further description of TR.

Retained Roots

Radiographs may be taken, both diagnostically and intraoperatively, to evaluate retained roots (Fig. 11.32). The presence of lucency around the root may indicate a disease that needs to be treated. The radiograph should be evaluated to determine whether other oral structures have been compromised.

Neoplasia

The proliferation of bone, missing bone, and/or displacement of teeth are all radiographic signs of neoplasia. No tumor can be diagnosed based on imaging alone, and these signs are not exclusive to neoplasia. Fig. 11.33 demonstrates marked nasal bone loss of the right side secondary to a nasal adenocarcinoma. Note that there is a retained root, which does not show evidence of inflammation.

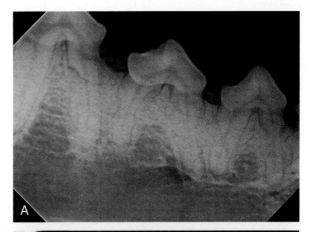

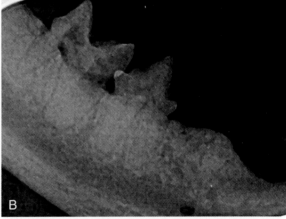

Fig. 11.31 (A) Canine tooth resorption (TR). The interface between the normal root and portion of the root with TR gives the appearance of a fracture. (B) Various stages of resorption of the right mandibular premolars and molar of a cat.

Unerupted or Impacted Teeth

In young patients, radiographs help the practitioner determine whether unerupted or impacted teeth are present. An impacted tooth is an unerupted or partially erupted tooth that is prevented from erupting further by any structure. Dental radiographs are taken in all patients to evaluate the status of the root and tooth when the tooth is missing or partly erupted. The practitioner may discover that the tooth is truly missing or may find an unerupted tooth. If an unerupted tooth is covered by bone, it is not likely to erupt. Additionally, an

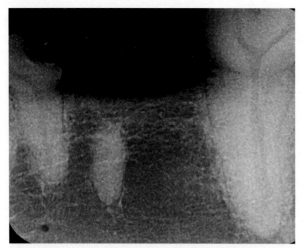

Fig. 11.32 Retained root of left mandibular fourth premolar in a dog. Note that there are no signs of inflammation.

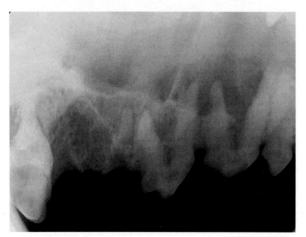

Fig. 11.33 Radiolucency associated with nasal adenocarcinoma.

unerupted tooth that is impacted by another tooth, cannot erupt without extraction of the tooth causing impaction and still may not erupt by extracting the impacting tooth.

Exodontics

Dental radiographs are indicated before extractions for diagnosis and evaluation of possible complications. Dental radiographs are obtained during the procedure to determine the presence of retained roots and other complications. Radiographs are indicated after extraction to ensure completeness of the procedure. Fig. 11.34A and B demonstrate a preextraction and postextraction radiograph.

RADIOGRAPHIC TRAINING

When it comes to actual application, a live patient is not the place to practice taking radiographs. Skulls or cadavers should be used to perfect the technique. The advantage of using a skull is that it is cleaner and can be used forever. It also allows better visualization of the bones and aids in understanding how to position for films. A disadvantage is that the temporomandibular joints are not connected by tissue and unless other materials are used, they become disarticulated. Additionally, it is not realistic that the trainee does not need to contend with cheeks and the tongue. This is where the use of cadavers is advantageous. However, cadavers are messy, have a finite lifespan, and can be displeasing to some trainees. Utilization of both is most beneficial.

CONE BEAM COMPUTED TOMOGRAPHY

Cone beam computed tomography (CBCT) is becoming widely used in veterinary dentistry. CBCT uses repeated X-ray exposure with an X-ray generator on one side of a rotating apparatus and a detector on the opposite to construct a three-dimensional view of the subject. Some of these machines can be rolled to the operatory table (Fig. 11.35).

Once the data is collected from the scan, the software can use the axial slices to reconstruct the sagittal and coronal slices. The result is three coordinated views showing the same point of interest known as *multiplanar reconstruction* (MPR).

The data can be reconstructed into a tridimensional image. This image can be manipulated in three dimensions, allowing rotation and sectioning. Three-dimensional images may aid in the reconstruction of maxillofacial trauma, treatment planning for resective surgeries, and evaluation of

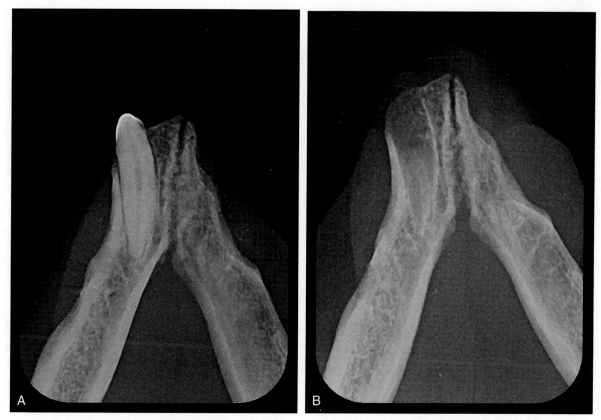

Fig. 11.34 (A) Preextraction radiograph of the right mandibular canine tooth of a cat. (B) Postextraction radiographs are necessary to demonstrate complete extraction of tooth without evidence of iatrogenic trauma.

the TMJs. There are limitations, and these images should not be used solely but as a supplement to the MPR.

The data can also be exported into special software connected to three-dimensional printers to create study models and surgical guides (Fig. 11.36). As technology allows, some medical devices may be created as well.

Panoramic studies can also be created. These can be used as a survey study of the premolars and molars and are like radiographs, and hence more "familiar" to the practitioner who is familiar with radiographs. As this software is more suited to image human mouths, there can be distortion of the canine teeth and incisors.

The time to acquire a full-mouth study is less for CBCT compared to dental radiographs. Overall, the information obtained from CBCT is superior to that obtained from dental radiographs. The ability to see the subject in three dimensions improves the assessment of periodontal bone loss. For example, loss of interradicular bone of the mesial roots of the maxillary fourth premolar is more apparent (Fig. 11.37), and vertical bone defects can be truly visualized if one is considering guided tissue regeneration. Oronasal fistulas associated with intact maxillary teeth are apparent (Fig. 11.38). Endodontic disease is much more apparent as periapical changes are obvious (Fig. 11.39), root fractures are simpler to detect, and necrotic pulp may

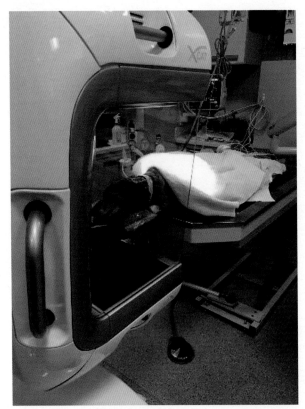

Fig. 11.35 An anesthetized patient in a position such that the head is in the Cone beam computed tomography unit. (Courtesy Dental Focus.)

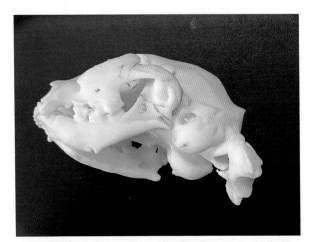

Fig. 11.36 Study model for preplanning of surgical procedure. The images were obtained with Cone beam computed tomography and printed with a 3D printer.

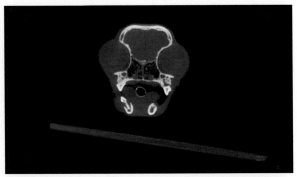

Fig. 11.37 Interradicular bone loss of the mesial roots of the left maxillary fourth premolar.

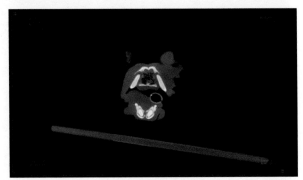

Fig. 11.38 Loss of alveolar bone palatal to the maxillary canine teeth leading to oronasal fistula.

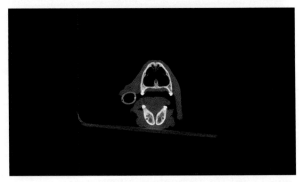

Fig. 11.39 Large periapical lucency of left mandibular canine tooth.

be obvious due to gas production within the root canal (Fig. 11.40).

Surgical planning of extractions is improved as the practitioner can visualize the relationship between teeth and adjacent structures such as the nasal sinus and mandibular canal (Fig. 11.41).

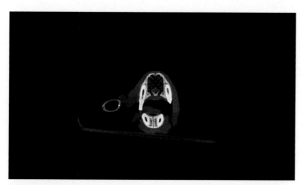

Fig. 11.40 Air attenuation of the right maxillary and both mandibular canine tooth root canals indicating gas presence.

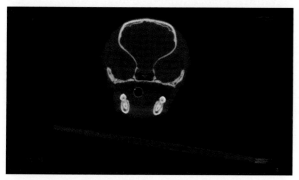

Fig. 11.41 The mandibular canal is located buccal to the mandibular first molar roots in this patient. This is valuable knowledge if these teeth were to be extracted.

Cone beam computed tomography is a considerably more expensive investment compared to dental radiography. Additionally, it does not eliminate the need for dental radiographs as radiographs are still necessary for intraoperative and postoperative images. The physical footprint of the equipment is a consideration as well. The patient will either need to be brought to the machine or there will be ample room needed for the machine to be placed at the head of the operatory table.

Cone beam computed tomography provides superior images of mineralized tissue compared to conventional CT but does not equal it in soft tissue imaging. Some manufacturers have units available that are superior for soft tissue as compared to other CBCT units. However, in the case of oral tumors and other soft tissue lesions, multidetector CT is still recommended.

Not all CBCT units are large enough to image the full head of larger canine patients. In these cases, two scans are necessary to image the TMJs and caudal portion of the skull. Some software does allow "stitching" of the studies to make a complete study.

As these machines produce more radiation than radiographs, additional safety measures may be required. The practice should consult both the manufacturer and state physicist regarding what safety measures are necessary for their unit.

The learning curve for interpreting CBCT images is substantial compared to dental radiographs. The same principles of interpretation of radiographs apply to CBCT images (albeit the terminology is slightly different) with the added challenge of understanding the three-dimensional picture and recognizing the associated anatomic structures. It is not that these structures are not present in radiographs, but they are more obvious with CBCT. This should be considered an advantage over dental radiographs.

The veterinarian is encouraged to review the normal anatomy of the head as well as normal CT findings. Making full-mouth dental radiographs of the patient to compare with CT findings is useful early in training. This gives the veterinarian a familiar comparison.

CHAPTER 11 WORKSHEET (ANSWERS ARE ON PAGE 296)

1. Personnel should be protected by use of _____, _____, and/or safe _____.
2. The minimum safe distance for safety is _____ feet positioned _____ degrees from the primary beam.
3. The only contraindication to performing dental radiographs is _____.
4. At least _____ millimeters of tissue away from the apex should be included in the radiograph.

5. The parallel technique is indicated for radiographs to evaluate _____ in the dog.
6. The _____ is used when parallel projections cannot be made.
7. If the radiographic machine is aimed more at the sensor/plate, the X-rays may miss the tooth. A distorted tooth by _____ is the complication with this approach.
8. The canine teeth are best evaluated by placing the X-ray generator head _____ degrees from the front of the patient and _____ degrees from the side of the patient.
9. CBCT is superior to standard CT when imaging _____.
10. _____ is a digital technology that uses a phosphor line polyester plate that has to be scanned.

FURTHER READING

Verstraete FJ, Kass PH, Terpak CH. Diagnostic value of full-mouth radiography in dogs. *Am J Vet Res.* 1998;59(6):686–691.

Verstraete FJ, Kass PH, Terpak CH. Diagnostic value of full-mouth radiography in cats. *Am J Vet Res.* 1998;59(6):692–695.

Exodontics (Extractions)

LEARNING OBJECTIVES

When you have completed this chapter, you will be able to:

- Define exodontic and describe indications for this type of treatment.
- Discuss legal concerns related to performance of tooth extractions by veterinary technicians.
- List the instruments used for performing dental extractions and describe the function of each.

- Describe the procedure for removal of a single-rooted tooth.
- Describe the procedure for removal of a multirooted tooth.
- List and describe potential complications to tooth extraction.

KEY TERMS

Closed extraction

Open extraction

Short finger stop technique

Vertical releasing incision

Although the objective of veterinary dentistry is to save teeth, extraction often becomes necessary. Exodontics is the branch of dentistry that involves tooth extraction. This chapter's intent is to familiarize the reader with indications, equipment, and techniques for exodontics. It is not a substitute for proper hands-on training given by experts to those legally authorized to do so.

INDICATIONS FOR EXODONTICS

Exodontics is indicated when the tooth cannot be salvaged or the client is unable or unwilling to perform home care.

The client should be consulted for authorization before any teeth are extracted. This allows for informed consent, making the client aware of potential complications and possible alternatives to extractions. Informed consent also prevents financial surprises and may lessen the emotional impact. Tooth extraction is a surgical procedure with potential for severe complications if performed poorly.

THE TECHNICIAN AND EXTRACTIONS

Regarding tooth extraction, laws vary from state to state. In all states, if extraction by someone other than a veterinarian is permitted, the extraction must be performed under a veterinarian's supervision. Some state regulations are contradictory. For example, in some states, registered veterinary technicians are permitted to perform extractions. However, the law forbids registered veterinary technicians from performing surgery. All extractions are surgery in the purest definition of the word. This presents a conflict for the technician. Further, there may be insurance issues concerning whether the veterinarian can allow unauthorized individuals to perform procedures for which they are not authorized by law or regulation.

The American Veterinary Dental College (AVDC), which represents board-certified veterinary dental specialists throughout the world, has evaluated the duties of veterinarians, registered veterinary technicians, and unlicensed individuals in practice. As a result, the AVDC developed a position statement stipulating that only veterinarians should provide extraction services. As per the position statement, "The AVDC considers the extraction of teeth to be included in the practice of veterinary dentistry. Decision making is the responsibility of the supervising veterinarian, with the consent of the pet owner, when electing to extract teeth. Only veterinarians shall determine as to which teeth are to be extracted and perform extraction procedures." Roles of veterinary professionals and dental procedures are listed in Box 12.1.

EXODONTIC PRINCIPLES

As with any surgical procedure, all extractions should be performed in a way that trauma to the patient is minimalized. Teeth are extracted by cutting, stretching, and tearing the periodontal ligament fibers and by slightly deforming the alveolus or tooth socket. The tooth should be eased out of the socket rather than forced. The complete root should be removed, except in the rare instance when more root retrieval would cause more damage. Portions of the root that have been replaced by bone do not need to be extracted. Neither of these exceptions should be considered lightly. With any extraction procedure, dental radiographs help ensure that all the root tissue has been removed. Finally, with few exceptions, the soft tissue is opposed to allow for more rapid healing.

Exodontic Technique

A methodical approach in the exodontic technique is important. Practitioners must always remember that the object is to remove the tooth with as little trauma as possible. Some basic principles apply to every extraction and certain extractions require additional steps. As with all surgical techniques, variations exist and are often operator dependent. However, it is the responsibility of the operator to understand which variations in technique are appropriate.

After proper diagnostics, the first step in every tooth extraction is to sever the gingival attachment from the tooth. This is initiated via a sulcular incision with a scalpel (Fig. 12.1), followed by the use of a periosteal elevator.

Closed Extraction Versus Open Extraction

After the gingival attachment is severed from the tooth, the process of tooth luxation and elevation commences when performing *closed extractions*, or extractions performed without utilizing a mucoperiosteal flap. The closed extraction technique is appropriate for small, single rooted teeth. In the dog this typically includes the incisors, first premolars, and mandibular third molar; in the cat, this typically includes the incisors and maxillary second premolar. The cat's maxillary first molar may be treated as a single-rooted tooth even though it has more than one root.

Larger teeth such as the canine teeth and multi-rooted teeth are typically extracted using the open extraction technique. An *open extraction* involves the development of a mucoperiosteal flap that aids single-rooted teeth in tooth sectioning, alveolar bone removal, and primary wound closure. The flap designs typically used for open tooth extraction are envelope flaps without a vertical releasing incision, three-cornered flaps with a single (typically mesial) vertical releasing incision and four-cornered flaps with both a mesial and distal vertical releasing incision. A *vertical releasing incision* is an incision in a coronal/apical direction at one or both buccal line angles of the tooth. It typically extends into the mucosa (Fig. 12.2).

The next step when performing open extractions is to remove buccal cortical bone if necessary (Fig. 12.3). This is accomplished using a water-cooled, highspeed bur, most commonly round or pear-shaped burs. The size of bur depends on the size of the patient and operator preference. The operator should remove adequate bone to allow for extraction without causing root fracture or undue force on the jaws while attempting to conserve bone. There is no standard rule as to how much bone should be removed. This varies based on the patient,

BOX 12.1   Roles of Veterinary Professionals and Dental Procedures

Veterinary Dental Healthcare Providers

The AVDC has developed this position statement as a means to safeguard the veterinary dental patient and to ensure the qualifications of persons performing veterinary dental procedures.

Primary Responsibility for Veterinary Dental Care

The AVDC defines veterinary dentistry as the art and practice of oral health care in animals other than humans. It is a discipline of veterinary medicine and surgery. The diagnosis, treatment, and management of veterinary oral health care are to be provided and supervised by licensed veterinarians or by veterinarians working within a university or industry.

Who May Provide Veterinarian-Supervised Dental Care?

The AVDC accepts that the following healthcare workers may assist the supervising veterinarian in dental procedures or perform professional dental cleanings (cleaning the surfaces of the teeth with an ultrasonic scaler and/ or hand tools and polishing the teeth with pumice or fluoride paste while the patient is under anesthesia) while under direct supervision by a veterinarian if permitted by local law: licensed, certified, or registered veterinary technician or a veterinary assistant with advanced dental training, a human dentist, or registered dental hygienist.

Operative Dentistry and Oral Surgery

The AVDC considers operative dentistry to be any dental procedure that invades the hard or soft oral tissue including, but not limited to, a procedure that alters the structure of one or more teeth or repairs damaged and diseased teeth. Only a veterinarian should perform operative dentistry and oral surgery.

Extraction of Teeth

The AVDC considers the extraction of teeth to be included in the practice of veterinary dentistry. Decision making is the responsibility of the supervising veterinarian, with the consent of the pet owner, when electing to extract teeth. Only veterinarians shall determine which teeth are to be extracted and perform extraction procedures.

Dental Tasks Performed by Veterinary Technicians

The AVDC considers it appropriate for a veterinarian to delegate maintenance dental care and certain dental tasks to a veterinary technician. Tasks appropriately performed by a technician include professional dental cleanings and certain procedures that do not result in altering the shape, structure, or positional location of teeth in the dental arch. The veterinarian may direct an appropriately trained veterinary technician to perform these tasks providing that the veterinarian is physically present and supervising the treatment.

Veterinary Technician Dental Training

The AVDC supports the advanced training of veterinary technicians to perform additional ancillary dental services: taking impressions, making models, charting veterinary dental pathology, taking, and developing dental radiographs, and performing nonsurgical subgingival root scaling and periodontal debridement, provided that they do not alter the structure of the tooth.

Further the AVDC does not support Diplomates training nonlicensed veterinarians, veterinary assistants, or veterinary technicians to perform oral surgery, including surgical extraction techniques.

Tasks That May Be Performed by Veterinary Assistants (Not Registered, Certified, or Licensed)

The AVDC supports the appropriate training of veterinary assistants to perform the following dental services: supragingival scaling and polishing, taking and developing dental radiographs, directly assisting the veterinarian in oral surgical and dental procedures, and making impressions and models.

Tasks That May Be Performed by Human Dentists, Registered Dental Hygienists, and Other Dental Healthcare Providers

The AVDC recognizes that human dentists, registered dental hygienists, and other dental healthcare providers in good standing may perform those procedures for which they have been qualified under the direct supervision of the veterinarian. The supervising veterinarian will be responsible for the welfare of the veterinary patient and any treatment performed on the patient.

The AVDC understands that individual states have regulations that govern the practice of veterinary medicine. This position statement is intended to be a model for veterinary dental practice and does not replace the existing law.

Adopted by the Board of Directors April 1998, revised October 1999, revised September 2006, revised 2022.

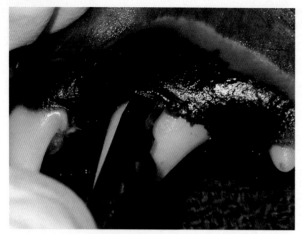

Fig. 12.1 Sulcular incision in preparation for extraction of the left maxillary canine tooth of a dog.

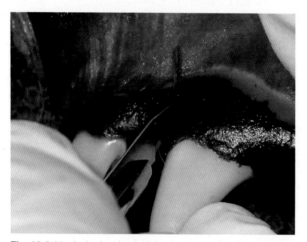

Fig. 12.2 Vertical releasing incision in preparation for extraction of left maxillary canine tooth in a dog.

tooth extracted, and operator. There are guidelines that should be followed. These include removing only alveolar bone and not removing structure bone, avoiding soft tissue with the bur, and not compromising the integrity of the mandible.

Tooth Sectioning

Multi-rooted teeth are typically sectioned into individual root components before extraction with few exceptions. Separating a tooth into individual roots decreases the risk of root and bone fracture and reduces surgical time. It may be tempting to attempt to extract a multi-rooted tooth that is mobile before sectioning. This increases the risk of root fracture.

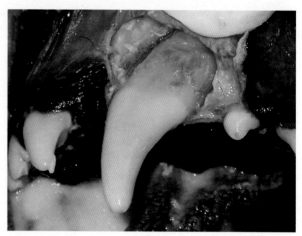

Fig. 12.3 Buccal cortical bone removal in preparation for extraction of left maxillary canine tooth.

Teeth are typically sectioned using a side cutting bur such as a 700 or 550 series carbide bur. These burs cut on the side. Keep in mind, it will take longer to cut through larger teeth. Trying to force the bur through the tooth can cause the bur to stall, in turn causing damage to the handpiece and possible thermal trauma to the patient. Instead, the bur is pressed against the tooth in a pulsatile fashion using 2 seconds of pressure against the tooth with a second of no pressure until the bur completely separates the tooth.

When possible, sectioning should start at the furcation of the tooth and progress coronally (Fig. 12.4). If this is not possible due to the furcation not being visible, the location of the furcation is estimated via imaging and anatomic landmarks.

Root Extraction

Roots are mobilized for extraction via severing the periodontal ligament, deforming the alveolus, and pushing the tooth from the alveolus using several techniques and instruments.

Short Finger Stop Technique

When dental luxators and elevators are being pushed toward the root apex, the *short finger stop technique* should be used. This is accomplished by keeping the end of the index finger near the cutting end of the instrument (Fig. 12.5). If the instrument were to slip, the index finger acts as a break or stop to prevent the instrument from penetrating further than desired and reducing the risk of injury to the patient.

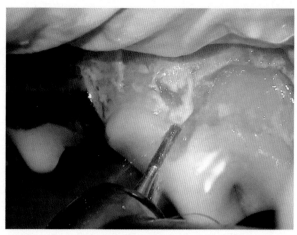

Fig. 12.4 Sectioning of left maxillary fourth premolar with a 557 bur. Note that the sectioning begins at the furcation.

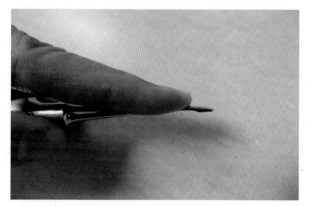

Fig. 12.5 The short finger stop technique is recommended to reduce the risk of iatrogenic trauma.

General Movements

Luxator and luxating periotome use. Luxators and luxating periotomes are used to severe the periodontal ligament by pushing the instrument between the alveolar bone and tooth in an apical direction. Not only does this cut the periodontal ligament, but it also acts as a wedge that expands the alveolus, allowing for easier extraction. A twisting motion or turning along the instrument's access should be avoided, as this may break the instrument.

Elevator use. Dental elevators can be used as a luxator when kept sharp. However, these instruments are typically thicker and difficult to wedge into the small space between the tooth and the bone. Thus, the use of elevators is typically limited to vertical rotation and horizontal rotation. Other elevator movements are beyond the scope of this book and are more appropriately covered in oral surgery textbooks.

Vertical rotation. In vertical rotation, the elevator is used parallel to the root (Fig. 12.6). An elevator, whose curve approximates that of the tooth, is inserted into the space between the tooth and the alveolus. The instrument is rotated along its axis using slow, steady pressure. The pressure is maintained for 5 to 15 seconds. This will break down the periodontal ligament and further deform the alveolus. Initially, the direction of the force is toward the window of bone removal if performed.

Horizontal rotation. Horizontal rotation, also known as the wheel and axle principle, utilizes a fulcrum (bone or adjacent toot/tooth root) to deliver force on a root in a coronal direction. With this technique, the elevator is placed perpendicular to the crown and tooth root with the working face (concave side) of the elevator facing the portion of the tooth to be extracted. The nonworking face (convex side) is rested against the alveolar bone or an adjacent tooth root. The elevator is rotated to push the target root in a coronal direction. Care should be taken not to luxate the tooth that is acting as a fulcrum or damage the bone used as a fulcrum (Fig. 12.7).

The practitioner should work all the way around the tooth and remember to be patient.

Tooth delivery. In some cases, the tooth will "fall out" after elevation. In most cases, extraction forceps are required to deliver the tooth from the alveolus. The beak of the instrument is placed past the crown of the tooth to engage the root (Fig. 12.8). While avoiding crushing the tooth with the forceps, the tooth is pulled in a coronal direction while using gentle rotational forces. Bending

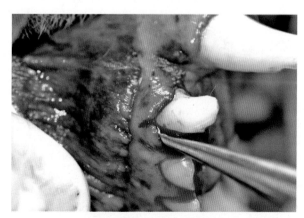

Fig. 12.6 Vertical rotation.

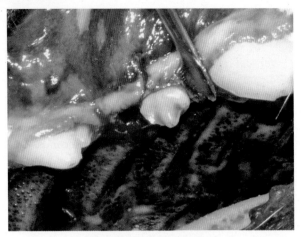

Fig. 12.7 Horizontal rotation.

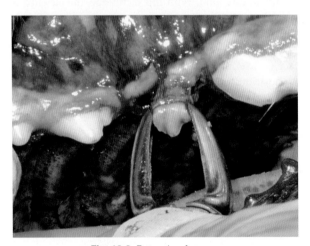

Fig. 12.8 Extraction forceps.

in the direction of root curvature may help deliver the tooth from the alveolus. Bending of the tooth in other directions or bending forces against a straight root is avoided as this can fracture the root. A dental radiograph is made to confirm and document the entire tooth has been extracted.

Preparation for closure. Any rough or sharp bone is smoothed (typically with a diamond bur). The mucosa at the edges of the alveolus (and any region to be sutured) is elevated from the bone approximately 3 mm to allow the suture needle to pass through the mucosa at a right angle. Larger mucoperiosteal flaps have a mucoperiosteal release performed, incising the periosteum while keeping the mucosa intact. The alveolus is irrigated with sterile saline.

Suturing. Finally, the gingiva is sutured using 3-0, 4-0, or 5-0 synthetic suture material. Monocryl is recommended because it dissolves or becomes untied and falls out in several weeks. A variety of suture patterns may be employed. The most used is the simple interrupted (Fig. 12.9A). It has the advantage of multiple knots so that if one fails the entire suture line does not fail. Cross-pattern mattress sutures have the advantage of speed (Fig. 12.9B), but the disadvantage is the larger suture mass as compared to a continuous interlocking pattern. A continuous interlocking pattern has the advantage of the speed and less suture mass in the extraction sites (Fig. 12.9C). Also, there may be less irritation to the patient from multiple knots. The disadvantage is that if one knot fails, the entire suture line can dehisce.

EXTRACTION OF SPECIFIC TEETH

Maxillary Fourth Premolar

The maxillary fourth premolar should be separated between the furcation and the crown of each of the three roots. The first cut is made between the cusps over the two mesial roots and distal root. This allows mobilization of the distal root, using a horizontal technique with the mesial roots acting as the fulcrum. Next, the second cut is made to separate the mesiobuccal and mesiopalatal roots (Fig. 12.10). After the mesiobuccal root is extracted, the interradicular bone between the two mesial roots is removed and the mesiopalatal root can be elevated and extracted (Fig. 12.11), followed by the distal root. The distal root is reserved as the last extraction as it can serve as a fulcrum to extract the two mesial roots.

Maxillary First and Second Molars

In dogs, a T-shaped cut can be made on the maxillary first and second molars. This T should first split off the mesial and distal roots from the palatine root and then separate the mesial and distal roots. Once the crown has been split, each individual root is treated as a separate tooth and extracted. It should be noted that the distobuccal root and palatal root of the second molar are sometimes fused in dogs. This is not always apparent on radiographs but may be apparent on computed tomographay (CT).

COMPLICATIONS OF EXTRACTIONS

The most common complications of extractions are dehiscence of the surgical site and retained roots.

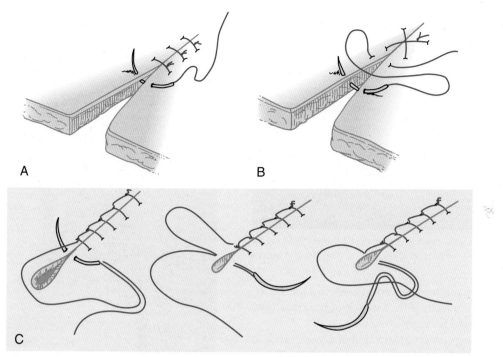

Fig. 12.9 Suture patterns. (A) Simple interrupted. (B) Cruciate pattern mattress. (C) Continuous interlock. (From Fossum TW. *Small Animal Surgery*. 3rd ed. St. Louis, MO: Mosby; 2007).

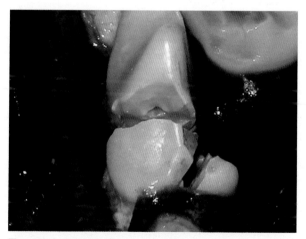

Fig. 12.10 Sectioning cuts needed to extract left maxillary fourth premolar.

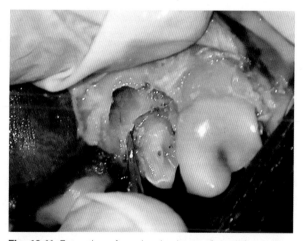

Fig. 12.11 Extraction of mesiopalatal root of the left maxillary fourth premolar with mesiobuccal root removed and interradicular bone removal.

Surgical dehiscence is often preventable with careful design of mucoperiosteal flaps, meticulous suturing, and assuring there is no tension on the sutures. Dehiscence can delay healing and lead to the formation of an oronasal fistula.

Fractured and retained roots are often the result of impatience during extraction and the use of improper instruments. If instruments are sharp, the technique is sound, and the operator is careful, retained roots can be avoided. If left in the alveolus, continued inflammation and pain can occur.

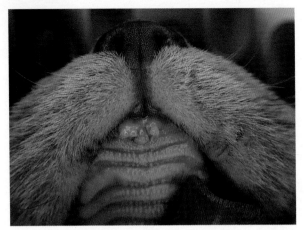

Fig. 12.12 Occlusal trauma of superior lip from mandibular canine teeth after extraction of maxillary canine teeth in a cat.

Other complications of extractions include occlusal trauma from teeth at the location of the extraction, hemorrhage, and iatrogenic trauma.

Most common to cats, extraction of a tooth can lead to traumatic occlusion from the opposing teeth. This is most seen after extraction of the maxillary canine teeth (Fig. 12.12) but can occur with premolar and molar extractions as well (Fig. 12.13).

During extraction, mild to moderate hemorrhage can occur from incision of minor vessels and bone removal. It can also occur as a complication due to inadvertent damage to larger vessels such as the mandibular, middle mental, and infraorbital vessels.

The first step in controlling hemorrhage is to apply pressure with a gauze sponge. When applying pressure, the gauze sponge should be rolled onto the wound. After 1 to 2 minutes of pressure, the gauze sponge should be carefully rolled off. This rolling action is continued until the bleeding stops. If a hemostat is necessary to control hemorrhage, it is applied, then pressure with a gauze sponge should be rolled or applied onto the wound and hemorrhage checked in a similar fashion.

Products such as HemaBlock, Gelfoam, Vetigel, and Vetspon can be used to control hemorrhage. These can be a source of inflammation and infection if left in the alveolus or other cavities.

If an elevator or luxator slips while being improperly held, the working end may be pushed into a nearby structure such as the eye or a sinus (Fig. 12.14). This is prevented with the short finger stop grip. When extracting fractured roots of premolars and molars, if apical pressure is placed ON the root and not ALONG the root,

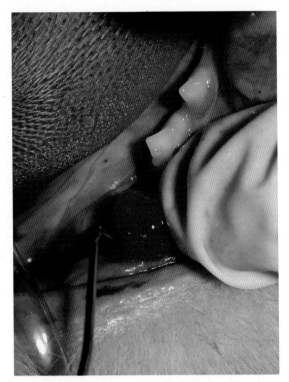

Fig. 12.13 Occlusal trauma of right mandible of a cat from maxillary fourth premolar tooth.

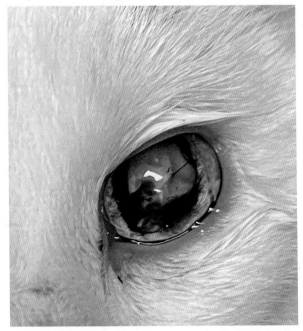

Fig. 12.14 Cataract caused by penetration of dental elevator into the eye.

the root may be inadvertently pushed into an adjacent structure such as the nasal sinus or mandibular canal. Retrieval of these roots can be difficult and risky. If any doubt exists as to if it can be removed safely, referral to a board-certified dentist is recommended.

With excessive force during elevation, iatrogenic fractures of the mandible occur. This often necessitates referral for fracture repair. In most cases, this is avoidable with proper technique. In some cases, the risk is high (Fig. 12.15) Table 12.1.

CONCLUSION

Extractions are a complex surgical procedure and if not performed well, there are several serious sequelae. Extractions should only be performed by licensed veterinarians with ample training and using the right equipment.

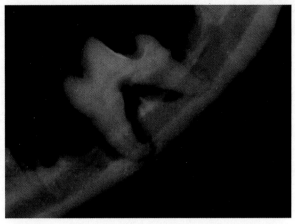

Fig. 12.15 Even in experienced hands, some extractions are associated with a high risk of mandibular fracture.

TABLE 12.1 Potential Complications of Tooth Extraction	Location	Consequence
Retained Roots	Any extraction	Ongoing inflammation, pain, and infection
Dehiscence of Mucoperiosteal Flap	Any extraction	• Delayed healing • Oronasal fistula (maxilary teeth)
Oronasal Fistula	Any maxillary extraction, more likely with extraction of canine teeth and premolars	Rhinitis
Jaw Fracture	Any extraction, more likely with extraction of mandibular canine teeth or first molars	• Pain • Dysphagia • Malocclusion
Occlusal Trauma	Extraction of maxillary canine teeth or mandibular first molar in cat	• Lip entrapment • Pyogenic granuloma
Root Displacement or Transportation Into Neighboring Structures	• Mandibular premolars or molars into mandibular canal • Maxillary premolars into nasal sinus	Inflammation of associated structure

CHAPTER 12 WORKSHEET (ANSWERS ARE ON PAGE 296)

1. Exodontics may be indicated if the tooth is judged nonsalvageable or if the client is unable or unwilling to perform _____.
2. The client should be consulted for _____ before any teeth are extracted.
3. As extractions are a surgical procedure, only _____ should perform extractions.
4. _____ are used to grasp the tooth and remove it from the socket.
5. Sectioning _____ teeth before extracting them is almost always the easiest method.

6. A _____ -shaped cut can be made on the maxillary first molar.
7. An _____ extraction involves the development of a mucoperiosteal flap and alveolar bone removal.
8. Using the _____ helps reduce the risk of slipping and injury to the patient.
9. _____ fracture of the mandible can occur when excessive force is used during extraction.
10. Hemostatic sponges may cause _____.

Advanced Veterinary Dental and Oral Surgery Procedures: Periodontal Surgery, Endodontics, Restorations, Orthodontics, and Maxillofacial Surgery

CHAPTER OUTLINE

LEARNING OBJECTIVES

When you have completed this chapter, you will be able to:

- Describe indications for periodontal surgery.
- Discuss indications, contraindications, and general procedure for performing gingivoplasty.

- Define oronasal fistula and list three techniques used to repair this condition.
- Define endodontics and describe equipment and supplies needed to perform these procedures.

- List and describe commonly performed endodontic procedures.
- Describe the general procedure for performing conventional, nonsurgical root canal therapy.

- List and describe restorative materials used in veterinary dentistry.

KEY TERMS

Absorbent points
Apicoectomy
Barbed broach
Bone augmentation
Dental composites
Dentinal bridge
Direct pulp capping
Endodontic therapy

File separation
Guided tissue regeneration
Gingivectomy
Gingivoplasty
Gutta-percha
Indirect pulp capping
Intrinsic staining
Plugger

Resective osseous surgery
Restorative dentistry
Root canal sealant
Sodium hypochlorite
Spreader
Surgical root canal therapy
Vital pulpotomy
Working length

The availability of more advanced dental procedures has increased over the past decade. Although not all practices have the resources to perform advanced procedures, the veterinary staff should have an idea of the range of procedures that can be performed to save teeth, what each procedure entails, and the type of equipment necessary. Some practices may perform many advanced dental procedures, and this chapter briefly addresses the most common ones. It is imperative that the operator be well trained before taking these cases on.

PERIODONTAL SURGICAL TECHNIQUES

Periodontal surgical techniques are employed after more conservative measures, such as closed periodontal debridement, have been attempted without success or when conservative means are not expected to succeed. This would include treatment of periodontal pockets that are greater than 5 mm in depth when new bone regeneration is desired or when trying to regain gingiva in areas of recession. In periodontal surgery, mucogingival flaps

are created to expose the tooth root and associated bone. The bone may be reshaped or augmented, and the gingiva may be sutured back to the initial position. Alternatively, the gingival height may be changed apically by gingival or bone surgery to decrease the pocket or coronally with guided tissue regeneration to increase the height of attachment. Finally, periodontal surgery may include gingival grafts to replace lost gingiva.

Evaluation for Procedure

Appropriate case selection is crucial, meaning the appropriate form of therapy should be chosen for the pathology, patient, and client. A combination of examination with a dental probe, evaluation of dental imaging, and assessment of the adjacent teeth is important to decide which treatments are possible. Just as important, the patient's health status, willingness to accept homecare, and the owner's ability to provide homecare and follow-up must be taken into consideration if the therapy is to be successful.

Goal of Periodontal Surgery

The goal of periodontal surgery is to eliminate pockets harboring subgingival plaque and calculus

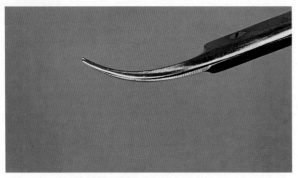

Fig. 13.1 LaGrange scissors with a serrated edge. The serrations help grip tissue while cutting.

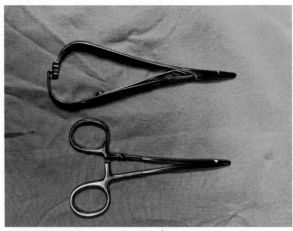

Fig. 13.2 Mathieu (*top*) needle drivers and Deaf (*bottom*) needle drivers are smaller and allow access to oral tissues. Mathieu needle drivers may allow more fine movement as there are no finger rings.

and to maintain adequate periodontal tissues to preserve periodontal health. The aim is to prevent subgingival plaque and calculus from returning and in turn reduce periodontal inflammation.

Instruments and Materials

Periodontal surgery requires various instruments and materials. Specific instrumentation is often operator preference, but the ultimate function of the instruments is the same across all operators. The following is for reference. The No. 3 handle is the standard type for scalpels. The No. 15c blade is extremely fine and therefore useful in periodontal surgical procedures. Some practitioners will utilize No. 12 blades and beaver tail blades at times. In addition, small tissue scissors, such as LaGrange scissors (Fig. 13.1), are helpful in trimming periodontal tissue. Often scissors are available with one serrated edge that can help grip small tissue tags during cutting.

Periosteal elevators are used to lift the gingiva away from the bone. Several types are available. The Molt elevator is one type; the Molt No. 9 is particularly popular. Many practitioners also like the ST-No. 7 instrument. Having a variety of periodontal surgical instruments available makes treating various anatomic and pathologic conditions less difficult.

Tissue forceps and needle holders are necessary for suturing. Needle holders should be small and should provide good tactile feedback. Derf,

Mathieu, or Castroviejo needle holders are smaller needle holders that are all utilized in oral surgery (Fig. 13.2).

Materials used in periodontal surgery include various irrigation and cleansing solutions, materials for creating new bone, local antibiotics, and sutures.

Chlorhexidine is used in a 0.1% to 0.2% solution and is available in two forms: diacetate and gluconate. Gluconate is preferred. The practice of using only premade chlorhexidine oral rinses is encouraged as errors in mixing have been shown to cause severe oral trauma. Chlorhexidine solutions are good for the initial disinfection of oral soft tissues before initiating surgical therapy. It can also inhibit the regeneration of new periodontal tissue and may not be appropriate for guided tissue regeneration. Sterile isotonic saline can be used freely to irrigate exposed connective tissue without the worry of iatrogenic trauma.

There are several materials available to the veterinary market for creating new periodontal bone. These include synthetic materials, natural nonbone materials, and natural bone. Each of these has benefits and concerns and the choice of which to use should be seriously considered based on study and not anecdotal recommendations. The astute practitioner may note that some products used on humans have initial studies performed on dogs. Although not labeled for use in dogs and cats, they may provide an alternative to the veterinary products.

When attempting to regain lost periodontal bone, a barrier is often recommended to prevent healing epithelium from displacing the bone graft and preventing new bone formation. Both synthetic and natural products are available. Some of these barriers, such as polytetrafluoroethylene (Teflon) are nonabsorbable and need to be surgically removed after the new bone has formed. Some are absorbable. Doxirobe gel has been proposed as a potential absorbable membrane based on the successful use of a similar carrier and the publication of a case series.

As with all oral surgery, poliglecaprone-type sutures are typically preferred. In the case of periodontal surgery, 5-0 or 4-0 is an appropriate size. The needle size is operator and situation present. Larger radius needles are often useful when treating lesions in the rostral oral cavity of medium-sized or larger dogs. With small dogs, cats, or situations that present less room for movement of the needle drivers, a smaller radius needle may be preferred.

Treatment Techniques
Gingival Hyperplasia
Gingivectomy is the removal of gingival tissue. *Gingivoplasty* is the reshaping of gingiva to its native shape. These therapies are typically used together to treat gingival hyperplasia. Gingivectomy should not be used for the treatment of deep periodontal pockets or as part of the routine prophy. This procedure is contraindicated when the attached gingiva is minimal or absent or bone loss is present apical to the mucogingival junction.

When hyperplastic gingiva is present, it can create a *pseudopocket* or an increased probing depth, not due to apical migration of the sulcus but due to the growth of the gingiva in a coronal direction. Pseudopockets may collect plaque, calculus,

and other debris, which can lead to periodontal abscesses and periodontitis.

Gingivectomy/gingivoplasty technique. The purpose of gingivectomy and gingivoplasty is to remove the pseudopocket and to reestablish normal periodontal anatomy and gingival shape. The pocket depth and contour are determined by inserting a probe into the depth of the pocket at several areas around the tooth. The corresponding depth is measured on the outside of the gingiva, also with the probe. A bleeding point is made by placing the tip of the probe perpendicular to the gingiva and applying slight pressure to make a small hole or by using a small-gauge needle. Bleeding points are made around the contour of the pocket and are used as a guide for the gingivectomy. Alternatively, a pocket marking probe can be used to create bleeding points. The gingivectomy incision is made at an angle apical to the bleeding point to create a beveled margin. At least 2 mm of healthy, attached gingiva must be present apical to the base of the incision. A diamond bur, multi-fluted bur, laser, scalpel blade, or electrosurgery blade is used to excise the gingiva by cutting below the bleeding points, with the instrument held at approximately a 45-degree angle and the tip of the blade toward the crown. The ends of the excision should be tapered into the surrounding gingiva to create the normal scalloped contour, particularly if several adjacent teeth are treated. Small gingival tags can be removed with the blade or a sharp curette. The exposed tooth and root surface can now be scaled and planed smoothly. Hemorrhage is controlled by applying pressure with wet gauze pads or hemostatic agents. If electrosurgery is being performed, caution must be exercised because the collateral damage may extend past the desired surgical line. This may result in damage to the periodontal bone or tooth and ultimately require extraction of the tooth and removal of nonvital bone. In Fig. 13.3, a periodontal probe is used to measure and mark the pocket depth. Once marked, a scalpel blade is used to perform the gingivoplasty.

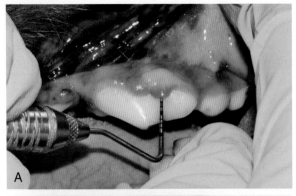

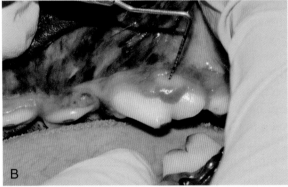

Fig. 13.3 (A) Periodontal probe gingivoplasty measurement. (B) Periodontal gingivoplasty probe marking the pocket depth.

Periodontal Pocket

The treatment of periodontal pockets beyond the range of closed periodontal debridement requires either the extraction of the tooth or the creation of a periodontal flap and then treatment. These pockets include any pocket with a depth greater than 5 mm or any other pocket that cannot be fully visualized. The flap allows visualization of subgingival tissues, calculus, and inflamed tissue. By creating a flap and reflecting the periodontal tissues off the tooth surface, the practitioner can see the tooth surface where periodontal debridement or root planing is being performed.

Open flap and root planing technique. The gingiva is disinfected. An incision should be made that follows the contour of the tooth within the sulcus. Releasing incisions may be created, starting at the line angle of the teeth mesial and distal to

the surgery site. In some cases, the flap can be created with an envelope flap if the anatomy allows, and the flap is to be repositioned into its original position. The gingiva is elevated with a periosteal elevator lingually/palatally and labially/buccally. If root planing alone is to be performed, the alveolar bone need not be exposed. If the underlying alveolar bone needs to be treated or bone grafting performed, the bone must be exposed. The exposed root surfaces are scaled to remove calculus and if disease cementum or imbedded calculus is present, the roots are planed. Before closure, the area is irrigated with saline. The flap is repositioned and sutured with interrupted sutures placed interdentally, and a direct pressure is placed on the tissue to eliminate dead space.

Resective osseous surgery. *Resective osseous surgery* is the removal of bone to eliminate disease and reduce disease recurrence. This is typically performed in cases of infraeruption when the tooth crown is partly buried in periodontal bone or in cases of bony enlargement such as alveolar bone expansion. It is also utilized in some cases of alveolar bone expansion if enough periodontal attachment is present. This is performed with a variety of periodontal chisels such as a Fedi (Fig. 13.4) or Ochsenbein or piezoelectric-powered instruments.

Bone augmentation. *Bone augmentation* is the addition of a bone-grafting material (Table 13.1) to areas of periodontal bone loss in an attempt to regain lost alveolar bone (Fig. 13.5A–C). As mentioned before, typically the periodontal epithelial tissues will migrate into the bone graft, and a barrier must be placed to allow the new bone and periodontal ligament to form before the migration of the epithelial tissues. This process is known as *guided tissue regeneration.*

Oronasal Fistula

An *oronasal fistula* (ONF) is an abnormal opening between the oral and nasal cavities. These can occur secondary to periodontal disease and after the dehiscence of gingiva on the extraction of maxillary incisors, the canine tooth, and premolars.

These may also occur secondary to trauma and other inflammatory diseases.

Several techniques are used for ONF repair. The most common is a simple, apical-based vestibular flap. The margins of the fistula are debrided of necrotic and epithelialized tissue around the entire circumference of the lesion so that one is suturing fresh, bleeding connective tissue to fresh, bleeding connective tissue. Vertical releasing incisions are created mesial

and distal to the defect, creating a flap that is wider than the defect and preferably wider than its length.

The flap is elevated and undermined such that the wound edges can be brought together and sutured in a tension-free manner. The flap is sutured with simple interrupted sutures, typically of 4-0 poliglecaprone. If the simple flap fails or the defect does not allow for this type of closure, other more advanced techniques are available but beyond the scope of this text.

Postoperative care of ONF is very important. Home-care instructions should include soft food for 2 weeks and not handling the mouth for 2 weeks. If possible, medications should be administered voluntarily via a food treat. If there is any chance of pawing, an Elizabethan Collar should be placed to prevent pawing and rubbing. The client should be made aware that some minor nasal bleeding on the operated side may be noted for 24 hours.

Follow-Up Recommendations for All Periodontal Surgery

After the surgery, the patient should be given a soft diet for 7 to 14 days. Oral antibiotics are administered, as appropriate. The oral cavity may be flushed once or twice daily with chlorhexidine rinse for 2 weeks. After the postoperative phase home care must be continued. Daily plaque removal is extremely important for a successful long-term outcome. Postsurgical checkups are important to monitor the patient's progress. A minimum of two follow-up appointments should be scheduled for 10 days and 1 month after the procedure. Additional appointments may be scheduled,

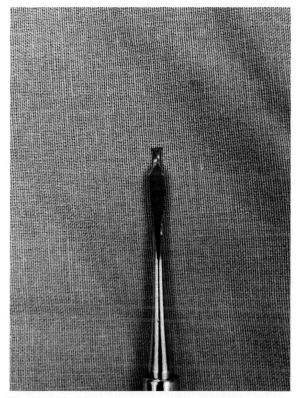

Fig. 13.4 Fedi bone chisel used in resective osseous surgery.

TABLE 13.1 Bone Grafting Materials		
Product	**Type of Graft**	**How Supplied**
Patient Harvested Bone Graft	Autograft	Obtained during surgical procedure
Decalcified Freeze-Dried Bone Graft	Natural xenograft or allograft	Supplied as dry bone particulate
Synthetic	Alloplast	Supplied as particulate or powder
	• Hydroxyapatite	
	• Calcium phosphate	
	• Bioglass	

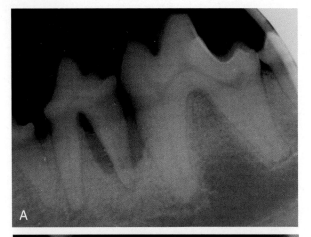

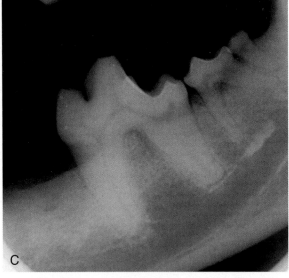

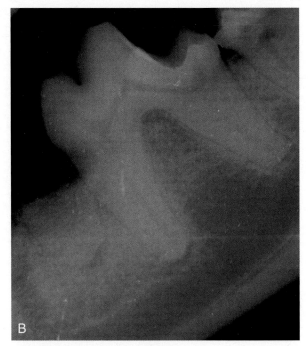

Fig. 13.5 (A) Vertical bone loss associated with teeth 308 and 309. (B) Bone augmentation with artificial bone graft. (C) Same patient in Fig. 5A and B after new bone has formed.

if necessary. Because these patients sometimes experience a relapse due to the disease process or noncompliance, monthly or quarterly follow-up visits may be necessary.

Periodontal probing after surgery should typically be delayed for 3 months, allowing the new gingival attachments to heal. Serial dental imaging is important for these cases.

ENDODONTICS

Fortunately, most veterinarians now recognize the need to treat fractured teeth and other endodontically compromised teeth, and many are aware of the treatment beyond extraction. Endodontic therapy provides a less invasive option for to extraction of these teeth. *Endodontic therapy* is a general term for the treatment of dental pulp that may be used to save living pulp, remove live or dead pulp, and prevent or treat infection. Endodontic therapy includes procedures beyond standard root canal therapy (RCT), and these procedures are summarized in Table 13.2.

Indications for Endodontic Therapy

The rationale for endodontic treatment is to maintain optimal health while salvaging the function of the tooth and avoiding the trauma of extraction.

TABLE 13.2	**Endodontic Procedures**		
Endodontic Procedure	**Description**	**Indication**	**Guidelines for Follow-Up Imaging**
Indirect Pulp Capping (PCI)	Pulp-capping material (Ca[OH]$_2$, MTA) placed on dentinal surface less than 2 mm from pulp	Restorative dental procedures in which pink pulp can be seen through dentin without pulp exposure	6 months then yearly
Direct Pulp Capping	Pulp-capping material (Ca[OH]$_2$, MTA) placed directly on exposed living and healthy pulp	• Fresh fractures in dogs less than 24 months of age • As part of crown reduction for malocclusion • Inadvertent pulp exposure during restorative procedure	Every 6 months until dentinal bridge noted then yearly
RCT	Complete removal of tooth pulp and shaping of root canal followed by obturation of root canal	• Tooth fractures in dogs over 2 years of age • Tooth fracture with nonvital or compromised pulp in dogs with mature tooth apices	6 to 12 months postoperative then yearly
RCT	• Removal of apex of tooth root followed by placement of root-end filling • This procedure follows RCT	• When root apex cannot be accessed during root canal therapy • Root canal failure when retreatment is not feasible • Overfill of obturant during root canal therapy	6 months postoperative then yearly

RCT, Standard root canal therapy.

If a tooth is fractured, bacteria gain entry into the pulp chamber. This is always the case in a complicated crown fracture and can occur with uncomplicated crown fractures. If the pulp becomes infected, it becomes inflamed and edematous and dies. Then the bacteria move into the apical region of the tooth. From this area, the bacteria spread through the canals in the apical delta of the tooth, which formerly served as tunnels for the nerves and blood vessels. Once the bacteria enter the apical bone, inflammation starts. The periapical inflammation often starts as a periapical granuloma and less commonly a periapical abscess or a periapical cyst. In more advanced cases, osteomyelitis and cellulitis can occur. It is not uncommon to find draining sinus tracts associated with periapical inflammation. This is most noted as the suborbital swelling often associated with pulpitis of the maxillary fourth premolar (although other teeth can cause this) and less commonly with mandibular teeth such as the mandibular canine or first molar.

It is important to recognize the signs of a patient with an endodontically compromised tooth. With a recent injury, the pulp is vital and painful. Often dogs and cats will not demonstrate obvious signs of pain. Once pulpal death occurs, most dogs and cats do not show pain. However, some animals chew food only on the side of the mouth opposite the traumatized tooth, or they drool and produce increased calculus on the injured side. Hunting dogs may refuse their training dummies; utility dogs may refuse their dumbbells; and apprehension dogs may either hesitate or bite and release repetitively because of the pain (this is referred to as *typewriting*).

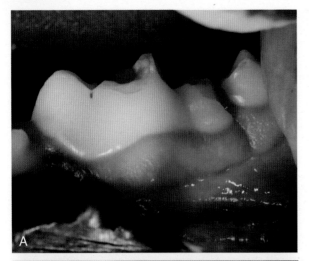

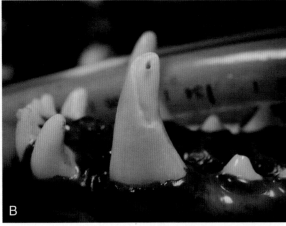

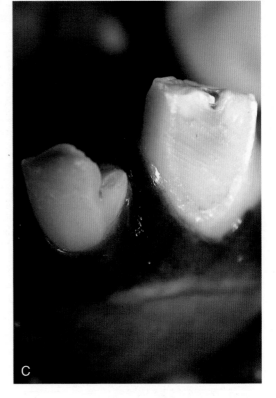

Fig. 13.6 (A) CCF with red bleeding pulp. (B) CCF with black necrotic pulp. (C) CCF with no visible pulp.

Because we cannot depend on dogs and cats to indicate when they have a painful tooth, the veterinary team needs to be able to recognize teeth that may have a compromised pulp. This includes fractured teeth, discolored teeth, and other subtle signs of endodontic disease.

The most common indication for root canal therapy is fractured teeth. In the case of a complicated fracture (T/FX/CCF), the pulp is exposed. This may appear as visible red or pink pulp, black discoloration within the exposure pulp chamber, or an open hole without visible pulp (Fig. 13.6A–C). Sometimes the open pulp chamber is too small to easily see, and anesthetized evaluation is necessary.

In the case of an uncomplicated fracture (T/FX/UCF), there is potential of the pulp dying due to direct trauma or due to the movement of bacteria into the pulp through dentinal tubules. These teeth should always be evaluated radiographically, and if evidence of pulp necrosis or pulpitis exists, they should be treated (Fig. 13.7A and B). In some uncomplicated fractures, the pulp is visible through the dentin but is not exposed. This is known as *near pulp exposure* (T/NE). The treatment of these teeth is always indicated.

A worn tooth, with a brown covering in the area where the pulp chamber was, indicates that the wear has occurred slowly enough that secondary dentin was deposited by the odontoblasts lining

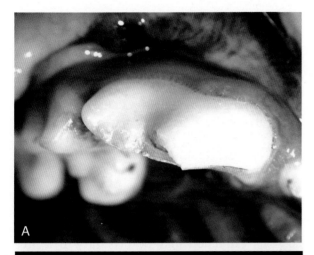

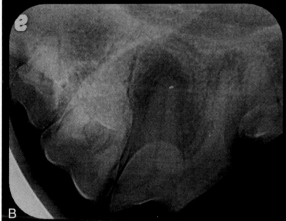

Fig. 13.7 (A) Fractured right maxillary fourth premolar without pulp exposure. (B) Radiograph of tooth in Fig. 7A demonstrating periapical lucency.

the root canal and pulp chamber. In this case, the tooth should be evaluated radiographically as the wear may have caused pulpitis and subsequent pulp necrosis.

Discolored teeth, especially those that are pink or purple, indicate pulpal hemorrhage. Pulp tissue responds to such physical trauma like any other bodily tissue—inflammation, pain, and swelling. If the apex of the tooth is completely developed, the swelling of the pulp is restricted by the confines of the hard dental tissue. The blood flowing into and out of the pulp through the apical delta of the tooth is limited. As a result, inflammatory swelling within

the pulp results in compressive strangulation of the blood vessels in the pulp, and tissue ischemia results. Red blood cells begin to break apart, and hemosiderin and other blood-breakdown products leach into the dentin of the tooth to cause discoloration. This discoloration arising from the deeper tissues of the tooth (pulp and dentin) is known as *intrinsic staining*. When the entire crown is discolored, it is likely that the pulp tissue is completely not vital. In one study, it was noted that 92.2% of intrinsically stained teeth in dogs demonstrated visual evidence of pulp necrosis when the pulp was mechanically entered. A second study looked at the pulp of dog teeth with intrinsic staining histologically. This study demonstrated that 87.6% of intrinsically stained teeth had histologically confirmed necrotic pulp with two-thirds not showing evidence of inflammation. If inflammation is present, even without bacterial contamination, periapical disease can occur. It is thought that bacteria in the blood may enter the dead pulp via a process called anachoresis. This is currently a controversial topic. Regardless, since pulp inflammation and subsequent periapical inflammation can occur in nonvital teeth, careful evaluation and client counseling are warranted.

Treatment considerations are dependent on the age of the patient and when the discoloration occurred. If the patient is between approximately 6 and 15 months of age, the pulp chamber and root canal are relatively large, meaning there may be less potential for pulpal congestion and more potential for pulpal healing. Therefore it is possible that the tooth may recover from this traumatic event and that the death of pulp tissue might only be restricted to the most coronal portion of the pulp. If the event that caused the pulpal hemorrhage is witnessed or the client is very astute and recognizes the injury right away, nonsteroidal anti-inflammatories might be beneficial. Intraoral imaging should be made as a baseline. This allows comparison of the width of the pulp cavity of the affected tooth and similar teeth, specifically its contralateral counterpart. If the teeth appear nearly identical, the radiographs should be followed up in 4 to 6 months. If the pulp cavity of the affected tooth is relatively wide to the contralateral tooth, this likely indicates pulp necrosis and the tooth should be treated.

With subsequent radiographs, if the discolored tooth remains vital, continued maturation will be seen. If the discolored tooth is nonvital, further maturation will not occur and the tooth will have a wider pulp cavity, and thinner dentinal walls compared to the other teeth. Recalling that necrotic pulp may become inflamed, root canal therapy or extraction should be discussed with the pet owner. If at any time, evidence of pulpitis is present, treatment is necessary.

An immature dead tooth has a poor prognosis, and depending on wall thickness, exodontics may be the only alternative. If the tooth has developed further and the wall is developed, endodontic therapy may be the best treatment as it is much less traumatic for the patient, and the function of the tooth is retained.

An older patient may present with a discolored tooth for a different reason—the odontoblasts throughout the life of the tooth have created dentin. Eventually, this dentin may occlude the apex of the tooth, walling it off from the rest of the body. The tooth may be dead but without the inflammatory process previously discussed. Radiographs of these teeth in patients more than 10 years of age may show a wisp of a pulp chamber and normal bone around the apex of the tooth.

Cats are particularly susceptible to pulpitis secondary to canine tooth fracture. The pulp chamber extends close to the tip, and any exposure of dentin allows bacteria into the pulp chamber. Chronic abscess of the canine teeth is extremely common in cats; all fractured teeth necessitate root canal therapy, extraction, or close monitoring.

Endodontic Therapy Versus Extraction

Endodontic therapy is a less invasive treatment option for teeth with compromised pulp. It also maintains the function of the tooth. In cases in which extraction may lead to iatrogenic trauma

or compromise the patient (such as mandibular canine teeth and mandibular first molars), it may be the best option, even when much of the crown is missing. As it is less invasive, it allows for a quicker return to function, which is an important factor when treating working dogs. Client desires should also be considered as many pet owners are not comfortable with the notion of their pet losing a tooth.

There are cases in which the root canal is contraindicated. If the tooth is compromised in a way that standard endodontics will not be successful and surgical root canal therapy (RCT/S) is not possible, extraction may be necessary. If a prolonged anesthetic is not prudent due to significant underlying comorbidities, the shorter anesthetic time associated with extraction may be desirable. If the clinician is not capable of performing endodontic therapy and the client will not accept a referral, endodontic therapy should not be performed. Finally, not treating a tooth with an obviously compromised pulp in lieu of extraction is not acceptable.

Endodontic Procedures
Vital Pulp Therapy

Vital pulp therapy (VPT) is indicated for recent fractures and iatrogenic pulp exposure to preserve healthy dental pulp in the dog. In the case of fracture, this procedure is classically reserved for injuries that occurred within 48 hours. There is evidence suggesting this window can be extended for up to 10 days in the right circumstances. The procedure is not typically recommended in the cat.

A vital pulpotomy is performed by removing the exposed, contaminated pulp and gently disinfecting the remaining pulp and access site. Hemorrhage of the pulp is controlled with cotton pellets or absorbent paper points. Calcium hydroxide $(Ca[OH]_2)$ or mineral trioxide aggregate (MTA) is placed over the entirety of the exposed pulp with a retro filler or a carrier (Fig. 13.8), with care not to overextend the material into the pulp. The placement of the material on top of the pulp is known

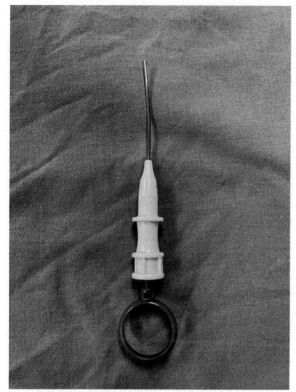

Fig. 13.8 Carrier used to deliver MTA to pulp during vital pulp therapy.

as *direct pulp capping*. Finally, the tooth is restored. The goal is the formation of a new dentin across the exposed pulp and maintaining a healthy, living pulp. This new dentin formed across the pulp is known as a *dentinal bridge* and is one of the hallmarks of successful VPT.

Ca(OH)$_2$ had been the preferred material to place on the exposed pulp until recent years. MTA is the preferred material currently. When comparing the two materials as pulp-capping materials, VPT performed with MTA was shown to be successful in 92% of treatments compared to 58% when performed with Ca(OH)$_2$. Ca(OH)$_2$ is associated with more cell death of the pulp and defects within the newly formed dentin compared to MTA.

Direct pulp capping can also be performed in cases of purposeful or accidental iatrogenic pulp exposure. Most commonly, this variation is performed on one or both mandibular canines to relieve traumatic penetration of the upper gingiva or palate due to malocclusion. This procedure is performed aseptically. The materials installed are the same as those used in a vital pulpotomy. However, the pulp does not require disinfecting because the teeth are invaded in a sterile manner.

Indirect Pulp Capping

Indirect pulp capping (PCI) is a restorative procedure performed when the preparation of a lesion does not penetrate the pulp but is perilously close (0.5 mm) to it. For such incidences, a therapeutic and insulating base layer is placed to protect the pulp. Materials for this include modified Ca(OH)$_2$, MTA, and certain glass ionomers. It is followed by the preparation for and the installation of an appropriate restoration.

Standard Root Canal Therapy

Standard root canal therapy is the act of complete removal of the pulp or *pulpectomy*, the shaping and disinfection of the root canal, and the application of a sealant to seal the apex from infection or reinfection. Access to the root canal is through either the fracture site or one or more created access openings. These access openings are created with high-speed burs to establish more direct access through the crown to the root canal apex. The need to create an access opening separate from the fracture site is dependent on anatomy, the fracture, and the type of root canal file used.

Standard root canal therapy is indicated for adult teeth that have exposed pulp or evidence of pulp death. It is the alternative to VPT when long-term pulp viability is in question. Comparing four different veterinary studies, the failure rate of root canal therapy in dogs ranges between 0% and 7%. The rate of failure of root canal therapy in cats has been shown to be 19%.

The radiograph in Fig. 13.9A, taken at the time of root canal therapy, shows a lytic area of bone around the apex of the tooth. The radiograph taken 3 years later (Fig. 13.9B) shows resolution

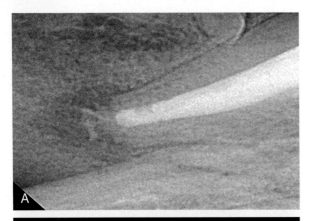

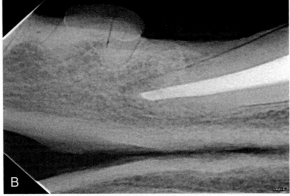

Fig. 13.9 (A) Postoperative radiograph. (B) Three-year follow-up radiograph.

of the lytic area. The endodontic procedure was successful.

Often, the basic steps of RCT are categorized using the ISO acronym. This stands for instrumentation, sterilization, and obturation. Each step can fit into one of these categories, although there is some overlap. Each step must be performed well for the subsequent steps to be successful.

Standard root canal therapy begins in the instrumentation phase by establishing access to the pulp cavity through the fracture site or an access opening as stated earlier. Once the root canal system is entered, the pulp may be removed straight away with the use of a barbed broach. Next, the walls of the canal are instrumented with endodontic files and reamers. This process removes diseased dentin and establishes a tapered or parallel shape to

the canal (dependent on the file type and operator preference). A tapered preparation aids in the irrigation and filling of the canal by taking advantage of the physics of fluid dynamics. The goal of the instrumentation phase is to remove all pulpal remnants and diseased dentin from the root canal system and to shape the canal to allow complete filling of the root canal with the obturation material.

Sterilization involves the use of irrigating solutions to flush debris from the canal and to dissolve or neutralize organic material and pathogens. In addition to sterilizing the canal, the irrigating solution maintains a patent canal and allows the files and reamers to work efficiently. In this way, the irrigating solutions have a place in the "instrumentation" phase just as the files and reamers have a place in the "sterilization" phase due to removing diseased material. Typically, sterilization overlaps instrumentation.

Once the canal has been completely instrumented and sterilized, it is dried and the obturation phase begins. Obturation involves the filling of the root canal with a material that seals the apex, ideally allowing the immune system to heal the inflammation and infection in the bone around the apex. The obturation material should also prevent bacterial leakage from the crown to the apex.

After the ISO steps are complete, the pulp chamber is cleaned of sealant and gutta-percha, and all access openings and openings caused by fracture are prepared for restoration and the appropriate restoration placed.

Endodontic Equipment

Endodontic therapy requires various instruments and materials. The equipment required includes barbed broaches, reamers, files, irrigating needles, mixing slab (or paper pad), spatula, pluggers, and spreaders. These are summarized in box 13.1.

Barbed Broaches

A *barbed broach* (Fig. 13.10) is manufactured by making angular cuts in a soft iron wire, creating flared barbs. This instrument is not strong, but it is

BOX 13.1 Endodontic Equipment, Instruments, and Materials

Pear or round carbide burs for making access openings (appropriate size based on tooth and file size)

Barbed broaches

Orifice wideners
- Gates Glidden
- Peeso Reamers
- Mueller Bur

Hand files
- K-files
- K-reamers
- Hedström files
- Sizes 15–140 with appropriate lengths for species (Sizes above 80 not typically available in 31, 35, 45 mm lengths)
- Endodontic "pathfinders"

Endodontic stops

File organizer

Endodontic ring

RC-Prep: Premier, PA, USA.

Canal irrigant
- Sodium Hypochlorite
- EDTA
- Saline

Irrigation needles of appropriate length

Syringes

Mixing slab and spatula

Paper absorbent points: Similar size to files

Root canal sealer: different types should be available dependent on case

Gutta-percha

Endodontic point forceps: Cotton or college pliers

Lentulo spiral fillers

Pluggers and spreaders: Short and long length

Restorative materials

Finishing disks, points, or stones

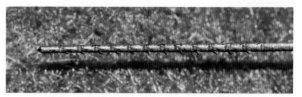

Fig. 13.10 Close-up of a barbed broach.

useful in removing intact pulp. The broach can also be used to remove from the root canal absorbent points, cotton pellets, separated file tips, and other foreign materials such as dirt, gravel, and grass.

Endodontic Files and Reamers

Files and reamers are used to clean dead material from the canal, remove diseased dentin, and shape the canal. These instruments may be operated by hand (hand files) or powered (rotary files). Several types of files exist, and understanding the function and limitations of each file is critical to successful treatment.

Files and reamers have two dimensions: length and diameter. A millimeter notation indicates the length. Usually, two lengths are needed: 25 mm and 31 mm for incisors, premolars, and molars and 45 mm and 55 or 60 mm for canines. The diameter is indicated by a number only, which represents the diameter of the file at the working end. A No. 10 file is 0.1 mm at the working end, and a No. 100 file is 1.0 mm at the working end.

Files and reamers are color coded to identify them by size. However, the numbers are repeated, so caution is necessary to prevent files of similar color but different size from being confused. The color-coding system is as follows:

Grey: 08

Purple: 10

White: 15, 45, 90, 150

Yellow: 20, 50, 100

Red: 25, 55, 110

Blue: 30, 60, 120

Green: 35, 70, 130

Black: 40, 80, 140

Some specific brands of files are available that increase by a percentage rather than by 0.05 mm or 0.1 mm. These files have their own color-coding systems, which must be identified by the manufacturer.

Most files taper from the handle to the working tip of the file, with the tip being narrower. The typical taper is a .02 taper. This means that for every millimeter from the tip, the file widens by 0.02 mm. This taper typically ends 16 mm from the working end at a point called D16. For reference, D0 is the working tip of the file, D1 is one millimeter from the tip and so on until the D16 is reached. The D16 of a .02 taper file is 0.32 mm wider than the D0. Thus a 45 file is 0.45 mm wide at the working tip and 0.72 mm wide at the D16. Other tapers include .04 and .08 tapers. If file tapers are mixed without the operator's knowledge, procedural complications can occur.

Some of the powered file systems do not have a taper or an atypical taper and will be discussed later.

The following is not an exhaustive list of the types of files available but describes some of the files more often encountered in veterinary dentistry.

Hand Files

K-files and reamers are created by twisting a square, rhomboid, or triangular rod, creating cutting flutes. These were first manufactured by Kerr, hence the name. Reamers are twisted with fewer flutes (or twists) per millimeter than on a file. Reamers are used with rotational force only, compared to the rotation and pulling motion used for K-files. With fewer twists than the file, the reamer has wider flutes between cutting edges, allowing more dentin to be augured from the canal. K-files produce a clean, smooth canal wall and, because of their design, are best used to cleanse and shape the apical portion of the canal. If excessive rotational force is applied, the file can be lodged into the canal. This can cause fracture of the instrument (see section regarding complications), which typically happens when twisting counterclockwise.

A Hedström file or H-file is created when a spiral groove is machined into the rod. It is weaker than a K-file because its core has been reduced in diameter by the machine. The shape of a Hedström file is that of inner-stacked cones. Its carrier effect is produced by a straight pull of the file. It does not cut on the push stroke. Hedström files should not be rotated in the canal as this can auger the file into the dentin, resulting in file breaking. Hedström files produce a clean but not cylindrical or smooth wall. They are used to cleanse and shape the coronal or incisal portion of the canal. An example of these three instruments is shown in Fig. 13.11.

Because an endodontic file is a cutting instrument, it operates most efficiently when sharp. The smaller sizes are delicate and prone to bending. They may also unravel, manifested by a shiny area between two cutting flutes, with repeated or improper use. Breakage occurs soon after a file has begun to unravel or after a file has been bent and subsequently straightened by the clinician as

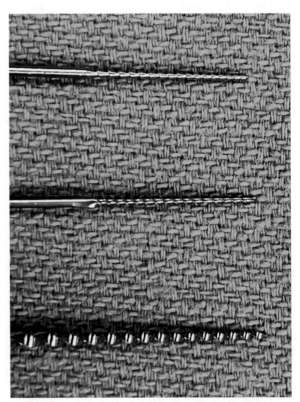

Fig. 13.11 H file on top, K-file in middle, K-reamer on bottom

it dulls and may become damaged, files need to be disposed of and new files added based on file type.

Rotary Files

Hand files are powered by the operator's fingers, which allows fine, controlled movement while providing tactile feedback. This is at the cost of potential operator fatigue. Rotary files are powered instruments in which a specialized handpiece turns the file in a 360-degree rotation or an oscillating motion. What these files lose in tactile feedback, they gain in reduced fatigue and possible reduced procedural time. The most used rotary file in veterinary medicine is the LSX file from Lightspeed (Fig. 13.12). The LSX file is a nontapered file that cuts only on the working end with a dull tip that reduces the risk of penetration past the canal. It cuts in a 360-degree rotation with two cutting edges engaging the canal and creating a circular shape to the canal. The file is made of nickel titanium (NiTi) which allows it to

flex more than the standard stainless-steel files and can allow it to be used with caution in canine teeth through the fracture opening without creating an additional access opening. The popularity of this file in veterinary medicine is likely due to the availability of both a 31 mm and 50 mm long file. Because it creates a round, nontapered cut, it is designed to be used with a nontapered proprietary gutta-percha "plug" called SimpliFill. Techniques do exist to create a taper and use standard gutta-percha cones.

Recently, iM3 has released a tapered NiTi rotary file that is like a K-reamer. The motion of this file is reciprocating compared to a constant rotary motion. Due to its taper, it is to be used with standard gutta-percha points.

Rotary files are typically powered by specific endodontic motors. Each type of file is designed to be used at a specific speed and torque. The endodontic motor may allow programming for these settings. Using rotary files with improper speed and torque can lead to file breakage.

The operator should be comfortable and proficient with several file types and methods of instrumentation as no file can instrument every canal type and file types may become obsolete and not be available.

File Storage

Files are stored in endodontic organizers (Fig. 13.13). These keep like files together and in

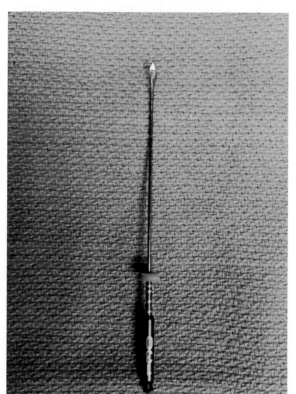

Fig. 13.12 LSX rotary file.

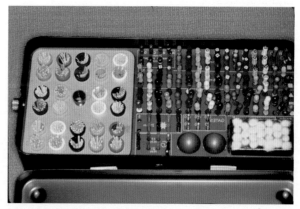

Fig. 13.13 This tray provides compact storage for materials.

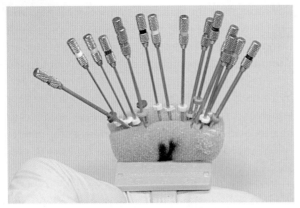

Fig. 13.14 An Endo-ring with files.

order of increasing diameter. Due to the different techniques used with different files, it is critical to not mix file times inadvertently, which may lead to instrument breakage.

As file are pulled out and used, they may be stored (and cleaned) intraoperatively with an Endo-ring. An Endo-ring is a metal or plastic instrument that fits around the finger (Fig. 13.14). An attached disposable sponge, in which the files can be placed in ascending order of size, helps organize the files during the procedure. In addition, the sponge helps clean the files during the endodontic procedure.

Regardless of if an endodontic sponge is used intra-operatively, all files should be cleaned and sterilized before use.

Endodontic Stops

Endodontic stops are pieces of rubber material placed on the file or reamer to aid in marking the distance from the root apex to the access opening. This measurement is known as *working length*. To find the apical working length, smaller files are placed in the canal, the stop is moved to the point where the file has entered the tooth, and a radiograph is taken. Once evaluated, the placement of the stop is adjusted so that the tip of the file reaches the apex when the stop just touches the access point. This distance is measured in millimeters and recorded. This is a critical step in the root canal process as working short of the working length will leave diseased material at the apex and working long of the working depth will cause the file to penetrate past the root canal and into the surrounding preapical tissues. Endodontic stops may be circular, tear drop shaped, circular with a marker, or polygonal. Some of these different shapes aid in not only measuring working length but also can indicate the rotational position of the file if desired.

Irrigation Materials

Irrigating solutions are introduced into the canal by means of a blunt-tipped endodontic needle. Typically, these needs have a port on the side so when the irrigating solution is delivered to the root canal, pressure does not push the irrigating solution through the apex, but the pressure is directed to the side. These needles are typically 27 gauge, but other sizes have been used. Due to the lack of availability of 50 mm and longer endodontic needles, the veterinary profession has been forced to find alternatives. One alternative is needles used to deliver plastic surgery fillers (Fig. 13.15). Several gauges and lengths are available.

Several irrigation solutions are available. The most used is *sodium hypochlorite* (NaOCl). Sodium hypochlorite helps break down and remove the organic material. The strength of NaOCl solution used varies from 0.5% to 6%. Higher concentrations are more effective in dissolving organic debris but present a bigger risk to injury to the patient. Most operators prefer a ¼ or ½ strength solution. Using 6% NaOCl (typical household bleach), the solution is diluted either 1:2 or 1:4 with water. Note that not all available bleach is 6% and some have unwanted additives and are not fit for use in root canal therapy. Please note that NaOCl in any concentration is caustic and can harm the patient and operator if the solution is not kept within the root canal.

Ethylenediaminetetraacetic acid (EDTA) is a chelating agent which helps break down and sequester inorganic material. This aids in removing dentin particles from the dentinal tubules in the canal and clearing the canal of fine dentinal

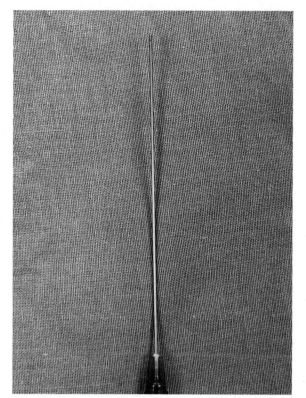

Fig. 13.15 Plastic surgery filler needle used as extended-length endodontic needle.

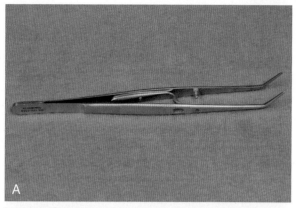

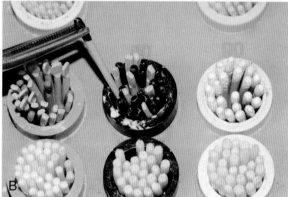

Fig. 13.16 (A) Cotton pliers. (B) Cotton pliers picking gutta-percha.

shavings not picked up by instrumentation. It is available in a 17% aqueous solution. It is often used alternating with NaOCl to enhance the ability of NaOCl to penetrate the dentinal tubules. It is also available in a semisolid (RC Prep) form which includes glycol, urea peroxide, and EDTA. This product can be inserted into narrow canals with a small endodontic file, helping lubricate the canal. In addition to other antibacterial properties, when this product is mixed with NaOCl, it produces oxygen, which can help push debris from the canal via effervescence.

Often saline is used as a final irrigation solution to remove the other irrigating solutions. Other irrigating solutions are available, and each has its own benefits and potential complications. It is advised to research interactions before comixing irrigating solutions in a canal as interactions can occur.

Cotton or College Pliers

Locking cotton, also known as *college pliers,* are used to pick up paper points or gutta-percha without contaminating the container or points (Fig. 13.16).

Endodontic Materials

Absorbent points or paper points are used for drying the pulp canal after it has been instrumented and irrigated. Absorbent points are tightly rolled, tapered paper available in sizes 15 to 140, which correspond to file sizes. They are available in lengths which correspond to the files used (Fig. 13.17). Absorbent points are disposable. Each size can be purchased in lots of 200 or fewer points, or they can be ordered in assorted sizes in conveniently organized packages.

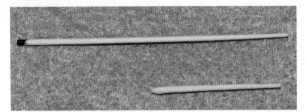

Fig. 13.17 Absorbent point lengths: 55-mm and 31-mm paper points.

The root canal is sealed to prevent bacteria from entering the canal. This is performed with a combination of root canal sealant and core material used to drive the sealant to the root apex and walls of the root canal. *Root canal sealants* are used to seal the apical delta and dentinal tubules that radiate from the walls of the canal. There are several root canal sealants available. The first sealant widely used by veterinary dentists was made of zinc oxide–eugenol (ZOE). It is best known for providing a long working time and being a good, nonirritating antimicrobial agent. Some dentists criticize it as being a temporary sealant because ZOE cements disintegrate after 5 to 8 years in the oral cavity. For most purposes, however, it is quite adequate for veterinary use because the life span of a dog or cat is much shorter than that of a person. The sealer is mixed by a figure-8 mixing motion on a glass slab or paper mixing pad. ZOE is incompatible with composite resins, requiring the use of an intermediate restorative layer between the two.

Noneugenol sealers appear to be more widely accepted among veterinary dentists. Other sealants include glass ionomer–based, resin-based, calcium hydroxide–based, silicone-based, and MTA-based sealants. There is no truly "best choice" in sealants. Some practitioners prefer to have several choices available, and the choice may depend on several factors. The ideal sealant would be easy to work with, seal the canal, not stain the tooth, be radiopaque, be biocompatible, be bacteriostatic, and not shrink on setting.

Mixing of these products may be similar to mixing ZOE or the product may mix in an automix syringe (Fig. 13.18).

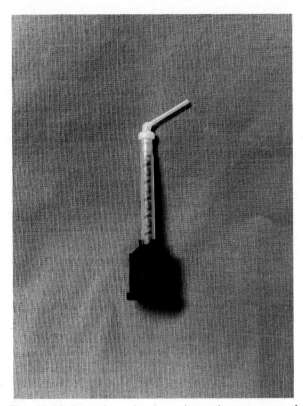

Fig. 13.18 Automix syringe used to mix two parts of endodontic sealant.

Gutta-percha is the most popular core material used by veterinary practitioners. It is made of natural resins with additives to make it radiodense. It does not irritate the periapical tissues and is highly compactible. It is used to help remove voids in the canal sealer and provide a better seal of the apex and openings to the dentinal tubules that radiate from the walls of the canal. Gutta-percha points, like absorbent points, are supplied in sizes 15 to 140 and in lengths to correspond with file sizes (Fig. 13.19). Gutta-percha is harvested from a rubber-type tree and is more commonly used in the softened beta form, which is more flexible and less brittle than the natural alpha form. Distributed to the clinician in the beta form, the material transforms to the less flexible and more brittle alpha form as its shelf-life expires.

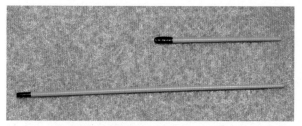

Fig. 13.19 Gutta-percha points.

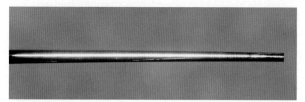

Fig. 13.20 Close-up of a plugger (*note the blunt tip*).

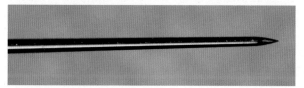

Fig. 13.21 Close-up of a spreader (*note the pointed tip*).

Pluggers and Spreaders

A plugger is used to obtain vertical (apical) compaction. Pluggers have blunted tips (Fig. 13.20). They are used to push gutta-percha (and sealant) apically to eliminate voids within the obturation material. Various lengths and diameters are available, including those specially designed for veterinary medicine.

Spreaders have a tapered, round shaft with a pointed tip. They are used to compact gutta-percha laterally and force sealant into dentinal tubules. By spreading the gutta-percha laterally, they make room for additional gutta-percha. Compared with the plugger, the spreader has a pointed tip (Fig. 13.21).

Heated pluggers are used for cutting and softening gutta-percha to better conform it to the pulp chamber (Fig. 13.22).

Radiographs

Radiographs must be made throughout the entire endodontic procedure. They are taken initially for

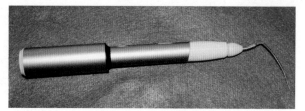

Fig. 13.22 Heated plugger.

diagnostic purposes. Once the operator believes he or she has reached the apical terminus of the root canal, the endodontic stop is advanced to the toot and a radiograph made to assure the file reaches the apex without over extension. When final filing of the canal is nearly complete, radiographs help the practitioner determine shape of the canal, assuring the walls are parallel or taper to the apex. This also aids in assessing if the file fills the root canal apex. Before the canal has been filled (obturated), a radiograph of the first cone placed an assure it fills the apex of the canal. After the canal has been obturated, radiographs help the practitioner evaluate the seal and fill of the canal. If an apical seal is not obtained, the gutta-percha should be either compacted to seal or remove and the filling started over again. Finally, a radiograph is made after the final restoration (filling) to assure there are no voids between the obturation and restoration. In total, at least six radiographs are needed to meet these purposes.

Surgical Root Canal Therapy

Surgical root canal therapy is the approach to the root apex (AP/X) through the alveolar bone, excision of the root apex, known as *apicoectomy*, removal of the apical obturation, and filling of the exposed root canal with a product such as MTA. It is indicated when blockages do not allow for completion of RCT and after failure of RCT when retreatment is not a viable option. The failure rate of RCT/S has been shown to be approximately 6%. This procedure is only an option for teeth in which the apex can be surgical accessed with minimal trauma to surrounding tissues.

Root Canal Complications

Complications of root canal therapy include instrument breakage, canal penetration, over fill of the canal, and idiopathic failure. Breakage of endodontic instruments within the canal, often called *file separation,* is often due to using damaged instruments and improper technique. When possible, the instrument should be retrieved from the canal. If it cannot be retrieved, it may be possible to obturate past the instrument. If not, surgical root canal may be required. Improper filing technique can also lead to penetration of the file through the root canal into the periodontal and periapical tissues. This may be repairable with MTA. If not, bleeding into the canal and inability to obtain a sealed root canal necessitates tooth extraction. Overfill of the canal may be minor at the apex, sometimes called apical blush. It may be excessive and depending on the obturation material used, inflammation of the periapical tissues can occur. Even with careful technique, root canal therapy can still fail, leading to continued or new inflammation of the periapical tissues. The cause may not be apparent, but the operator should consider the quality of each step performed to improve on the next procedure.

Follow-Up for Endodontic Therapy

After endodontic therapy, periodic follow-up is required to monitor the health of the treated tooth. This includes inspection of the restoration and radiographs to assess for continued endodontic viability if performing VPT and assuring there is evidence periapical inflammation is resolving or not progressing with all endodontic therapy. In the case of VPT, follow-up radiographs should be made every 6 months until pulp viability can be confirmed. This is often 2 years post treatment. In the case of RCT, follow-up radiographs should be made 6 to 12 months post treatment, favoring an earlier re-evaluation if procedure complications were noted. With all endodontic therapy, radiographs should be repeated with every dental cleaning.

RESTORATIVE DENTISTRY

Restorative dentistry involves the replacement of dental tissue lost to disease or injury. This includes the use of composite resins and the preparation and placement of dental crowns. Restoration alone should not be performed on teeth with exposed or necrotic pulp as this does not treat the primary pathology. Restorations should be placed in a manner that reduces the risk of future pathology. On the same note, restoration is a critical piece of endodontic treatment and a thorough knowledge of restorative dentistry is necessary if one is to undertake endodontic therapy.

A restoration protects the integrity of the crown and returns the tooth to its previous form and function. The restoration must be confluent with the margin of the defect and have the smoothest surface possible; this delays the formation of plaque and calculus on the surface of the restoration and prevents moisture leakage at its margins.

Instruments for Restoration

A light curing unit (Fig. 13.23) emits high-intensity light in the wavelength of 450 to 490 nm. Classically these units were quartz tungsten halogen type which require a filter and produce more heat than

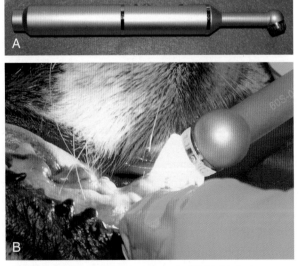

Fig. 13.23 (A) Light-cure gun. (B) Light curing.

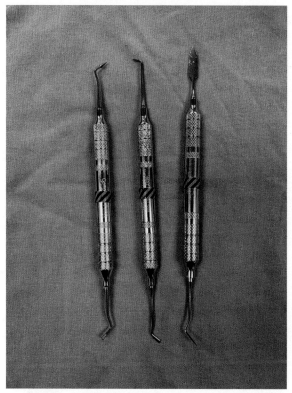

Fig. 13.24 Coated metal composite instruments used to shape composite before curing.

the new LED lights that do not require a filter. LED lights are also more intense and may cure deeper than the classic 2 mm depth of the quartz tungsten halogen type. Both types of light function by activating an initiator in the monomer resin that initiates the polymerization process. Laser-based light curing units are now available. While these may cure the surface of the material more quickly, the depth of cure appears to be less and the cost of the units may be prohibitive. It is important not to look at the light-cure gun or tooth without special glasses or filters covering the light-curing process.

Composite instruments may be as simple as plastic spatulas but also include coated metal instruments (Fig. 13.24) to aid in carrying and shaping composite. Other instruments include composite carriers, fine brushes, and an assortment of burs and polishing disks to shape and smooth the restoration.

Composite Restoration

Dental composite is a restorative material designed to mimic the natural tooth in appearance and durability. It consists of a resin, inorganic filler (silicates, quartz), and an agent that couples the resin and filler. Most composites used today are light curable but some special use composites are cured via mixing two separate parts of the composite. Composites used in veterinary dentistry, like other dental restoratives, are manufactured for use in humans. However, dogs have a bite that is three times as powerful as that of humans. Dogs also abuse their teeth more than humans do. Therefore, the right type of composite should be chosen to reduce the chance of damage to the restoration, often sacrificing smoothness and easy application of the composite for strength. Regardless, composites may not withstand the forces dogs place on the restoration and other types of restorations such as crowns are necessary.

Composites do not cure in a moist environment such as blood, saliva, or water. Even the oil from the operator's fingertips or contaminated water or air sprays will negatively affect the setting properties of composite resin. The site must be rinsed to remove the pumice residue and then air-dried.

The composites used in veterinary medicine typically require use of a conditioner or acid etchant and a bonding agent as well as the composite. The basic process is outlined below.

The restoration site is prepared using a bur of the appropriate size and shape. As little of the tooth structure is removed as possible to prevent weakening but still allow for mechanical retention with the restorative material while removing diseased tissue and debris.

The site is cleaned with flour pumice to remove any surface oils that would interfere with adhesion to the composite resin.

A conditioner or acid etchant (typically phosphoric acid) is applied with a disposable brush or directly to the tooth to remove the powdered tooth debris (smear layer), 1 to 5 microns thick, created by the cutting bur (Fig. 13.25A). The conditioner

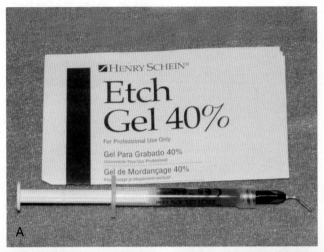

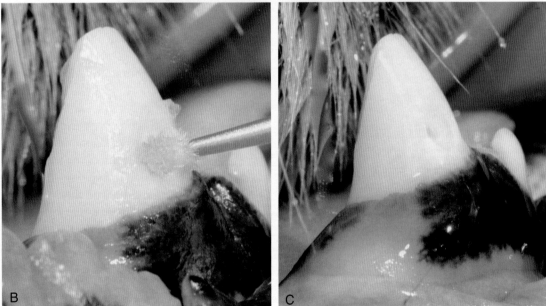

Fig. 13.25 (A) Acid-etch gel. (B) The acid-etch gel is placed on the tooth before placement of the restoration. (C) The dry enamel appears chalky *white*.

makes tiny etches in the tooth's surface by removing mineral. Etching permits bonding agents to later penetrate into the etch-induced micro-irregularities and thereby form interlocking tags (Fig. 13.25B).

After application, the acid etchant is thoroughly rinsed with water from the air-water syringe. After rinsing, the tooth is gently air-dried with air from a three-way syringe. Once dry, the enamel will appear chalky white (Fig. 13.25C).

Next, a bonding agent is applied to the tooth (Fig. 13.26A and B). The bonding agent often contains unfilled resin and a hydrophilic agent, an agent that will attract water and aid in the evaporation of water from the restoration surface. It will have a photo initiator as composite does. After applying the bonding agent, the area is gently blown dry with air from a three-way syringe and light-cured according to the

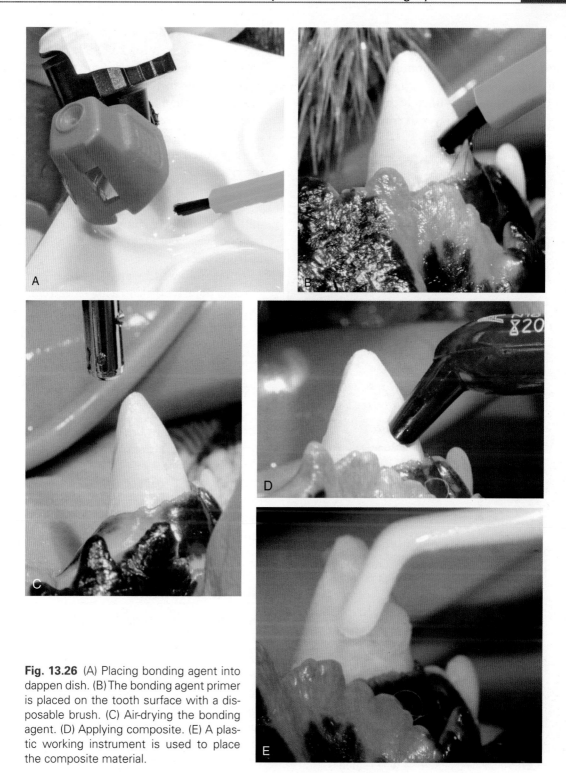

Fig. 13.26 (A) Placing bonding agent into dappen dish. (B) The bonding agent primer is placed on the tooth surface with a disposable brush. (C) Air-drying the bonding agent. (D) Applying composite. (E) A plastic working instrument is used to place the composite material.

manufacturer's recommendations, usually 10 to 20 seconds (Fig. 13.26C). This will initiate polymerization of the bonding agent from a monomer to a polymer.

Finally, the defect is filled with composite, leaving no voids. First, a layer of composite no more than 2 to 3 mm thick is applied (Fig. 13.26D). This layer is light-cured for 20 to 60 seconds, according to the manufacturer's instructions. Layering continues in this manner until the defect is slightly overfilled and the composite overlaps the margins of the defect. A composite instrument is used to smooth out the composite before the final layer is cured in preparation for the final finishing (Fig. 13.26E). Once contoured, the final layer of composite is light-cured.

The restored tooth is finished, or smoothed, until its surface is shiny and flawless. Finishing methods vary and include the use of the following instruments:

1. A fine, followed by an extra-fine, garnet sandpaper abrasive disk on a low-speed contra-angle (Fig. 13.27A).
2. A composite finishing green stone followed by a white Arkansas stone bur (Fig. 13.27B) on a low- or high-speed handpiece.
3. 12-, 16-, and then 30-fluted finishing burs. Finishing disks work best for fairly flat, broad surfaces. Rotating stones are useful when working close to the gingival margin or when recreating a developmental groove in the tooth's surface.

Some choose to place a final layer of an unfilled resin on the restoration, extending to the natural tooth. This can help fill small defects created by finishing the restoration and makes the final restoration smoother.

GLASS IONOMER

One alternative to a full composite restoration is to apply a base layer of glass ionomer prior to placing the composite restoration. This technique must be used when the older ZOE endodontic sealers are placed. It is also used as a base layer to place on top of the pulp capping material before restoring a tooth being treated with VPT. Glass ionomer tends to be softer than composite and bonds to dentin better. As it is softer than composite, it is not often used as a stand-alone restorative agent.

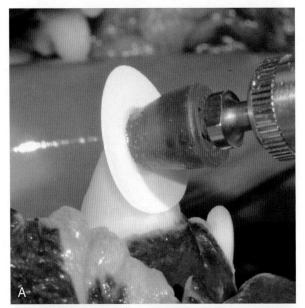

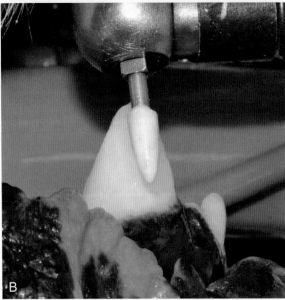

Fig. 13.27 (A) Sanding disk. (B) A *white* stone is used to shape and smooth the cured composite resin.

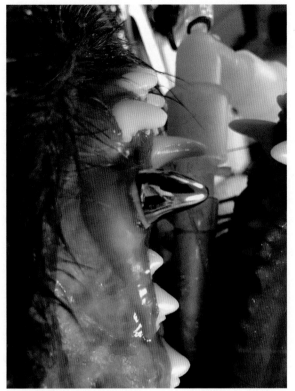

Fig. 13.28 Full coverage metal crown of right maxillary canine tooth.

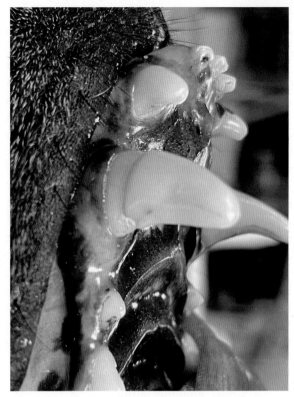

Fig. 13.29 Ceramic crown that has fractured after 2 years.

Crown Restorations

Full-coverage metal crowns (Fig. 13.28) are used to protect the surface of the endodontically treated tooth from further injury and to provide renewed height, shape, and function of severely deformed, fractured teeth. However, preparing the tooth to receive the crown may weaken the tooth. The metal alloys of these vary and the choice of alloy may depend on several factors, including if a metal crown is already in place. If so, like metals should be used as the electric potential difference between unlike metals can lead to corrosion of the metals among other complications.

Porcelain-fused-to-metal (PFM) crowns are more cosmetically pleasing than metal crowns. With any type of full-coverage crown, careful evaluation of tooth size, stage of tooth development, and oral habits of the patient is imperative to achieve successful results. In many patients, installing full-coverage crowns, whether metal or PFM, is unwise.

Ceramic crowns provide an aesthetic alternative. This material is known to crack over time, necessitating repair or replacement of the material. As with PFM crowns, it may not be the best material to use for crown therapy in dogs. There are many reports of ceramic crowns fracturing after placement (Fig. 13.29).

Crown therapy may be the best choice for restoration of the caudal, chewing teeth. The creation of a metal shield around the tooth protects it from chip fractures but does not prevent "catastrophic" fractures. Crowns require a great deal of effort in terms of design and preparation; installing a crown is therefore an advanced procedure.

Although metal crowns may provide renewed shape and function to the tooth, the clinician must be careful to avoid building the crown too high or torque forces will accumulate. Metal crowns are custom-made and require preparation of the tooth and construction of a model. This is typically constructed off impressions made of silicone-based material. One technique for creating an impression with these materials is called a *putty wash technique.* An appropriately sized rigid tray is selected. A putty-type impression material is used as the base of the impression. This is a two-part material like modeling clay. Equal parts are mixed until the material has a uniform color. This is done with ungloved and clean hands as the impression material may be negatively affected by latex. The putty is placed into the tray, and the teeth are carefully pushed into the material. The impression is carefully removed before setting and the impression of the tooth of interest is slightly widened. A lighter-bodied material is then put into the impression, carefully to avoid air bubbles and onto the tooth of interest. The impression is replaced onto the teeth and held with gentle pressure until cured. This is all done while avoiding fluids such as saliva and blood from contaminating the impression. The result is a near-identical negative representation of the tooth, which can be used for creating a stone model. At a minimum, the opposing teeth should have an impression made as well as a bite registration.

These are all submitted to a prosthodontic lab, which can create an accurate stone model of the tooth to create the crown. It is important to communicate with the lab regarding which tooth was prepared if the preparation is coronal or apical to the gingival margin, the type of metal to consider, and any other details that may help produce the best crown possible. This may include photographs. At a minimum, a written prescription with these details should be submitted (Fig. 13.30).

A three-fourths metal crown may be elected for the treatment of abrasion of the distal surface of the canine teeth (Fig. 13.31). These crowns leave the mesial surface of the canine tooth exposed for access to root canal therapy at a later date if it is discovered the pulp has died. Additionally, there is less metal in the region of occlusal contact between the maxillary third incisor, mandibular canine, and maxillary canine, which may lead to better occlusion.

Although metal crowns are the most durable restoration available, dogs who continue destructive habits can wear through the metal (Fig. 13.32).

"Bonded Sealants"

Some practitioners recommend placing a "bonded sealant" over areas of exposed dentin. This consists of odontoplasty to smoothen the tooth, applying an acid etchant to the prepared area followed by the application of a bonding agent and unfilled resin. The theory of this treatment is that the bonding agent and unfilled resin fill the exposed dentinal tubules with the goal of preventing pulpal inflammation.

This procedure must not be performed on teeth with exposed pulp, irreversible pulpitis, or dead pulp. Those teeth would require endodontic therapy and application of a bonded sealant alone, at best, does not treat the primary problem.

It is unclear if this practice is effective. If dentin is exposed and immediately restored, most can agree it is a beneficial procedure. However, if the duration of trauma is several weeks old, the pulp side of the dentin may be already occluded by reparative dentin. It does not mean that applying the restoration is bad practice if the principles of restorative dentistry are maintained.

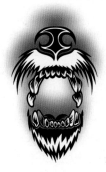

CREATURE CROWNS

1857 TEANAWAY DR
POST FALLS, ID 83854
360.513.1194
CREATURECROWNS1@GMAIL.COM

CLINIC _____   DR. _____   DATE _____ / _____ / _____

ADDRESS _____   CITY _____

STATE _____   ZIP _____   PHONE _____

PATIENT _____   DUE DATE _____

DOG/CAT BREED _____

ALLOY: ☐ Argen Platinum Plus   ☐ Argen Y+   ☐ Talladium   ☐ Full Zirconia

Additional Instructions

CREATURECOWNS.COM

Maxillary Left
Quadrant

Mandibular Left
Quadrant

Maxillary Right
Quadrant

Mandibular Right
Quadrant

Fig. 13.30 Example of prescription for communication with prosthodontics lab.

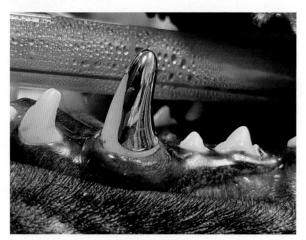

Fig. 13.31 Three-fourths coverage metal crown.

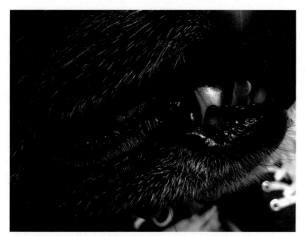

Fig. 13.32 This patient continued destructive habits, leading to wear through the metal crowns.

ORTHODONTICS

The term *orthodontics* refers to the correction of dental malocclusions. Before accepting the patient for orthodontic correction, the practitioner must advise the client of the potential legal and ethical implications of these procedures. Orthodontic procedures should not be performed on animals intended for breeding or show, and whenever possible, animals should be neutered prior to the procedure.

Bite Evaluation

Orthodontic diagnosis and management require a three-dimensional evaluation of the relationships between the bone, teeth, and soft tissue structures within and between the dental arches. Although the incisor relationship is important, bite evaluation entails more than just observing the incisor relationship. Some commonly used lay terms such as "overbite" or "underbite" are not universally defined and can be interpreted differently. It is best to use scientific nomenclature that has been carefully worded and defined by the AVDC. The classes of occlusion are normal, class 1, class 2, class 3, and class 4. Normal occlusion is a scissor bite in which the lower incisors occlude on the cingulum on the palatal surface of the upper incisors. The upper and lower premolars are in an interdigitated relationship with the maxillary teeth buccal to the mandibular teeth. The upper and lower arches are symmetric. The reader is referred to Chapter 2 for the classes of malocclusion.

Good-quality photographs, taken with the macro setting that show the arrangement of the rostral teeth and side view of the caudal maxillary and mandibular teeth with the mouth held closed and the lips retracted, are often helpful for evaluation and consultation.

Interceptive Orthodontics

It is recommended that deciduous teeth be selectively extracted as treatment of malocclusions for several reasons:

1. The patient currently is feeling pain as the sharp crown cusp of the deciduous mandibular canine tooth penetrates the palatal tissue whenever the mouth is closed. Patients with malocclusion tend to be more "mouthy" than other animals because they would rather have a shoe or piece of furniture in their mouth than having that misaligned tooth or teeth penetrate their soft tissues and cause them pain.
2. An abnormally displaced deciduous tooth can interfere with jaw development by interlocking and preventing forward and side-to-side jaw

growth. The four arches grow independently from the growth centers located in the caudal regions of the mandible and maxilla. The time the deciduous teeth are present corresponds to the most active period of growth. Although the arches are not physically joined together, they grow in a coordinated fashion owing to the interdigitation of the teeth. With soft tissue penetration on one side or even both sides, free forward and side-to-side growth can be inhibited, leading to a more serious malocclusion as the permanent teeth erupt.

3. The pointed crown cusp of a deciduous mandibular canine tooth will penetrate the palatal tissue in the location of the nonerupted and developing crown of the permanent, maxillary canine tooth and can lead to developmental damage.

Interceptive orthodontics does not cause the jaws to grow more, but it can allow the full genetic potential of the jaws to develop.

Dental Models

Dental models are made for orthodontic evaluation and treatment and the manufacture of restorative crowns. The following section includes a fundamental technique that provides basic information on the creation of a model. All techniques require instruction and practice.

Orthodontic correction usually requires a three-stage process. In the first stage, an impression and dental model are made. An appliance is created from the model. In the second stage, the appliance is placed in the patient's mouth using orthodontic cement. Once the appliance is in place, the patient is carefully monitored at home and is returned to the practice for periodic rechecks. The third stage is the removal of the appliance after treatment is complete.

Materials for Making Models

Impression trays may be purchased from commercial sources (Fig. 13.33). Trays designed specifically for dogs and cats should be used, although impression trays used in human dentistry will work for some veterinary impressions. Custom trays may be made from plastic materials.

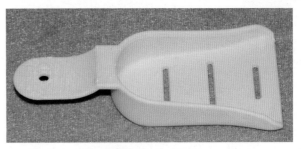

Fig. 13.33 Impression tray.

When mixed with water, alginate forms an agar suspension that hardens to a gel in minutes. The actual rate of this process depends on the chemical formulation. Fast-setting and normal-setting varieties of alginate are available. Fast-setting alginate hardens in 1 to 2 minutes and is also known as type I alginate. Normal-setting alginate sets in 2 to 4.5 minutes and is known as type II alginate. The setting rate of alginate also varies according to water and environmental temperatures. Heat speeds up the setting rate, whereas coldness slows it down. The trays should be tested in the mouth to make sure they fit before the alginate is mixed.

Alginate is mixed in flexible rubber mixing bowls. Either metal or plastic spatulas are used for stirring. Dental stone is hardened gypsum stone. The material is mixed, allowed to set, crushed, mixed, allowed to set once more, and then crushed again several times. Its hardness and resistance to shrinkage distinguish dental stone from plaster of Paris, which is also frequently used. A dental vibrator is used to agitate the mixed dental stone material so that bubbles emerge and escape before hardening. Also, this vibration causes the material to flow more readily.

Technique for Making Models

Before alginate is mixed, the trays should be tested in the mouth. Specific product directions should always be consulted beforehand. The alginate jar should first be lightly shaken to "fluff up" the material and give it a uniform volume. Alginate is measured by volume with the measuring spoon provided (Fig. 13.34a). The alginate is then placed in a mixing

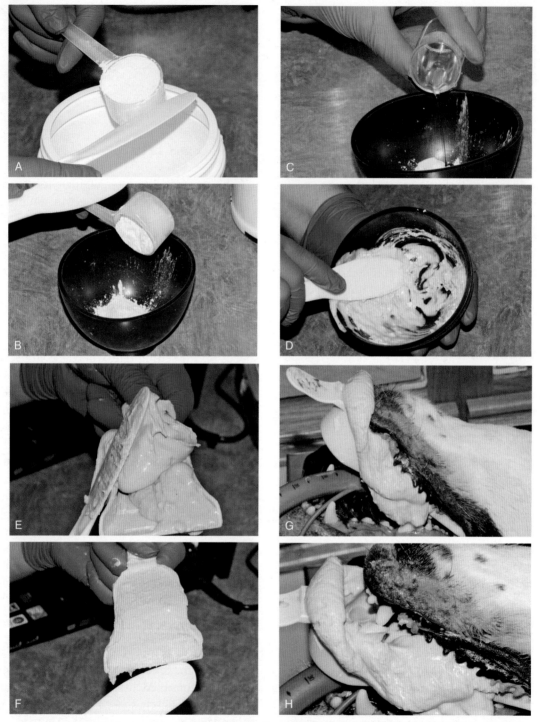

Fig. 13.34 (A) A dry spatula is used to level the amount of alginate in the measuring spoon. (B) The alginate is placed in the rubber mixing bowl. (C) The directions on the alginate bottle should always be followed; usually, one scoop of alginate requires one measure of water. (D) A spatula is used to transfer the alginate into the tray. (E) Transferring to tray. (F) A spatula is used to smooth the alginate before placing it in the mouth. (G) An alginate tray is placed in the mouth and held steady until the alginate hardens. (H) Removing alginate from the mouth.

bowl (Fig. 13.34B). A measuring cup for the water is provided with the alginate (Fig. 13.34C).

Next, the water is added to the bowl. Measuring systems are available in various sizes. The correct ratio of alginate to water is important, so the vessels should be marked if alginate from different manufacturers is being used. The alginate is mixed in a figure-8 mixing motion with a metal or plastic spatula. The bowl is rotated during mixing to ensure uniformity (Fig. 13.34D). The mixed alginate is transferred by spatula to a tray of appropriate size. The alginate must be mixed, poured, and quickly placed because it will harden in only a few minutes. Once the alginate reaches a smooth consistency, it is transferred to the tray (Fig. 13.34E). Spreading the material evenly in the tray with a spatula before inserting it into the mouth helps prevent the formation of air pockets and bubbles in the impression (Fig. 13.34F). The tray is placed in the posterior portion of the mouth first, and the anterior portion of the tray is rotated forward and held in position until it sets (Fig. 13.34G and H).

The last step is to have the patient take a bite registration. Two types of materials are used: bite wax and two-part bite-registration compounds. The two models (maxillary and mandibular) can be matched up with a bite registration. Bite-registration material assists the laboratory in lining up the occlusion before laboratory work (Fig. 13.35).

The next step is pouring the stone model: measurement of the powder and liquid is important in the mixing process. Most dental stones are measured by weight as opposed to volume (Fig. 13.36). The measured water is placed in the bowl, and the dental stone is mixed. A vibrator is used to assist in the flow of the dental stone and to remove bubbles (Fig. 13.37). A base may be poured. This adds

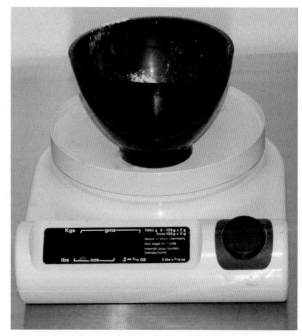

Fig. 13.36 A gram scale is used to measure the powder portion of the dental stone.

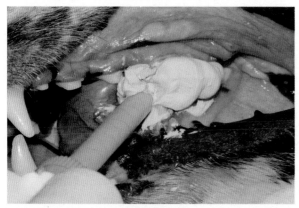

Fig. 13.35 Bite-registration material is placed in the mouth and allowed to harden.

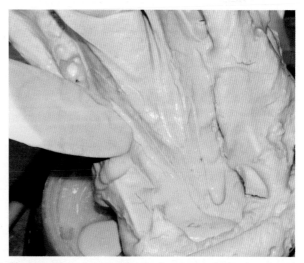

Fig. 13.37 A dental vibrator is used to help the dental stone to flow into the impression more readily.

thickness to the model and may allow for easier removal of the model from the impression.

The model should be removed from the impression as soon as it has hardened. It is important that the alginate remains moist; if the models are not removed immediately, the model, alginate, and tray should be kept wrapped with damp towels in a plastic bag. Removing the tray before the alginate is removed from the model may be helpful. Care should be taken not to break the teeth as the alginate is being removed.

CHAPTER 13 WORKSHEET (ANSWERS ARE ON PAGE 296)

1. _____ is only performed in cases where hyperplastic gingiva is present.

2. _____ is a general statement indicating the treatment of the dental pulp.

3. Intrinsic staining of a tooth likely indicates _____.

4. _____ therapy is indicated for adult teeth that are discolored and endodontically dead or that have been contaminated with long-standing infection.

5. _____ files are powered and reduce operator fatigue.

6. Files and reamers have two dimensions: _____ and _____.

7. _____ have blunted tips. They are used to vertically compact gutta-percha.

8. _____ is a pulp-capping material that appears to be superior to calcium hydroxide.

9. The surgical removal of the root apex is called _____.

10. _____ are used to indicate the working length of a file.

FURTHER READING

Adrian AI, Balke M, Lynch R, Fink L. Radiographic outcome of the endodontic treatment of 55 fractured Canine teeth in 43 dogs (2013–2018). *J Vet Dent.* 2022;39(3):250–256. doi:10.1177/08987564221101091.

Alterman JB, Huff JF. Guided tissue regeneration in four teeth using a liquid polymer membrane: a case series. *J Vet Dent.* 2016;33(3):185–194. doi:10.1177/0898756416676564.

Feigin K, Bell C, Shope B, Henzel S, Snyder C. Analysis and assessment of pulp vitality of 102 intrinsically stained teeth in dogs. *J Vet Dent.* 2022;39(1):21–33. doi:10.1177/08987564211060387.

Hale FA. Localized intrinsic staining of teeth due to pulpitis and pulp necrosis in dogs. *J Vet Dent.* 2001;18(1):14–20. doi:10.1177/089875640101800102.

Kuntsi-Vaattovaara H, Verstraete FJ, Kass PH. Results of root canal treatment in dogs: 127 cases (1995–2000). *J Am Vet Med Assoc.* 2002;220(6):775–780. doi:10.2460/javma.2002.220.775.

Lee DB, Arzi B, Kass PH, Verstraete FJM. Radiographic outcome of root canal treatment in dogs: 281 teeth in 204 dogs (2001–2018). *J Am Vet Med Assoc.* 2022;260(5):535–542. doi:10.2460/javma.21.03.0127.

Luotonen N, Kuntsi-Vaattovaara H, Sarkiala-Kessel E, Junnila JJT, Laitinen-Vapaavuori O, Verstraete FJM. Vital pulp therapy in dogs: 190 cases (2001–2011). *J Am Vet Med Assoc.* 2014;244(4):449–459. doi:10.2460/javma.244.4.449.

Strøm PC, Arzi B, Lommer MJ, et al. Radiographic outcome of root canal treatment of canine teeth in cats: 32 cases (1998–2016). *J Am Vet Med Assoc.* 2018;252(5):572–580. doi:10.2460/javma.252.5.572.

Lagomorph, Rodent, and Ferret Dentistry

Alexander M. Reiter and Ana C. Castejon-Gonzalez

CHAPTER OUTLINE

LEARNING OBJECTIVES

When you have completed this chapter, you will be able to:

- Define the term heterodont dentition and explain how it applies to lagomorphs, rodents, and ferrets.
- Define the terms aradicular hypsodont and brachyodont and explain how they apply to lagomorphs, rodents, and ferrets.
- List the dental formulas of the adult rabbit, hare, guinea pig, chinchilla, degu, rat, hamster, gerbil, squirrel, and ferret.
- List the equipment needed for dental care of lagomorphs, rodents, and ferrets.
- List and describe common oral problems and diseases and treatments in lagomorphs and rodents.
- List and describe common oral problems and diseases and treatments in ferrets.

KEY TERMS

Abrasion
Anisognathic jaw relationship
Aradicular hypsodont
Atraumatic malocclusion
Attrition
Blind intubation
Bone substitute
Brachyodont
Buccotomy
Calcium hydroxide
Caries
Carnivore
Cheek pouch impaction
Cheek retractors
Chinchilla
Diastema
Enamel hypomineralization
Endoscopic intubation
Endotracheal intubation
Ferret
Files

Floating
Gingivitis
Guinea pig
Herbivore
Heterodont dentition
Intermediate plexus
Intubation
Isoflurane
Ketamine
Lagomorph
Laryngoscope
Mandible/mandibular
Manipulation
Maxilla/maxillary
Mouth gag
Occlusal equilibration
Odontoplasty
Omnivore
Otoscope
Palpation
Patency

Periodontal abscess
Periodontal disease
Periodontal-endodontic
    abscess
Periodontitis
Rabbit
Rasps
Retrograde intubation
Rodent
Scurvy
Sevoflurane
Slobbers
Stethoscope-aided intubation
Stomatitis
Tongue entrapment
Tongue retractors
Tooth elongation
Tracheotomy intubation
Traumatic malocclusion
Vital pulp therapy

This chapter discusses the basics of lagomorph, rodent, and ferret dentistry, including equipment, supplies, and techniques for oral examination, diagnosis, and treatment. Relevant anatomy is reviewed.

GENERAL INFORMATION

Lagomorphs

Lagomorphs are the species of the order *Lagomorpha*. The order *Lagomorpha* includes the domestic rabbit, hare, and cottontail. Lagomorphs were once grouped with rodents; a separate order was later created owing to distinct differences in the number of incisor teeth. The rabbit is the only member of this order commonly kept as a family pet. Adult rabbits have between 26 and 28 teeth.

Rodents

The term "rodent" comes from the Latin word *rodere,* meaning "to gnaw." The order *Rodentia* is the largest order of the class *Mammalia* and contains a great diversity of species. Smaller animals within this order that are kept as pets are the rat, mouse, guinea pig, hamster, gerbil, chinchilla, gopher, squirrel, and prairie dog. Most adult pet rodents have between 12 and 22 teeth.

Ferrets

Ferrets belong to the order *Carnivora* and the family *Mustelidae*. Ferrets have deciduous and permanent dentitions. Adult ferrets have 34 teeth.

DENTAL ANATOMY

Dentition in the Lagomorph, Rodent, and Ferret

All lagomorphs and most rodents are *herbivores*, eating leaves, grass, and other lush green plants; however, some rodents are *omnivores*, eating plants and other animals. Lagomorphs and rodents have a dental formula that features variation in tooth size and shape among the incisors (I), premolars (PM), and molars (M), known as a *heterodont dentition*. Lagomorphs and rodents do not have canine teeth (**C**) but instead have a long *diastema* (toothless area) (D) between the incisors and cheek teeth. Ferrets are *carnivores* or animals who have a diet primarily of meat, with a heterodont dentition consisting of incisors, canines, premolars, and molars. Lagomorphs differ from rodents in that they have two pairs of maxillary incisor teeth. The rostral row of incisors consists of two larger functional teeth; a second row of two rudimentary incisors (sometimes referred to as "peg" teeth) sits immediately behind the first row.

Type of Teeth in the Lagomorph

Both the incisors and cheek teeth of lagomorphs are of the aradicular hypsodont type (continuously growing and erupting throughout life, also referred to as elodont) (Fig. 14.1). These teeth have clinical crowns (CR/CC) visible intraorally and reserve crowns (CR/RC) submerged below the gingival margin. They continue to grow and erupt as the teeth undergo normal wear. These teeth never form roots (RO).

Type of Teeth in the Rodent

Two basic types of teeth are found in the rodent: the *aradicular hypsodont* (continuously growing and erupting) incisors and cheek teeth and, in some species, aradicular hypsodont incisors and brachyodont cheek teeth. The *brachyodont* cheek tooth is the same type of tooth found in humans, cats, and dogs (i.e., a tooth with a true distinction between crown and root structure that no longer grows once fully erupted). Guinea pigs (Fig. 14.2) and chinchillas (Fig. 14.3) have aradicular hypsodont incisors and cheek teeth, whereas mice and rats have aradicular hypsodont incisors and brachyodont cheek teeth.

Type of Teeth in the Ferret

Ferrets have long, thin canine teeth, with the mandibular canine teeth occluding into the space between the maxillary third incisors and

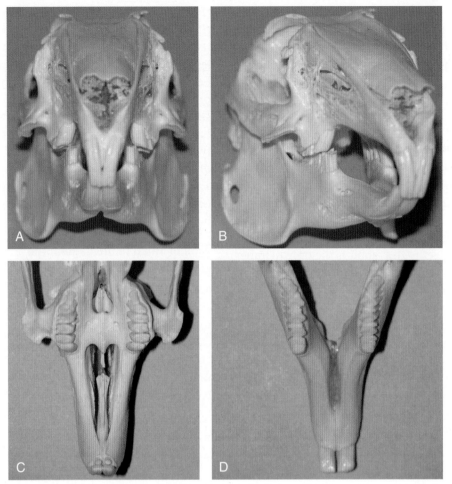

Fig. 14.1 Rabbit skull. (A) Frontal view. (B) Frontolateral view. (C) Upper jaw occlusal view. (D) Lower jaw occlusal view. (Copyright 2025, Alexander M. Reiter.)

canines, thus forming a tight dental interlock when the mouth is closed. Incisor teeth are small, with three incisors in each quadrant. The maxillary fourth premolar and mandibular first molar teeth are sectorial, closing in a scissor-like fashion. Hourglass-shaped maxillary first molar teeth are a common dental finding of the family *Mustelidae* (Fig. 14.4). The relatively small size of the teeth and oral cavity, coupled with the animal's active nature, makes it difficult to thoroughly assess oral health in conscious ferrets, and therefore oral pathology can easily be overlooked without sedation or anesthesia.

Ferrets, being carnivores, have a highly specialized brachyodont dentition.

Incisor Teeth of Lagomorphs and Rodents

The maxillary and mandibular incisor teeth of lagomorphs and rodents, with the exception of the peg teeth of lagomorphs, come to a chisel-like point. These teeth have enamel (E) on the front and lateral sides but typically just cementum and dentin on the palatal/lingual surface. Cementum and dentin wear much faster than enamel, resulting in a chisel edge that is longer labially. The enamel of incisors in most rodents takes on a yellow-orange color—an

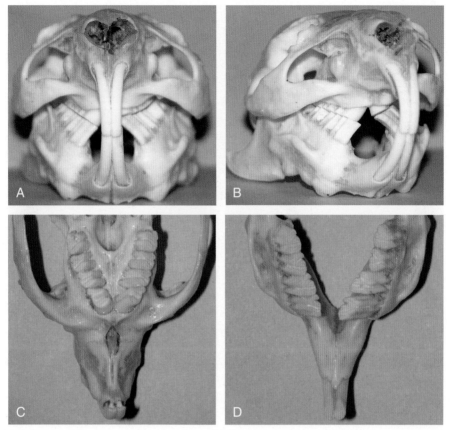

Fig. 14.2 Guinea pig skull. (A) Frontal view. (B) Frontolateral view. (C) Upper jaw occlusal view. (D) Lower jaw occlusal view. There is elongation of the clinical crowns (intraorally) and reserve crowns (periapically; note the bony bumps at the ventrolateral aspect of both mandibles and medial aspect of the left orbit) of the cheek teeth. (Copyright 2025, Alexander M. Reiter.)

exception is seen in the guinea pig. Incisor teeth are very long and curved. The location of the apex of these teeth varies with the species of animal. In most species, the apex of the maxillary incisor teeth lies in the area of the diastema. However, in rats and mice, the mandibular incisor apices are distal to the roots of the last cheek tooth, whereas rabbits and chinchillas usually have their mandibular incisor apices near the mesial surfaces of the first cheek teeth.

Hypsodont Cheek Teeth of Lagomorphs and Rodents

Because of their unique function, hypsodont cheek teeth often have an angled rather than a flat occlusal table surface. The highest point of the chisel tip

of the maxillary cheek teeth is on the labial side, angling dorsally toward the soft tissue of the hard palate. The bevel of the mandibular cheek teeth goes in the opposite direction. The chisel point of the mandibular cheek teeth is on the lingual side, and the tooth's occlusal table angles toward the soft tissue of the cheek. These wear patterns are owing to the fact that the maxillary cheek teeth are spread wider apart from the midline than the mandibular teeth. This is known as an *anisognathic jaw relationship*, or naturally unequal, jaw relationship, in which the upper dental arch is slightly wider than the lower dental arch. Healthy rabbits have only a very slight angulation to the occlusal plane of the cheek teeth (~10-degree angle from dorsolingual

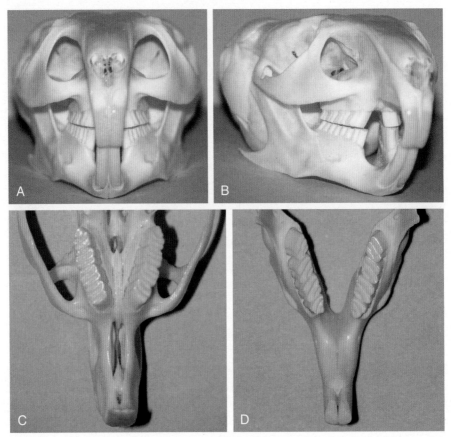

Fig. 14.3 Chinchilla skull. (A) Frontal view. (B) Frontolateral view. (C) Upper jaw occlusal view. (D) Lower jaw occlusal view. (Copyright 2025, Alexander M. Reiter.)

to ventrobuccal), healthy guinea pigs have a relatively steep angulation (~30-degree angle from dorsobuccal to ventrolingual), and healthy chinchillas have a level occlusal plane.

Periodontal Ligament

The periodontal ligament of permanent aradicular hypsodont teeth may differ from that of permanent brachyodont teeth owing to the presence of an intermediate plexus between its tooth and bone attachments. An *intermediate plexus* is a middle zone of the periodontal membrane situated between the cemental group of fibers attached to the root of the tooth and the alveolar group of fibers attached to the alveolar bone. This structure may allow continuously growing teeth to move coronally as they grow. This adaptation of hypsodont teeth is thought to explain how the periodontal ligament allows for continued eruption, although the presence of the intermediate plexus has been debated.

Adult Lagomorph Dental Formulas

Rabbit: 2 × (I 2/1, C 0/0, P 3/2, M 2-3/3) = 26 to 28 total teeth

Hare: 2 × (I 2/1, C 0/0, P 3/2, M 3/3) = 28 total teeth

Adult Rodent Dental Formulas

Guinea pig and chinchilla: 2 × (I 1/1, C 0/0, P 1/1, M 3/3) = 20 total teeth

Degu: 2 × (I 1/1, C 0/0, P 1/1, M 3/3) = 20 total teeth

Rat: 2 × (I 1/1, C 0/0, P 0/0, M 2-3/2-3) = 12 to 16 total teeth

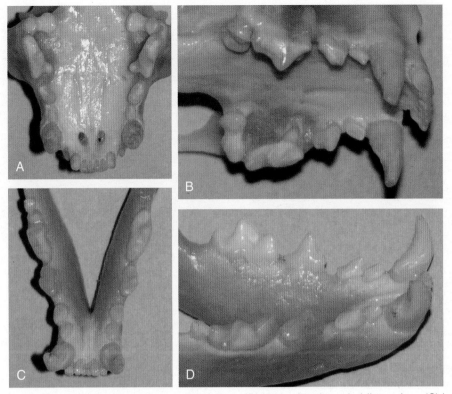

Fig. 14.4 Ferret skull. (A) Upper jaw occlusal view. (B) Upper jaw lateral oblique view. (C) Lower jaw occlusal view. (D) Lower jaw lateral oblique view. (Copyright 2025, Alexander M. Reiter.)

Hamster: 2 × (I 1/1, C 0/0, P 0/0, M 2-3/2-3) = 12 to 16 total teeth

Gerbil: 2 × (I 1/1, C 0/0, P 0/0, M 3/3) = 16 total teeth

Squirrel: 2 × (I 1/1, C 0/0, P 1-2/1, M 3/3) = 20 to 22 total teeth

Adult Ferret Dental Formula

Ferret: 2 × (I 3/3; C 1/1; P 3/3; M 1/2) = 34 total teeth

INSTRUMENTS AND EQUIPMENT USED TO TREAT LAGOMORPHS, RODENTS, AND FERRETS

The following instruments and equipment are used in the treatment of oral disorders in lagomorphs, rodents, and ferrets:

Towels are helpful for restraint and for maintaining normothermia during procedures.

Anesthesia is available in two forms: injectable and inhalant. Injectable medications such as ketamine and acepromazine usually result in a longer recovery time than inhalants. Some injectables are reversible. Inhalants such as isoflurane and sevoflurane are preferred for maintenance of anesthesia for most procedures. Anesthesia masks can be used for induction of anesthesia prior to intubation or for the maintenance of anesthesia using an off-and-on mask approach during the actual dental procedure. Induction may also be administered in an anesthesia chamber, although small mammals may hold their breath because of the odor of the inhalant. Anesthesia and oxygen may also be delivered through an endotracheal tube. A laryngoscope with a small pediatric straight blade is used for

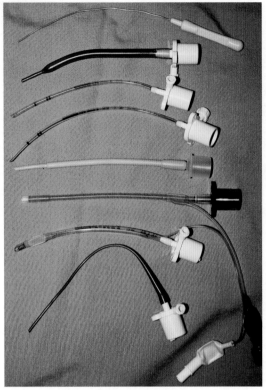

Fig. 14.5 Standard, Cole type, and handmade endotracheal tubes and a stylet for use during tube placement. (Copyright 2025, Alexander M. Reiter.)

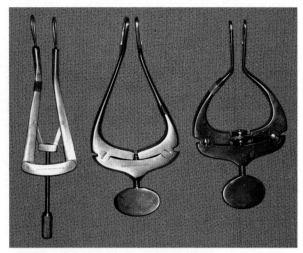

Fig. 14.6 Mechanical mouth gags. Care should be taken to avoid excessive force by opening the mouth only as wide as needed for visualization of the oral cavity. (Copyright 2025, Alexander M. Reiter.)

endotracheal intubation to maintain the airway and administer anesthesia. Endotracheal tubes in sizes 1.5, 2.0, 2.5, or 3.0 Cole or a standard endotracheal tube may be used, depending on the patient's size. A wire stylet placed in the tubes makes passage much easier (Fig. 14.5).

An **otoscope** with ear cones or a nasal speculum may be used to visualize the teeth and oral cavity of small mammals. In addition, these can be used as an aid in passing endotracheal tubes.

Intravenous (IV) catheters (12- to 14-gauge) can be used as an endotracheal tube for smaller rodents if the stylet is removed. These catheters can often be passed with the use of an otoscope as a laryngoscope.

Umbilical tape is used to anchor the endotracheal tube by snugly tying it to the tube and then behind the pet's head.

Cotton-tipped applicators are used during dental procedures to clear the oral cavity of food, saliva, and debris.

Explorers/probes are used to examine teeth and their attachment structures.

Handpieces (HPs), both high-speed and low-speed, can be used with burs to shape, trim, prepare, or extract teeth.

Mouth gags sit between the teeth and aid in keeping the mouth open during inspection and treatment. Most are spring activated, or they may expand with a screw device (Fig. 14.6).

Cheek retractors are single-bladed instruments that retract the cheek on a single side or double-bladed instruments with a spring wire that can spread apart both cheeks at the same time (Fig. 14.7).

Tongue retractors are generally instruments with a single, flat blade used to move the tongue away from the area to be inspected or treated (Fig. 14.8).

Burs are used for the removal of hard tissue. The most common types are diamond burs, carbide round burs, carbide tapered fissure burs, and white stone points (Fig. 14.9). A cylindrical diamond bur works well for incisors and cheek teeth. Carbide burs are more aggressive than diamond burs and white stones. Of the carbide burs, the 701 L tapered fissure and #1 and #2

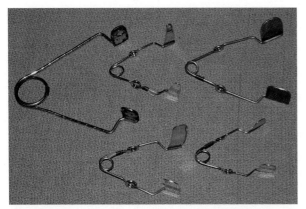

Fig. 14.7 Spring-loaded cheek retractors used to move the cheeks laterally for improved visualization of and access to the cheek teeth. (Copyright 2025, Alexander M. Reiter.)

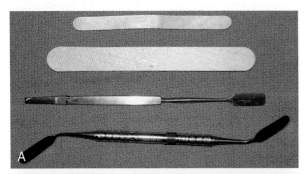

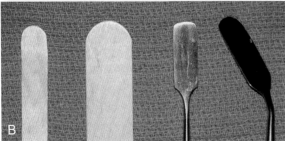

Fig. 14.8 (A) Handheld spatulas made from wood and metal for tongue and cheek retraction. (B) Close-up view of their working ends. (Copyright 2025, Alexander M. Reiter.)

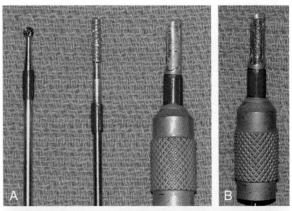

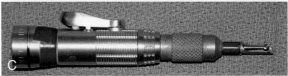

Fig. 14.9 Power tools for trimming overgrown teeth. (A) Round carbide bur, cylindrical diamond bur, and safety guard. (B) Cylindrical diamond bur within safety guard (note the opening on one side which will face the area of the tooth to be worked on). (C) Round carbide bur, safety guard, and low-speed handpiece. (Copyright 2025, Alexander M. Reiter.)

round ball burs are helpful. Of the white stone abrasive points, the flame-shaped point works well. Friction grip (FG) burs are used on high-speed HPs when working in the rostral oral cavity, but straight HP burs are necessary for use on the cheek teeth of most lagomorphs and rodents owing to poor accessibility with the high-speed HP. A safety guard can be used to effectively protect soft tissues from being traumatized by the bur. The use of a diamond disk without a safety guard is strongly discouraged.

Files/rasps (sometimes referred to as "floats") are instruments used to level an abnormally uneven occlusive table of the teeth or remove excess dental hard tissue causing trauma to adjacent soft tissue (Fig. 14.10). The hand floats used in the small mouths of lagomorphs and rodents are typically either modified bone files or rasps. The rasps cut both on the push and pull stroke, whereas the files typically cut only on the pull stroke. The rabbit molar file is a float specifically developed for use in rabbits. Most have a large handle for better control and a working end that is similar to a bone rasp. A smaller diamond-coated rasp works well for the final smoothing of jagged tooth surfaces after the use of a bur or larger file to reduce an overgrown tooth (Fig. 14.11).

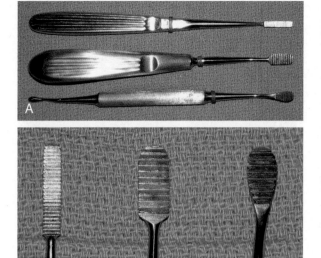

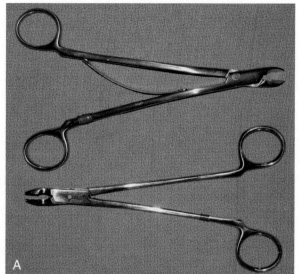

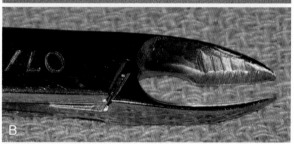

Fig. 14.10 (A) Files used for floating of teeth in lagomorphs and rodents. (B) Close-up view of their working ends. (Copyright 2025, Alexander M. Reiter.)

Fig. 14.12 (A) Tooth cutters used for removal of small spurs on the clinical crowns of lagomorph and rodent teeth. (B) Close-up view of the working end. (Copyright 2025, Alexander M. Reiter.)

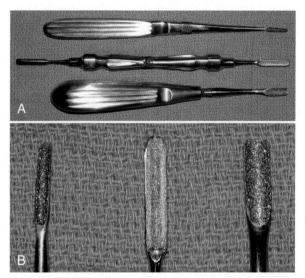

Fig. 14.11 (A) Diamond-coated rasps used for fine-contouring of teeth in lagomorphs and rodents. (B) Close-up view of their working ends. (Copyright 2025, Alexander M. Reiter.)

Tooth cutters may be modified hard-tissue nippers, pin, and wire cutting pliers, or side-cutting rongeurs (Fig. 14.12). However, some have been developed specifically for use in rabbits.

Luxators and elevators are used to work circumferentially around a tooth in the periodontal ligament space to aid in the tooth's removal (Fig. 14.13). Hypodermic needles, sizes 18- to 22-gauge (or smaller), can often be used for this function in lagomorphs and rodents (Fig. 14.14). However, standard elevators can also be used, such as No. 1 and 2 winged elevators, 301 apical elevators, and specific rabbit luxators.

Extraction forceps are used to grasp teeth loosened by elevation or severe disease. Most incisors can be handled with small animal extraction forceps. For the cheek teeth, a small 90-degree angled Halstead mosquito forceps or an angled root tip forceps can be useful. Some

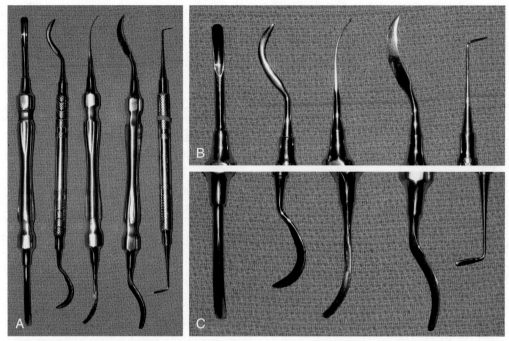

Fig. 14.13 (A) Luxators and elevators for use on lagomorph and rodent teeth. (B and C) Close-up views of their working ends. Note that the instrument on the right of each image is for luxation and elevation of cheek teeth, while all the others are for luxation and elevation of incisor teeth. (Copyright 2025, Alexander M. Reiter.)

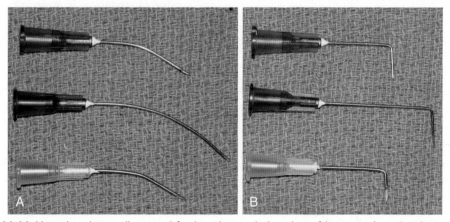

Fig. 14.14 Hypodermic needles used for luxation and elevation of lagomorph and rodent teeth. (A) Curved needles for incisor teeth. (B) Needles bent at a 90-degree angle for cheek teeth. (Copyright 2025, Alexander M. Reiter.)

extraction forceps are specifically designed for use in rabbits and rodents (Fig. 14.15).

Bone substitutes are placed into areas in which periodontal or endodontic disease has resulted in bone loss. These grafts may be combined with an antibiotic or other medicament when placed in a bony void.

Antibiotic-impregnated beads may be placed for treatment of refractory infections. They may be nonabsorbable, such as

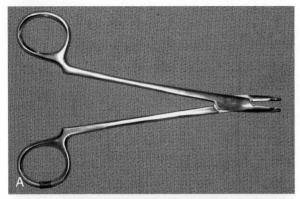

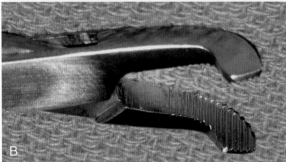

Fig. 14.15 (A) Extraction forceps for cheek teeth of lagomorphs and rodents. (B) Close-up view of the working end. (Copyright 2025, Alexander M. Reiter.)

polymethylmethacrylate beads. Polymethylmethacrylate releases heat during polymerization. Thus, a thermostable antibiotic (e.g., gentamicin) must be used. Calcium phosphate antibiotic-impregnated beads are typically absorbed within weeks after placement.

Paper points are commonly used to apply medicaments to exposed pulps (PU).

Calcium hydroxide is commonly used in either a powder or paste form. It is placed over the exposed pulp of a tooth in an attempt to maintain its vitality. Newer pulp-capping materials include mineral trioxide aggregate, biodentine, and nano-hydroxyapatite. The use of calcium hydroxide has also been described as packing material in infected draining abscesses, although severe soft tissue necrosis owing to its high pH could result.

Restoratives used in small mammals and exotic pets are ordinarily temporary filling materials, such as reinforced zinc oxide-eugenol cements or glass ionomer restorative materials.

COMMON ORAL PROBLEMS AND DISEASES IN LAGOMORPHS AND RODENTS

Common problems in lagomorphs and rodents are gingivitis, periodontitis, enamel hypomineralization (E/HP)/hypoplasia (E/H), caries, tooth fracture (T/FX), malocclusion (MAL), tongue entrapment, tooth overgrowth (elongation), jaw abscess, cheek pouch impaction, stomatitis, oral tumors, and slobbers.

Gingivitis

Gingivitis in the rostral mouth of lagomorphs and rodents is often owing to trauma caused by rough edges on watering devices and food bowls. Treatment includes removal, repair, or replacement of the defective device causing the trauma. Once the source of irritation is removed, most patients respond positively without further treatment. However, if the situation warrants, the lesion can be treated with multiple coats of tincture of myrrh and benzoin or topical antibiotic ointments.

Periodontitis

Periodontitis is generally found in the cheek teeth of animals with brachyodont teeth, such as mice and rats. Treatment consists of professional dental cleaning and, if warranted, tooth extractions. Chinchillas also frequently suffer from periodontitis. Periodontitis may develop secondary to tooth elongation (T/EL) and/or tooth resorption (TR) in aradicular hypsodont cheek teeth of rabbits, chinchillas, and guinea pigs.

Enamel Hypomineralization/Enamel Hypoplasia

Hypomineralized/hypoplastic areas of enamel may be seen occasionally on incisor teeth. This may

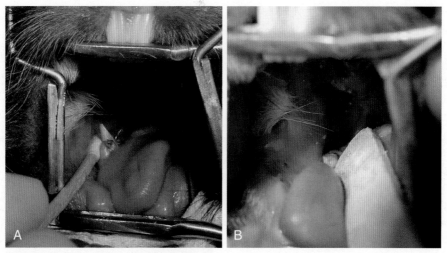

Fig. 14.16 Treatment of an overgrown (elongated) right mandibular cheek tooth in a rabbit. (A) Before treatment. (B) After occlusal equilibration and odontoplasty. (Copyright 2025, Alexander M. Reiter.)

appear as a chalky white or brown discoloration on the labial surface of the tooth. Enamel abnormalities generally result from either a nutritional imbalance, infection, or inflammation that temporarily decreases enamel production. Generally, the only treatment required is correction of the initiating cause. Trauma to and subsequent death of ameloblasts may result in long-term enamel defects. The teeth seldom require any direct treatment, unless the weakened area of the tooth results in T/FX.

Caries

True caries (CA) lesions are generally found in only the cheek teeth of rodents with brachyodont teeth. Caries is considered to be uncommon, but detection of this problem is challenging because cheek teeth are difficult to examine. Caries may be on the occlusal surface of the crown, but many lesions are found on the root surfaces, making them even more difficult to detect. The most common treatment is extraction, although removal of the diseased dental structure with a bur and glass ionomer restorations have been used in some cases in an attempt to maintain the teeth as vital and functional.

Malocclusion

Malocclusion can be classified into two basic categories: traumatic and atraumatic.

Traumatic Malocclusion

Traumatic injuries to the teeth can result in broken crowns, which may cause overgrowth (elongation) of the opposing tooth because of the lack of normal *attrition* (AT) (tooth-to-tooth wear). Overgrowth of teeth opposite to previously lost or extracted teeth may also fall into this category.

1. Treatment of the overgrown opposing tooth can generally be controlled by periodic odontoplasty (ODY) and is known as *occlusal equilibration* (Fig. 14.16).
2. Treatment of the fractured tooth includes initial inspection to determine if the tooth's pulp has been exposed. If the pulp is exposed and the tooth shows no clinical or radiographic evidence of not being vital, a vital pulp therapy should be performed to improve the chances of maintaining the tooth's vitality and return of normal occlusal interaction with the opposing tooth. If the tooth is nonvital, it and its opposing tooth may eventually require extraction (X, XS, or XXS).

Atraumatic Malocclusion

Atraumatic malocclusions are caused by hereditary factors or by nutritional or other atraumatic changes of the teeth, temporomandibular joints (TMJ), mandibular symphysis (SYM), or bone that result in improper tooth alignment. Atraumatic MAL is found in three basic forms:

1. Short maxillary diastema results in the maxillary incisor teeth failing to meet properly with the mandibular incisors. This results in the overgrowth of one or more of the incisor teeth. This condition typically manifests within the first year of the animal's life and is generally considered to be of autosomal recessive inheritance in rabbits resulting in a shortened maxillary diastema. Treatment involves control of the overgrowth by routine ODY of the incisor teeth.

2. Genetics, nutrition, or abnormal mandibular excursion may also result in MAL of the incisors or the cheek teeth. This condition usually manifests after 2 years of age. It has a poor long-term prognosis, and clients should be made aware of this fact. Treatment includes occlusal equilibration of the affected teeth, nutritional changes, and symptomatic treatment of secondary conditions that may arise. This may include the use of antiinflammatory medications and fluid therapy.

3. Improper wear is usually also a result of insufficient chewing from feeding the wrong diet. Treatment consists of dietary correction, if required, and the periodic ODY of overgrown teeth.

Tongue Entrapment

Tongue entrapment occurs when the clinical crowns of the mandibular cheek teeth elongate intraorally to meet at the midline, pinning the tongue in the intermandibular space (that is common in the guinea pig) (Fig. 14.17). Treatment involves trimming of the overgrown teeth to release the tongue and routine ODY of these teeth in the future to prevent recurrence. Antiinflammatory medication, fluids, hand feeding, and other supportive therapies may be required. Long-term prognosis may be poor.

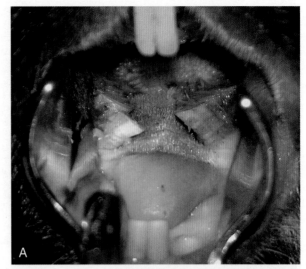

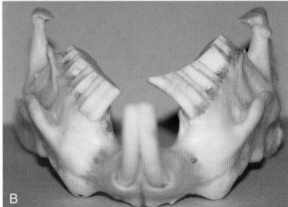

Fig. 14.17 Tongue entrapment in guinea pigs. (A), Clinical patient. (B) Dry specimen showing elongation of the clinical crowns of the mandibular cheek teeth. (Copyright 2025, Alexander M. Reiter.)

Incisor Tooth Overgrowth

When not complicated by cheek tooth involvement, incisor tooth overgrowth (elongation) (Fig. 14.18) can usually be treated and controlled by one of the following methods:

1. Odontoplasty, which reestablishes a functional occlusion.

2. Extraction, which removes the occlusal interference and trauma while establishing a functional occlusion.

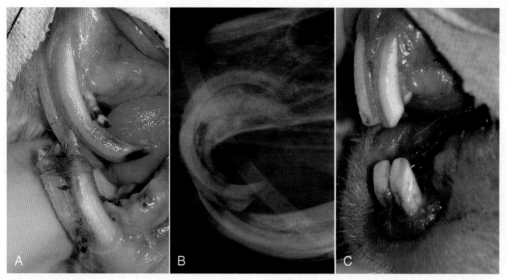

Fig. 14.18 Overgrowth (elongation) of incisors in a rabbit. (A) Before treatment. (B) Radiograph before treatment. (C) After treatment. (Copyright 2025, Alexander M. Reiter.)

Cheek Tooth Overgrowth

Once cheek tooth overgrowth (elongation) (Fig. 14.19) and periapical disease begin, a serious, life-threatening process ensues. Cheek tooth overgrowth results in a chronic inflammatory disease that causes gradual weight loss and many secondary health problems. The condition can be controlled by ODY, antibiotics, antiinflammatory medications, and supportive care.

Jaw Abscess

Teeth may develop abscesses as a result of periodontal or endodontic/periapical disease. Treatment may involve endodontic procedures, but extraction of the diseased tooth is generally necessary. The actual abscess may require excision, extraction of involved teeth, wound debridement, lavage, closure, or marsupialization (MAR).

Cheek Pouch Impaction

Occasionally, food becomes impacted in the cheek pouches, causing mild buccal irritation or stomatitis. This is known as *cheek pouch impaction*. Treatment consists of removal of the impacted material. In severe cases, antibiotic therapy may be warranted.

Stomatitis

Most cases of stomatitis are secondary to a nonoral cause, such as hypovitaminosis C, which results in *scurvy*. Scurvy leads to gingivitis, periodontitis, oral hemorrhage, mobile or lost teeth, anorexia, and loss of body weight. Treatment should be immediately initiated with vitamin C supplements and supportive care, which may include fluid therapy and tube feeding. The diet should be enhanced with fruits and vegetables rich in vitamin C. If a commercial diet is being used, its expiration date should be closely inspected because vitamin C in commercial diets gradually depletes with time. These diets are usually dated for safety.

Oral Tumors

Many oral tumor types can be seen in small mammals and exotic pets. Odontogenic tumors (odontoma, pseudo-odontoma, elodontoma) have been reported in lagomorphs and rodents. A diagnosis is made by means of incisional or excisional biopsy, and the choice of treatment greatly depends on histopathologic findings. In cases of odontoma, pseudo-odontoma, and elodontoma, radiographs are usually very suggestive of the disease.

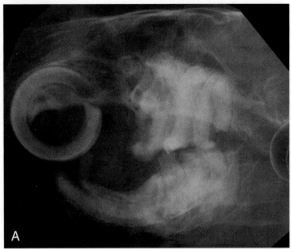

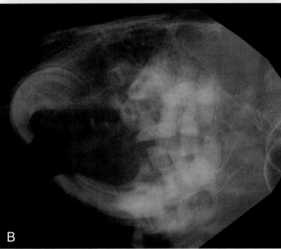

Fig. 14.19 Overgrowth (elongation) of incisors and cheek teeth in a chinchilla. (A) Radiograph before treatment. (B) Radiograph after treatment. (Copyright 2025, Alexander M. Reiter.)

However, the prognosis is often poor to guarded because the tumors tend to grow and invade adjacent structures.

Slobbers

Slobbers, or wet dewlap, is a condition in which excess drooling saliva results in a moist dermatitis and hair loss around the mouth, neck, and front limbs. Many of the previously described oral diseases may result in slobbers. Treatment includes

control of the initiating disease. Dermatitis is treated by clipping the hair, cleansing, and topical treatment with antibiotics, if secondary infection is present.

COMMON ORAL PROBLEMS AND DISEASES IN FERRETS

Common oral problems and diseases in ferrets include tooth extrusion, tooth abrasion, T/FX, endodontic and periapical disease, crowding of mandibular incisor teeth, and periodontal disease.

Tooth Extrusion

Tooth extrusion can be seen when the root surface is exposed in the absence of gingival recession. As is commonly seen in domestic cats, extrusion of the canine teeth results in a longer than normal clinical crown. Based on a study of 63 rescued ferrets, extrusion was seen in one or more of the canine teeth in 93.7% of ferrets. Although extrusion itself does not require treatment, it may predispose the extruded tooth to fracture or luxation.

Tooth Abrasion

Abrasion (AB) (wear owing to contact of a tooth with a nondental material) was seen in 76.2% of rescued ferrets and 63.2% of client-owned ferrets. AB can be seen in nearly every tooth, although the prevalence differs depending on the population investigated. AB is most commonly seen on the mandibular and maxillary third premolar teeth in rescued ferrets, whereas the rostral teeth were more affected in client-owned ferrets. The progression of AB may be slowed by minimizing exposure to hard toys, although ferrets will often still chew on housing and cage bars. AB can result in pulp exposure if the rate of wear occurs more rapidly than the odontoblasts on the inside of the tooth can produce tertiary dentin. If pulp exposure is not present and the tooth is not sensitive, treatment may not be required.

Tooth Fracture

Tooth fractures were seen in 31.7% of the rescued ferrets and 73.7% of the client-owned ferrets, with

60% of fractured teeth having evidence of pulp exposure, also referred to as a *complicated T/FX*. The most commonly affected tooth is the canine tooth. No treatment may be needed for uncomplicated fractures (without pulp exposure) other than monitoring. Complicated T/FXs will result in pulpitis, pulp necrosis, and periapical pathology (PA/P) (such as periapical granuloma [PA/G], periapical cyst [PA/C], or periapical abscess [PA/A]). Treatment of complicated T/FXs involves either extraction or endodontic therapy. Endodontic therapy is recommended overextraction for a fractured maxillary canine tooth to avoid upper lip ulceration owing to contact with the ipsilateral mandibular canine tooth.

Malocclusion

Malocclusion is rare in ferrets, with the exception of mild crowding of the mandibular incisors, which results in a more lingual position of the mandibular second incisors in 95.2% of rescued ferrets. This MAL does not require specific treatment, but any crowding of teeth may be associated with an increased risk of developing periodontal disease.

Periodontal Disease

Clinical evidence of periodontal disease was seen in 65.3% of rescued ferrets and 100% of client-owned ferrets. Periodontal pockets in ferrets are present if the probing depth of the gingival sulcus is >0.5 mm. Occasionally, facial swelling may be seen; this is caused by endodontic infection secondary to severe periodontal disease.

PREPARATION FOR PROCEDURES

Preanesthesia Examination

The preanesthesia examination has two parts. The first is a thorough general physical examination in preparation for anesthesia. The second is an examination of the oral cavity and associated structures to assess the type of problems that may be encountered so that appropriate equipment, instruments, and supplies can be prepared for further diagnostics and treatment. However, the conscious oral examination may not be particularly informative because of the small size of the oral cavity in small mammals and exotic pets. The use of an otoscope with an ear cone inserted into the mouth sometimes allows a degree of visualization of the teeth and surrounding tissues in tolerant lagomorph and rodent pets.

Preanesthesia Preparation

Preanesthesia preparation is an integral part of the procedure. The planned procedure and its risks are discussed with the client. An estimate of cost and procedure time should be provided so that clients do not become unnecessarily anxious during the procedure. If the client will not be present during the procedure, a contingency plan should be arranged in case any additional problems arise or are discovered during the procedure. If the client has failed to provide direction or cannot be contacted during a procedure, only the agreed-upon procedures and those necessary to maintain the patient should be performed. Antibiotics, if indicated, may be given before or during anesthesia. Preanesthesia restriction of food and water is often not required in lagomorphs or rodents because their digestive system does not ordinarily allow for the regurgitation of stomach contents. In compromised patients, even short-term nutritional restriction may be contraindicated.

Inhalant Anesthesia

Ether has been used in the past as an inhalant anesthetic, but because of its flammability and safety concerns, its use in general practice is not recommended. Isoflurane and sevoflurane are currently the inhalant anesthetics of choice for general usage in lagomorphs, rodents, and ferrets.

Anesthesia Induction

Induction of anesthesia is done in one of three ways: (1) restraint and use of injectable anesthetics, (2) restraint and masking with inhalant anesthetics, or (3) placement of the pet in an anesthesia chamber and use of inhalant anesthetics.

Anesthesia Maintenance

Maintenance of anesthesia is also typically accomplished in one of three ways: injectable anesthetics, alternating off/on masking of inhalants, or intubation for delivery of inhalants. Possible disadvantages of injectable anesthesia include administration site hair loss and abscess, prolonged recovery time, and sensitivity in chronically ill animals. The advantage of injectable anesthesia is the ability to administer it to almost any animal fairly easily. Disadvantages of strict inhalant anesthesia are potential for severe hypotension and airway irritation owing to higher concentrations of inhaled anesthetics. Once an animal is induced, the technique of alternating off/on masking, or keeping the nares covered with a small mask while working in the mouth, allows time for treatment of minor oral conditions and easily accessed incisors and other more rostrally located teeth. This technique can also be used for more complicated treatments in the mouth, but it is not necessarily recommended since it can greatly prolong procedure time because of waiting to reestablish the desired plane of anesthesia. Treatment in the oral cavity, especially the cheek teeth, is easier to perform, and recovery is usually rapid and uneventful when intubation can be accomplished.

Intubation

Intubation of lagomorphs and rodents can be difficult. Intubation of ferrets can be accomplished relatively easily with a cuffed endotracheal tube (inner diameter 2.5 mm). With practice, intubation can be accomplished in many of the small mammals and exotic pets. To avoid accidental extubation, one can also suture the endotracheal tube to the skin of the lip in addition to having it tied with umbilical tape behind the ears.

Blind Intubation

Used primarily in rabbits, chinchillas, and larger rodents, blind intubation is often the most simple and effective way of intubating these animals. The patient is usually placed in sternal recumbency. An endotracheal tube (inner diameter 2.0, 2.5, or 3.0 mm) is cut to the appropriate length depending on the animal to be intubated. A wire stylet is made with a loop on one end for easy removal from the connector end of the tube. The wire is cut so that it is approximately 1 to 2 mm short of the end of the tube. This reduces the chance of trauma to the soft tissues caused by the wire extending beyond the end of the tube. The wire is bent 1 cm from the beveled end of the endotracheal tube at a 45-degree angle. A section of umbilical tape is tied around the tube for its eventual anchorage. The tube is then inserted into the oral cavity with the bent tip contacting the roof of the mouth, causing the tip of the tube to enter the trachea. Typically, a light gagging reflex will be induced; with transparent tubes, condensation is visible with each breath. The umbilical tape should be tied behind the ears to anchor and stabilize the tube. Should the first attempt fail, another attempt should be made before attempting the next intubation technique.

Pediatric Laryngoscope

Pediatric laryngoscope blades may be used primarily in rabbits, chinchillas, larger rodents, and ferrets. The straight blade seems to provide the needed visualization for intubation more accurately than the angled blade. The lighted blade is first inserted into the mouth. The endotracheal tube with a wire stylet is introduced parallel to and outside of the blade track to maximize visualization of intubation. An alternative procedure, which is sometimes easier, is to first pass a No. 5 French urinary catheter into the trachea. The endotracheal tube is slid down over the urinary catheter, and finally, the urinary catheter is removed. The endotracheal tube should be secured by tying umbilical tape around the tube and behind the ears.

Otoscope or Endoscopic Intubation

Intubation using an otoscope with an endotracheal tube or IV catheter is primarily used with rats, hamsters, gerbils, chinchillas, and smaller lagomorphs and rodents. This form of intubation calls for the use of an ear cone in a size appropriate for the size and depth of the animal's oral cavity. The otoscope is advanced until the laryngeal area can be identified. An endotracheal tube can be advanced beside the otoscope and then into the trachea by visual placement. The plastic sheath of an IV catheter with the stylet removed may be advanced down the actual inside of the otoscope into the trachea. The otoscope and cone must then be removed without disturbing the positioning of the catheter. The use of IV catheters for intubation allows for a patent airway, but regulation of inhalant anesthesia through such small devices is suboptimal because they can quickly become blocked with mucus or debris. Therefore, their patency should be closely observed and maintained.

Stethoscope-Aided Intubation

An endotracheal tube is attached to a standard clinical stethoscope using an appropriate adapter. An elliptic hole is made in the stethoscope tubing near the attachment to the endotracheal tube. The animal is placed in sternal recumbency, and the neck is extended. The endotracheal tube is advanced into the mouth over the base of the tongue. Using the stethoscope, it is possible to identify the inspiratory and expiratory phases of respiration to accurately place the end of the tube over the epiglottis. The endotracheal tube is advanced into the trachea during inspiration. Proper placement results in a cough reflex, which is vented through the hole in the stethoscope tubing. The endotracheal tube is removed from the stethoscope and is attached to the anesthesia tubing.

Retrograde Intubation

Retrograde intubation can be used in all sizes of lagomorphs and rodents. However, this method can be traumatic and irritating to the trachea and should be used only when the two previously described techniques have failed. In this technique, a needle is inserted through the midventral neck region between two of the tracheal rings and directed toward the head. The needle should be stopped as soon as it penetrates the trachea. A monofilament suture is then passed through the needle into the trachea and gently pushed until it exits into the mouth. The end of the suture is then grasped and passed through the endotracheal tube. The tube is then slid down over the suture into the trachea. Both ends of the suture should be held firmly to provide a smooth, taut guideline for the tube. Once the tube is in the trachea, the suture and needle are removed from the neck and the endotracheal tube is adjusted to the appropriate depth.

Tracheotomy Intubation

Tracheotomy intubation may be performed in all sizes of lagomorphs and rodents. However, this method should be reserved only for special or critical cases in which intubation is absolutely required and more conservative techniques have failed. Proper clipping of the hair and disinfection of the site with surgical scrub solutions should be performed. A tracheotomy is performed by making a longitudinal skin incision over the trachea midway between the larynx and thoracic inlet. A stab incision is made between two of the tracheal rings, and the endotracheal tube is passed into the trachea and then anchored with umbilical tape, which is tied to the tube and then around the animal's neck to prevent accidental extubation.

Stabilization and Monitors

Starting at the time of premedication, the patient should be monitored closely. A spare endotracheal tube should be available for emergencies. Oxygen flow should be at a minimum of 500 mL/min, and isoflurane is set at approximately 1% to 2.5% for maintenance. Once every 2 minutes, the tube patency should be checked by light positive pressure ventilation. If moisture or mucus blocks the tube, the tube should be disconnected and an open-end tom cat catheter inserted down the tube. A syringe can be attached and light negative pressure used to remove the debris. Should patency not be immediately reestablished, the tube should be removed and the patient masked until the spare tube can be placed or the patient awakened. Pulse oximeters have been shown to be useful in lagomorphs and rodents. Knowledge of basic physiologic parameters is needed for proper monitoring (Table 14.1).

TABLE 14.1	Patient Physiologic Monitoring Data		
Species	Respiration (breaths/min)	Heart Rate (beats/min)	Body Temperature (°C)
Rabbit	32–60	130–325	38.0–39.6
Guinea pig	42–104	230–380	37.2–39.5
Chinchilla	40–65	40–100	36.1–37.8
Rat	70–115	250–450	35.9–37.5
Hamster	35–135	250–500	37.0–38.4
Gerbil	70–120	260–600	38.1–38.4

Complete Oral Examination

Once the patient has been anesthetized and monitors show the patient is stable, a detailed examination of the oral cavity is performed. This will confirm a diagnosis for an appropriate treatment plan. External palpation, jaw manipulation, and visual and radiographic examination—all play a part in an accurate diagnosis of the problem.

Palpation and Manipulation

Palpation of the head, face, jaws, neck, and throat should be carefully performed to locate any sites of swelling, discharge, or fluctuancy, which might indicate a pathologic condition. Subtle lumps under the ventrolateral aspect of the mandible can be a normal anatomic finding in some species, but prominent bony swellings may suggest periapical disease of the cheek teeth.

The jaws should be gently manipulated to examine for resistance to normal occlusal movements. Is there reasonable vertical movement, and do the edges of the maxillary and mandibular incisors meet in an appropriate scissors bite? When the lower jaw is moved from side to side in a horizontal movement, is the occlusion forced open on one side, or can crepitus be felt? If so, this suggests there is an overgrowth (elongation) of teeth on the side opposite the open bite.

Visual Examination and Aids

The use of a mouth gag, cheek retractor, tongue retractor, good lighting, and appropriate magnification can greatly enhance the visual examination (Fig. 14.20). When proper soft tissue retraction cannot be attained, visual inspection typically reveals little. While inspecting the teeth, the practitioner should look for hooks, vertical blades of enamel, uneven occlusal planes, general T/EL, increased interdental spaces between cheek teeth, gingival enlargement, and dental defects. It is common for cheek T/EL to be on the opposite side of the face to that of incisor T/EL.

Diagnostic Imaging Examination

Radiographs are highly useful diagnostic and monitoring tools for small mammals and exotic pets. The use of dental phosphor plates or sensor pads is more convenient and can give greater distinction of detail (even when used extraorally), but standard medial radiography can also be used. Helpful for small mammals and exotic pets are sizes 0, 1, 2, and 4. An intraoral technique can sometimes be used, depending on the size of the patient. A modification of the size 3 of the phosphor plates (slim plate) is useful for obtaining intraoral radiographs of the cheek teeth. The use of intraoral radiographs allows for isolation of incisor teeth and cheek teeth. The size 4 phosphor plates are used extraorally for dorsoventral or ventrodorsal, lateral, lateral oblique, and rostrocaudal views of the entire head, including dentition and TMJ. The lateral and lateral oblique views are most commonly diagnostic, revealing hooks, elongation, uneven occlusal planes, and PA/P.

Computed tomography (CT) and cone-beam CT (CT/CB) are other diagnostic imaging options for evaluation of diseases of the oral cavity and associated structures, allowing for the assessment of lesions without superimposition of other structures.

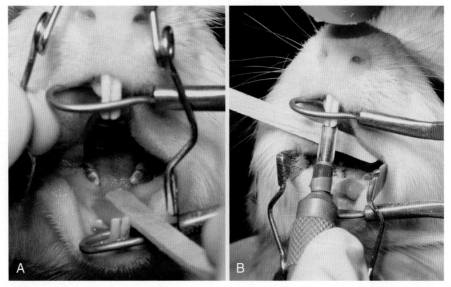

Fig. 14.20 Oral examination and occlusal equilibration in a guinea pig. (A) Mouth gag, cheek retractor, and tongue depressor allow for proper visualization of the oral cavity (odontoplasty had already been performed on the cheek teeth). (B) Low-speed handpiece, safety guard, and cylindrical diamond bur used to trim the maxillary incisors. (Copyright 2025, Alexander M. Reiter.)

However, in very small patients, CT might not have enough resolution to identify abnormalities. When CT/CB was compared to conventional CT, CT/CB was superior for the evaluation of dental structures. All of these diagnostic imaging modalities also allow for 3-D reconstruction that can make it easier to visualize lesions and explain them to the client.

CHARTING

All detected pathologic conditions should be recorded in an appropriate chart as thoroughly as possible. The use of charts customized to small mammal and exotic pet species can be helpful.

TREATMENT

Professional Dental Cleaning

Lagomorph, rodent, and ferret teeth can be cleaned in a fashion similar to that of most other species (see Chapter 7). Because of the small oral aperture and risks of fluids entering the respiratory tract, care should be taken when considering the use of water spray, particularly if the patient has not been intubated. Therefore, hand instruments or mechanical scalers that produce little heat are helpful; certain sonic scalers may meet this requirement. The teeth can be polished with a prophy cup on a low-speed HP except in very small patients where access is limited. Excess polish and debris should be cleaned from the mouth with cotton-tipped applicators.

Floating or Odontoplasty of Teeth

The term *floating* refers to creating a level occlusal surface; *occlusal equilibration* is the equivalent medical term. ODY refers to the process of recontouring a tooth surface, which is not limited to leveling an occlusal surface. Both terms are used almost interchangeably when referring to the adjustment of aradicular hypsodont teeth. Instruments used for adjustment of the teeth include tooth cutters, rasps, files, and various burs and abrasive points.

Tooth Cutters

Tooth cutters are available in two types: incisor cutters and molar cutters. They are typically either burs or edge-cutting hand instruments. The edge-cutting hand instruments should generally be used only for cutting tooth spurs and hooks at aradicular hypsodont teeth and not for attempting to actually reduce an elongated clinical crown. When used to cut teeth and reduce occlusal height, they are likely to break, crack, or shatter teeth. Dog toenail clippers should not be used for reducing tooth height.

Burs

When cutting incisors in lagomorphs and rodents, burs on a low- or high-speed HP provide a smooth, even cut, reestablishing the chisel-shaped edges, which slope caudally and toward the palatal and lingual gingiva. White stone flame-shaped points, fluted burs, carbide burs, and diamond burs all work well, although stones and diamond burs are inherently less aggressive and thus safer. Edge-cutting hand instruments should be used with caution because shattering and crushing of the teeth are common. These should be used on incisors only to remove spurs or hooks and not to reduce actual tooth height.

When dealing with cheek teeth in lagomorphs and rodents, high-speed HPs are difficult to use efficiently and safely because of the right angle and short shank of the bur. A low-speed HP with a straight HP carbide or diamond bur is useful with careful attention (using a safety guard) to avoid damage to the tongue, gingiva, or alveolar, sublingual, and buccal mucosa.

Rasps and files. Rasps and files can be used to gradually reduce the clinical crowns of cheek teeth in lagomorphs and rodents, while also recontouring them into a reasonable reestablishment of the proper occlusal table angulation (Fig. 14.21). Files cut primarily on the pull stroke. Rasps usually cut on both the push and pull strokes, which may result in a more rapid reduction of the tooth surface. Diamond-coated rasps are particularly helpful, although they do not cut as aggressively as other instruments. Care should be taken in the push stroke on mandibular cheek teeth, particularly in rabbits, where trauma to a branch of the

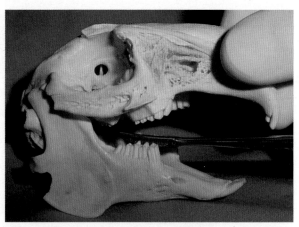

Fig. 14.21 Demonstration of a diamond-coated rasp being used on the right mandibular cheek teeth of a rabbit skull. (Copyright 2025, Alexander M. Reiter.)

inferior alveolar vessels can occur beneath the caudal oral mucosa, resulting in rapid and unexpected bleeding.

Abscess Treatment

Diseased teeth may develop jaw abscesses (periodontal, periapical, or a combination of periodontal-periapical abscesses). Medical therapy alone is extremely unlikely to result in a favorable long-term outcome. Most dental abscesses are detected by the clients usually on the face or lower jaw.

Periodontal Abscesses

Abscesses of this nature are typically caused by food or other debris being forced into the periodontal ligament space of a tooth. This results in an abscess along the gingival or alveolar mucosal surface adjacent to the tooth. The abscess is lanced and debrided, systemic antibiotics may be initiated, and the causative substances should be removed from the diet. Stemmy hays and roughage are often found within these lesions.

Periapical Abscesses

Periapical abscesses frequently result from some form of trauma that has exposed the pulp and resulted in devitalization of the tooth. Root canal therapy (RCT) can be performed on these teeth,

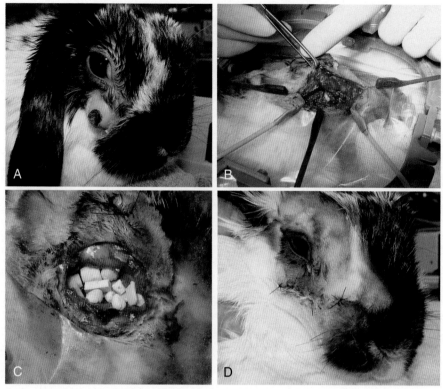

Fig. 14.22 Abscess in a rabbit. (A) Right-sided facial swelling. (B) Incision, removal of abscess capsule, and debridement and lavage of the wound. (C) Placement of antibiotic-impregnated beads. (D) Wound closure. (Copyright 2025, Alexander M. Reiter.)

but long-term success in aradicular hypsodont teeth is rare. Extraction is usually the most prudent approach to treatment. The tooth should be extracted and the fistulous tract debrided. In addition to the treatment of the tooth/teeth of origin, the treatment of the abscess includes removal of the abscess capsule, debridement and lavage of the wound, suturing of the intraoral tissues, and possibly leaving a portion of the surgical site open externally MAR to allow for postoperative lavage and second intention healing. In some cases, the abscess may have caused considerable bone loss, and fracture of the jaw is possible during extraction. Placement of antibiotic-impregnated beads may be considered in some cases where the surgical site is closed primarily (Fig. 14.22). If the wound is left open externally, a paste or slurry form of an antibiotic, such as ampicillin, clindamycin, tetracycline, doxycycline or minocycline, can be placed into the surgical site and replaced every 2 weeks until the defect heals from the inside out by second intention. The patient may be placed on postoperative antibiotics, especially if the surgical site is left open for drainage and flushing and if remaining bone is significantly diseased.

Periodontal-Periapical Abscesses

Periodontal-periapical abscesses occur owing to the extension of periodontal disease apically to enter the pulp of a fractured or worn tooth with pulp exposure. Treatment is similar to that described for periapical abscesses.

Extractions

Extractions can be broken down into two categories depending on whether the tooth is an incisor

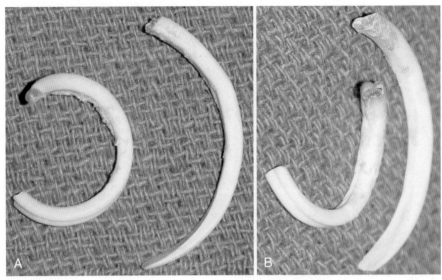

Fig. 14.23 Extracted rabbit first incisors. (A) Lateral view. (B) Apicolateral view. Note the difference in curvature of the maxillary incisor (on the left of each image) versus the mandibular incisor (on the right of each image). (Copyright 2025, Alexander M. Reiter.)

or a cheek tooth. Each type of extraction requires different techniques and equipment.

Incisor Teeth

Incisor teeth in ferrets usually are removed in a closed fashion (i.e., without creating a flap). Because of the highly curved reserve crown structure and the fragile nature of incisor teeth in lagomorphs and rodents, the use of appropriate technique and equipment is required (Fig. 14.23). Most of the strength of the periodontal ligament holding the tooth in place is found in the gingival third of the reserve crown and on the mesial surface. This means the primary area to be elevated is the reserve crown near the gingival surface. Curved hypodermic needles sometimes can be quite useful for this purpose. The 18- to 22-gauge 1½ inch needle has been used for many years in rabbits. However, the No. 1 and No. 2 winged elevators and specific ("Crossley") rabbit luxators are well designed for this function. Elevation of the tooth is achieved by pressing the elevator into the periodontal ligament space between the tooth and alveolar bone and gently rotating it. These incisor teeth are fragile, especially in the apical portion of their reserve crowns. Once the teeth are loosened, extraction forceps can be used to grasp the tooth and remove it. The operator should recall that the tooth curves in an arch and the extraction pull must be made in that same circular plane. Once the tooth has been extracted, the alveolus (A) is debrided and rinsed, and the gingiva is sutured with absorbable material.

Teeth broken during extraction must be evaluated carefully. They are generally categorized as nondiseased and diseased. Nondiseased teeth with no preexisting infection, such as teeth being extracted because of an atraumatic MAL, may have a growth center at the apex that is intact and active. If this is the case, the tooth will typically regrow in 1 to 4 months, and a second attempt at extraction can be made at that time, if still needed. Diseased teeth are characterized by preexisting infection, pulp exposure, abscess, or traumatic MAL. Most are associated with some form of trauma to the tooth or gums. Should an infected T/FX during extraction, every reasonable attempt should be made to retrieve the entire tooth because the remaining portion usually continues to cause problems. If the segment cannot be removed, local or systemic antibiotics may be warranted. If the retained piece of reserve crown continues to cause problems, a surgical approach will be necessary to remove it and debride the wound.

Canine Teeth in Ferrets

Canine teeth in ferrets are found on oral examination to exhibit fractures with pulp exposure owing to their long, thin crown shape. Fractured teeth with pulp exposure can be treated by performing RCT or extraction. RCT is performed through the fracture site and is preferred to extraction in ferrets, particularly for fractured maxillary canine teeth. Similar to cats, extraction of the maxillary canine tooth in a ferret allows the upper lip to fall into a more medial position, resulting in upper lip trauma from the sharp cusp of the ipsilateral mandibular canine tooth (Fig. 14.24). If extraction of

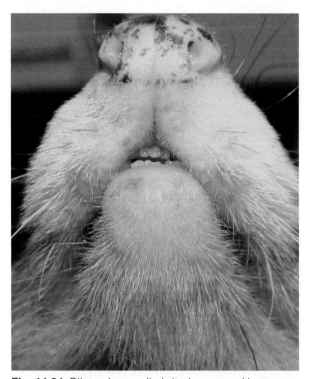

Fig. 14.24 Bilateral upper lip irritation caused by trauma from the opposing mandibular canine teeth noticed 24 hours after extraction of the maxillary canine teeth in a ferret. (Copyright 2025, Alexander M. Reiter.)

a ferret canine tooth is necessary, care is taken to raise a mucoperiosteal flap, and a stay suture is placed in the extremely thin flap to retract it and avoid trauma with forceps. Bone is removed over the labial aspect of the canine tooth with a No. 1 or 2 round carbide bur attached to a water-cooled high-speed HP. After elevation of the tooth, the alveolus is debrided, and the site is closed with 5-0 absorbable suture in a simple interrupted pattern. In the case of maxillary canine tooth extraction, careful ODY of the cusp of the ipsilateral mandibular canine tooth followed by sealing of exposed dentinal tubules may help to decrease trauma to the upper lip, but only approximately 1 mm may be removed before risking iatrogenic pulp exposure.

Cheek Teeth

Brachyodont cheek teeth of rats, mice, and ferrets are usually easier to extract than the aradicular hypsodont cheek teeth of lagomorphs, guinea pigs, and chinchillas. In ferrets, closed and open extraction techniques can be employed similar to what is done in cats (Fig. 14.25). In rats and mice, the No. 2 Molt surgical elevator and an 18- to 22-gauge 1½ inch needle bent at a 90-degree angle work reasonably well as elevators for intraoral extraction of brachyodont cheek teeth. Aradicular hypsodont cheek teeth have a more complex and deeper reserve crown structure compared to the roots of brachyodont teeth. Therefore, extractions are usually more difficult. However, the same basic techniques as previously described for brachyodont teeth can be used, but tooth repelling or even buccotomy (BUC) may also be required. BUC is a full-thickness incision through the skin, mucosa, and subcutaneous tissue to allow for direct visualization and the ability to treat cheek teeth. In many smaller rodents, suturing the extraction site may not be possible because of lack of access.

Tooth repelling (XSS/RPL) is the procedure of making an access hole below the tooth and pressing a small, blunt metal rod against the bottom of the tooth to push it into the oral cavity. Often with diseased teeth, only light hand pressure is required

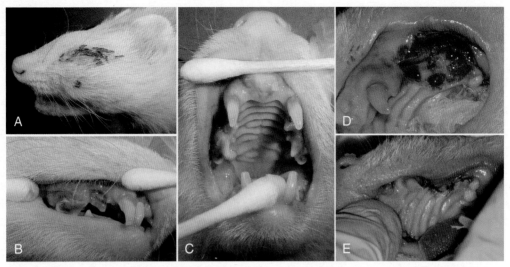

Fig. 14.25 Tooth extraction in a ferret. (A) Periorbital swelling/bleeding at the left eye and sinus tract formation at the left upper lip skin. (B and C) Note the use of cotton-tipped applicators to retract lips/cheeks and open the mouth for conscious oral examination. (D) Maxillary cheek teeth removed using an open extraction technique. (E) Wound closure. (Copyright 2025, Alexander M. Reiter.)

to accomplish the repelling of the tooth into the mouth. Alternatively, the cheek tooth can sometimes be retrieved through an extraoral incision through the skin, subcutaneous tissue, and oral mucosa, thus allowing tooth extraction by means of a commissurotomy (XSS/COM) or buccotomy (XSS/BUC) and if needed with alveolectomy (XSS/COM/ALV and XSS/BUC/ALV). This procedure can leave permanent scars, which some clients may find objectionable. Because many of these species actively use the cheek pouch during eating and may store food in the pouch, complications of infection and dehiscence of the suture line may occur.

Vital Pulp Therapy

Vital pulp therapy, performed to maintain tooth vitality, may be required when injury or iatrogenic action causes exposure of the pulp. Any instrument or material coming in contact with exposed pulp tissue must be sterile. The site of exposure should be cleaned with lactated Ringer's solution. The coronal portion of the pulp is removed with a small round carbide bur or a small round diamond bur on a high-speed HP (partial pulpectomy). A paper point is dipped into a dappen dish of lactated Ringer's solution. The moistened end is then dipped into a dappen dish of calcium hydroxide powder. The powder adheres to the paper point, which is then placed into the pulp chamber of the injured tooth until it contacts the pulp. The paper point is then gently tapped against the pulp to place a small coating of the calcium hydroxide on the pulp (direct pulp capping). Newer pulp capping materials include mineral trioxide aggregate, biodentine, and nano-hydroxyapatite. The walls of the access site are cleaned, and a restorative, such as a glass ionomer or reinforced zinc-oxide eugenol cement, is placed over the exposure to seal the tooth (restoration).

Tooth Fillings

Because of the small size of the teeth generally involved, restoratives that easily bond to enamel and dentin are preferred for fillings. Among these are materials, such as the glass ionomers, reinforced zinc-oxide eugenol cements, and composites.

Glass ionomers are used for restoration in lagomorphs and rodents. The dental lesions should be prepared and the glass ionomer applied according to the manufacturer's recommendations. Composites, when used with bonding agents, are also well suited for use in lagomorphs, rodents, and ferrets, although they are more technique-sensitive than glass ionomers. Composites that flow easily are often less difficult to apply in the restricted space of these small oral cavities. Reinforced or macro-fill composites should be avoided in lagomorphs and rodents because their wear pattern might be slower than that of the associated tooth structure.

Drug Treatment

Various antibiotics and other drugs are used in treatment the dosages of which must be calculated not only by weight but also by species. CAUTION: Some lagomorphs and rodents are sensitive to certain antibiotics; some drugs may even cause death. In rabbits, hamsters, and guinea pigs, the potential

of fatal colitis caused by the use of antibiotics, especially oral antibiotics, is always present. Therefore, antibiotics should be carefully selected and dosages checked before administering.

Home-Care Instructions

Clients should closely observe food and water intake during the first 4 hours after recovery from surgery in lagomorphs and rodents. Seriously ill patients may be reluctant to eat and drink after dental and oral surgical procedures. If the patient fails to ingest food and water within the first 4 hours after treatment, hand feeding with liquid concentrates and water should be instituted until normal intake resumes. Prolonged inappetence is generally an indication of a more severe secondary problem, which may require administration of fluids, antibiotics, antiinflammatory medications, and other supportive care and treatments.

CHAPTER 14 WORKSHEET (ANSWERS ARE ON PAGE 296)

1. Rabbits, chinchillas, and guinea pigs have _____ incisor and cheek teeth that continually grow and erupt throughout the animal's life and never form roots, whereas rats and mice may have _____ incisor and _____ cheek teeth.
2. Rabbits, chinchillas, and guinea pigs have a _____ dentition, consisting of _____, _____, and _____ teeth but no _____ teeth.
3. Continual growth and eruption of aradicular hypsodont teeth may be possible by a special anatomical feature of the periodontal ligament known as the _____.
4. _____ is a term describing the discrepancy of widths of the upper and lower dental arches.
5. Healthy _____ have a relatively steep angulation (~30 degrees from dorsobuccal to ventrolingual) to the occlusal plane of the cheek teeth, whereas healthy _____ have a level occlusal plane.
6. The _____ on the labial surfaces of the incisor teeth in most rodents takes on a yellow/orange color; an exception is seen in the _____.
7. Hourglass-shaped maxillary _____ are a common dental finding in the family of _____.
8. Malocclusions in lagomorphs and rodents are generally grouped into two categories: _____ or _____.
9. Tongue entrapment is commonly seen in the _____ when mandibular _____ elongate intraorally to meet in the midline.
10. The condition in which excess drooling saliva results in a moist dermatitis is often referred to as _____.
11. For how long should food and water be restricted in lagomorphs and rodents prior to anesthesia? ____ hours.
12. Carelessly pushing a rasp or file caudally along mandibular cheek teeth in _____ can cause trauma to the _____, resulting in profuse _____.

13. The extraction of a maxillary canine tooth in a ferret may result in long-term trauma to the ipsilateral _____.
14. When performing vital pulp therapy, any instrument or material contacting exposed pulp tissue must be _____.
15. If a lagomorph or rodent fails to ingest food and water within the first ____ hours after an anesthetic procedure, hand feeding with liquid concentrates and water should be instituted until normal intake resumes.

FURTHER READING

Benato L, Rooney NJ, Murrell JC. Pain and analgesia in pet rabbits within the veterinary environment: a review. *Vet Anaesth Analg*. 2019;46(2):151–162. doi:10.1016/j.vaa.2018.10.007.

Böhmer C, Böhmer E. Shape variation in the craniomandibular system and prevalence of dental problems in domestic rabbits: a case study in evolutionary veterinary science. *Vet Sci*. 2017;4(1):5. doi:10.3390/vetsci4010005.

Böhmer C, Böhmer E. Skull shape diversity in pet rabbits and the applicability of anatomical reference lines for objective interpretation of dental disease. *Vet Sci*. 2020;7(4):182. doi:10.3390/vetsci7040182.

Böhmer E, Crossley D. Objective interpretation of dental disease in rabbits, guinea pigs and chinchillas. Use of anatomical reference lines. *Tierarztl Prax*. 2009;37:250–260.

Böhmer E. *Dentistry in Rabbits and Rodents*. Ames, Iowa: John Wiley & Sons, Ltd. 2015.

Brown T, Beaufrère H, Brisson B, et al. Ventral rhinotomy in a pet rabbit (*Oryctolagus cuniculus*) with an odontogenic abscess and sub-obstructive rhinitis. *Can Vet J*. 2016;57(8):873–878.

Capello V, Cauduro A. Comparison of diagnostic consistency and diagnostic accuracy between survey radiography and computed tomography of the skull in 30 rabbits with dental disease. *J Exot Pet Med*. 2016;25:115–127.

Capello V, Gracis M, Lennox AM. *Rabbit and Rodent Dentistry Handbook*. Lake Forth, FL: Zoological Education Network; 2005.

Capello V, Lennox A, Ghisleni G. Elodontoma in two guinea pigs. *J Vet Dent*. 2015;32:111–119. doi:10.1177/089875641503200205.

Capello V, Lennox A. Advanced diagnostic imaging and surgical treatment of an odontogenic retromasseteric abscess in a guinea pig. *J Small Anim Pract*. 2015;56:134–137. doi:10.1111/jsap.12249.

Capello V. Diagnostic imaging of dental disease in pet rabbits and rodents. *Vet Clin Exot Anim*. 2016;19:757–782. doi:10.1016/j.cvex.2016.05.001.

Capello V. Intraoral treatment of dental disease in pet rabbits. *Vet Clin North Am Exot Anim Pract*. 2016;19:783–798. doi:10.1016/j.cvex.2016.05.002.

Capello V. Surgical treatment of facial abscesses and facial surgery in pet rabbits. *Vet Clin Exot Anim*. 2016;19:799–823. doi:10.1016/j.cvex.2016.04.010.

Cox PG, Fagan MJ, Rayfield EJ, et al. Finite element modelling of squirrel, guinea pig and rat skulls: using geometric morphometrics to assess sensitivity. *J Anat*. 2011;219:696–709. doi:10.1111/j.1469-7580.2011.01436.x.

Cox PG, Jeffery N. Reviewing the morphology of the jaw-closing musculature in squirrels, rats, and guinea pigs with contrast-enhanced microCT. *Anat Rec*. 2011;294:915–928. doi:10.1002/ar.21381.

Crossley DA, Dubielzig RR, Benson KG. Caries and odontoclastic resorptive lesions in a chinchilla (*Chinchilla lanigera*). *Vet Rec*. 1997;141:337–339. doi:10.1136/vr.141.13.337.

Crossley DA, Jackson A, Yates J, et al. Use of computed tomography to investigate cheek tooth abnormalities in chinchillas (*Chinchilla laniger*). *J Small Anim Pract*. 1998;39:385–389. doi:10.1111/j.1748-5827.1998.tb03737.x.

Crossley DA, Miguélez MM. Skull size and cheek-tooth length in wild-caught and captive-bred chinchillas. *Arch Oral Biol*. 2001;46:919–928. doi:10.1016/s0003-9969(01)00055-3.

Crossley DA. Clinical aspects of lagomorph dental anatomy: the rabbit (*Oryctolagus cuniculus*). *J Vet Dent*. 1995;12(4):137–140.

Crossley DA. Clinical aspects of rodent dental anatomy. *J Vet Dent*. 1995;12(4):131–135.

Crossley DA. Dental disease in chinchillas in the UK. *J Small Anim Pract*. 2001;42:12–19. doi:10.1111/j.1748-5827.2001.tb01977.x.

Crossley DA. Oral biology and disorders of lagomorphs. *Vet Clin North Am Exot Anim Pract.* 2003;6:629–659. doi:10.1016/s1094-9194(03)00034-3.

De Rycke LM, Boone MN, Van Caelenberg AI, et al. Micro-computed tomography of the head and dentition in cadavers of clinically normal rabbits. *Am J Vet Res.* 2012;73:227–232. doi:10.2460/ajvr.73.2.227.

Donnelly TM, Vella D. Anatomy, physiology and non-dental disorders of the mouth of pet rabbits. *Vet Clin Exot Anim.* 2016;19:737–756. doi:10.1016/j.cvex.2016.04.004.

d'Ovidio D, Rossi G, Meomartino L. Oral malignant melanoma in a ferret (*Mustela putorius furo*). *J Vet Dent.* 2016;33:108–111. doi:10.1177/0898756416654028.

Eroshin V, Reiter AM, Rosenthal K, et al. Oral examination results in rescued ferrets: clinical findings. *J Vet Dent.* 2011;28:8–15. doi:10.1177/089875641102800102.

Gardhouse S, Sanchez-Migallon Guzman D, Paul-Murphy J, et al. Bacterial isolates and antimicrobial susceptibilities from odontogenic abscesses in rabbits: 48 cases. *Vet Rec.* 2017;181(20):538. doi:10.1136/vr.103996.

Gardhouse S, Sanchez-Migallon Guzman D, Petritz OA, et al. Diagnosis and treatment of sialectasis in domestic rabbit (*Oryctolagus cuniculus*). *J Exot Pet Med.* 2016;25:72–79.

Gracis M. Clinical technique: normal dental radiography of rabbits, guinea pigs, and chinchillas. *J Exot Pet Med.* 2008;17:78–86.

Graham J, Fidel J, Mison M. Rostral maxillectomy and radiation therapy to manage squamous cell carcinoma in a ferret. *Vet Clin North Am Exot Anim Pract.* 2006;9:701–706. doi:10.1016/j.cvex.2006.05.008.

Hatai H, Kido N, Ochiai K. Multilobular tumor of bone on the forehead of a guinea pig. *J Vet Diagn Invest.* 2020;32:747–749. doi:10.1177/1040638720941507.

He T, Friede H, Kiliaridis S. Dental eruption and exfoliation chronology in the ferret (*Mustela putorius furo*). *Arch Oral Biol.* 2002;47:619–623. doi:10.1016/s0003-9969(02)00043-2.

He T, Friede H, Kiliaridis S. Macroscopic and roentgenographic anatomy of the skull of the ferret (*Mustela putorius furo*). *Lab Anim.* 2002;36:86–96. doi:10.1258/0023677021911795.

Hong IH, Lee HS, Park JK, et al. Actinomycosis in a pet rabbit. *J Vet Dent.* 2009;26:110–111. doi:10.1177/089875640902600206.

Jekl V, Gumpenberger M, Jeklova E, et al. Impact of pelleted diets with different mineral compositions on the crown size of mandibular cheek teeth and mandibular relative density in degus (*Octodon degus*). *Vet Rec.* 2011;168(24):641. doi:10.1136/vr.d2012.

Jekl V, Hauptman K, Jeklova E, et al. Dental eruption chronology in degus (*Octodon degus*). *J Vet Dent.* 2011;28:16–20. doi:10.1177/089875641102800103.

Jekl V, Hauptman K, Knotek Z. Quantitative and qualitative assessments of intraoral lesions in 180 small herbivorous mammals. *Vet Rec.* 2008;62:442–449. doi:10.1136/vr.162.14.442.

Jekl V, Knotek Z. Evaluation of a laryngoscope and a rigid endoscope for the examination of the oral cavity of small mammals. *Vet Rec.* 2007;160:9–13. doi:10.1136/vr.160.1.9.

Jekl V, Krejcirova L, Buchtova M, et al. Effect of high phosphorus diet on tooth microstructure of rodent incisors. *Bone.* 2011;49:479–484. doi:10.1016/j.bone.2011.04.021.

Jekl V, Redrobe S. Rabbit dental disease and calcium metabolism. The science behind divided opinions. *J Small Anim Pract.* 2013;54:481–490.

Johnson-Delaney CA. Anatomy and disorders of the oral cavity of ferrets and other exotic companion carnivores. *Vet Clin North Am Exot Anim Pract.* 2016;19:901–928. doi:10.1016/j.cvex.2016.04.009.

Kido N, Ono K, Omiya T, et al. Extraction of an incisor embedded within the nasal cavity in two guinea pigs. *J Vet Med Sci.* 2016;77:1651–1653. doi:10.1292/jvms.15-0283.

King AM, Cranfield F, Hall J, et al. Radiographic anatomy of the rabbit skull with particular reference to the tympanic bulla and temporomandibular joint: part 1: Lateral and long axis rotational angles. *Vet J.* 2010;186:232–243. doi:10.1016/j.tvjl.2009.09.002.

King AM, Cranfield F, Hall J, et al. Radiographic anatomy of the rabbit skull, with particular reference to the tympanic bulla and temporomandibular joint. Part 2: ventral and dorsal rotational angles. *Vet J.* 2010;186:244–251. doi:10.1016/j.tvjl.2009.07.022.

Legendre L. Anatomy and disorders of the oral cavity of guinea pigs. *Vet Clin Exot Anim.* 2016;16:825–842. doi:10.1016/j.cvex.2016.04.006.

Legendre L. Oral examination and occlusal equilibration in rodents and lagomorphs. *J Vet Dent.* 2011;28:52–57. doi:10.1177/089875641102800113.

Legendre L. Rodent and lagomorph tooth extractions. *J Vet Dent.* 2012;29:204–209. doi:10.1177/089875641202900315.

Legendre L. Treatment of oral abscesses in rodents and lagomorphs. *J Vet Dent.* 2011;28:30–33. doi:10.1177/089875641102800106.

Legendre LF. Malocclusions in guinea pigs, chinchillas and rabbits. *Can Vet J.* 2002;43:385–390.

Legendre LF. Oral disorders of exotic rodents. *Vet Clin North Am Exot Anim Pract.* 2003;6:601–628. doi:10.1016/s1094-9194(03)00041-0.

Long CV. Common dental disorders of the degu (*Octodon degus*). *J Vet Dent.* 2012;29:158–165. doi:10.1177/089875641202900304.

Mancinelli E, Capello V. Anatomy and disorders of the oral cavity of rat-like and squirrel-like rodents. *Vet Clin Exot Anim.* 2016;19:871–900. doi:10.1016/j.cvex.2016.04.008.

Mans C, Jekl V. Anatomy and disorders of the oral cavity of chinchillas and degus. *Vet Clin Exot Anim.* 2016;19:843–869. doi:10.1016/j.cvex.2016.04.007.

Martin LF, Winkler D, Tütken T, et al. The way wear goes: phytolith-based wear on the dentine-enamel system in guinea pigs (*Cavia porcellus*). *Proc Biol Sci.* 2019;286(1912):20191921. doi:10.1098/rspb.2019.1921.

Mehrani Y, Kazemi Mehrjerdi H, et al. Effects of probiotic *Lactobacilli plantarum* in treatment of experimentally induced periodontal disease in rabbits. *J Vet Dent.* 2024;41(3):210–216. doi:10.1177/08987564231163193.

Meredith AL, Prebble JL, Shaw DJ. Impact of diet on incisor growth and attrition and the development of dental disease in pet rabbits. *J Small Anim Pract.* 2015;56:377–382.

Minarikova A, Fictum P, Zikmund T, et al. Dental disease and periodontitis in a guinea pig (*Cavia porcellus*). *J Exot Pet Med.* 2016;25:150–156.

Minarikova A, Hauptman K, Jeklova E, et al. Diseases in pet guinea pigs: a retrospective study in 1000 animals. *Vet Rec.* 2015;177(8):200. doi:10.1136/vr.103053.

Minarikova A, Hauptman K, Knotek Z, Jekl V. Microbial flora of odontogenic abscesses in pet guinea pigs. *Vet Rec.* 2016;179(13):331. doi:10.1136/vr.103551.

Miwa Y, Nakata M, Takimoto H, et al. Spontaneous oral tumours in 18 rabbits (2005–2015). *J Small Anim Pract.* 2021;62:156–160. doi:10.1111/jsap.13082.

Müller J, Clauss M, Codron D, et al. Growth and wear of incisor and cheek teeth in domestic rabbits (*Oryctolagus cuniculus*) fed diets of different abrasiveness. *J Exp Zool.* 2014;321A:283–298. doi:10.1002/jez.1864.

Nemec A, Zadravec M, Raonik J. Oral and dental diseases in a population of domestic ferrets (*Mustela putorius furo*). *J Small Anim Pract.* 2016;57:553–560. doi:10.1111/jsap.12546.

Norman R, Wills A. An investigation into the relationship between owner knowledge, diet, and dental disease in guinea pig (*Cavia porcellus*). *Animals.* 2016;6:73. doi:10.3390/ani6110073.

Okuda A, Hori Y, Ichihara N, et al. Comparative observation of skeletal-dental abnormalities in wild, domestic, and laboratory rabbits. *J Vet Dent.* 2007;24:224–229. doi:10.1177/089875640702400403.

O'Neill DG, Craven HC, Brodbelt DC, et al. Morbidity and mortality of domestic rabbits (*Oryctolagus cuniculus*) under primary veterinary care in England. *Vet Rec.* 2020;186(14):451. doi:10.1136/vr.105592.

Primožič PK, Žagar Ž, Šmalc K, Račnik J, Švara T, Nemec A. Follow up on simple (closed) extraction of fractured maxillary canine teeth in domestic ferrets (*Mustela putorius furo*). *Front Vet Sci.* 2021;8:677680. doi:10.3389/fvets.2021.677680.

Regalado A, Legendre L. Full-mouth intraoral radiographic survey in rabbits. *J Vet Dent.* 2017;34:190–200. doi:10.1177/0898756417723145.

Reiter AM. Pathophysiology of dental disease in the rabbit, guinea pig and chinchilla. *J Exotic Pet Med.* 2008;17:70–77.

Riggs GG, Arzi B, Cissell, et al. Clinical application of cone-beam computed tomography of the rabbit head: part 1—normal dentition. *Front Vet Sci.* 2016;3:93. doi:10.3389/fvets.2016.00093.

Riggs GG, Cissell DD, Arzi B, et al. Clinical application of cone beam computed tomography of the rabbit head: part 2—dental disease. *Front Vet Sci.* 2017;4:5. doi:10.3389/fvets.2017.00005

Roux P. Extraction of the incisors in a dwarf rabbit. *Schweiz Arch Tierheilkd.* 2005;147:311–313. doi:10.1024/0036-7281.147.7.311.

Sasai H, Iwai H, Fujita D, et al. The use of micro-computed tomography in the diagnosis of dental and oral disease in rabbits. *BMC Vet Res.* 2014;10:209. doi:10.1186/s12917-014-0209-4.

Schulz E, Piotrowski V, Clauss M, Mau M, Merceron G, Kaiser TM. Dietary abrasiveness is associated with variability of microwear and dental surface texture in rabbits. *PLoS One.* 2013;8(2):e56167. doi:10.1371/journal.pone.0056167.

Schumacher M. Measurement of clinical crown length of incisor and premolar teeth in clinically healthy rabbits. *J Vet Dent.* 2011;28:90–95. doi:10.1177/089875641102800205.

Schweda MC, Hassan J, Böhler A, et al. The role of computed tomography in the assessment of dental disease in 66 guinea pigs. *Vet Rec.* 2014;175:538–543. doi:10.1136/vr.101469.

Steenkamp G, Crossley DA. Incisor tooth regrowth in a rabbit following complete extraction. *Vet Rec.* 1999;145:585–586. doi:10.1136/vr.145.20.585.

Tanaka M, Sawamoto O. Spontaneous ameloblastic fibroma in a young Guinea pig. *J Toxicol Pathol.* 2013;26:325–328. doi:10.1293/tox.26.325.

Taylor M, Beaufrere H, Mans C, et al. Long-term outcome of treatment of dental abscesses with a wound-packing technique in pet rabbits: 13 cases. *J Am Vet Med Assoc.* 2010;237:1444–1449. doi:10.2460/javma.237.12.1444.

Tyrrell KL, Citron DM, Jenkins JR, et al. Periodontal bacteria in rabbit mandibular and maxillary abscesses. *J Clin Microbiol.* 2002;40:1044–1047. doi:10.1128/JCM.40.3.1044-1047.2002.

Van Caelenberg A, De Rycke LM, Hermans K, et al. Comparison of radiography and CT to identify changes in the skulls of four rabbits. *J Vet Dent.* 2011;28:172–181. doi:10.1177/089875641102800304.

Van Caelenberg AI, De Rycke LM, Hermans K, et al. Computed tomography and cross-sectional anatomy of the head in healthy rabbits. *Am J Vet Res.* 2010;71:293–303. doi:10.2460/ajvr.71.3.293.

Van Caelenberg AI, De Rycke LM, Hermans K, et al. Low-field magnetic resonance imaging and cross-sectional anatomy of the rabbit head. *Vet J.* 2011;188:83–91. doi:10.1016/j.tvjl.2010.02.020.

Villano JS, Cooper TK. Mandibular fracture and necrotizing sialometaplasia in a rabbit. *Comp Med.* 2013;63:67–70.

Whitten KA, Popielarczyk MM, Belote DA, et al. Ossifying fibroma in a miniature rex rabbit (*Oryctolagus cuniculus*). *Vet Pathol.* 2006;43:62–64. doi:10.1354/vp.43-1-62.

Winkler DE, Schulz-Kornas E, Kaiser TM, et al. Forage silica and water content control dental surface texture in guinea pigs and provide implications for dietary reconstruction. *Proc Natl Acad Sci USA.* 2019;116:1325–1330. doi:10.1073/pnas.1814081116.

Winkler DE, Tütken T, Schulz-Kornas E, et al. Shape, size, and quantity of ingested external abrasives influence dental microwear texture formation in guinea pigs. *Proc Natl Acad Sci USA.* 2020;117:22264–22273. doi:10.1073/pnas.2008149117.

Witt S, Köstlinger S, Fehr M. Extraction of diseased mandibular incisors in the guinea pig (*Cavia porcellus*) via ventral mandibular trepanation. *Tierarztl Prax Ausg K Kleintiere Heimtiere.* 2021;49:415–424. doi:10.1055/a-1617-5180.

Wong HE, Hedley J, Stapleton N, et al. Odontoameloblastoma with extensive chondroid matrix deposition in a guinea pig. *J Vet Diagn Invest.* 2018;30:793–797. doi:10.1177/1040638718794784.

Wyss F, Muller J, Clauss M, et al. Measuring rabbit (*Oryctolagus cuniculus*) tooth growth and eruption by fluorescence markers and bur marks. *J Vet Dent.* 2016;33:39–46. doi:10.1177/0898756416640956.

Team Approach to Communication

KEY TERMS

ARA
check off list

informed consent
master problem list

SOAP format medical records

Teams who are excellent at communication tend to perform routine operations at a higher level and are better prepared when situations become nonroutine. Effective communication between all members of the veterinary team results in better patient care and fewer medical errors. Assuring communications with clients are clear and complete increases client satisfaction and improves medical compliance. Clear communication between medical care providers, such as between the general care provider and the specialist, prevents the loss of critical pieces of a patient's continued care.

VETERINARY TEAM COMMUNICATION

For the veterinary team to be able to communicate effectively regarding patient healthcare, each member needs to understand the basics of the disease process and the goals of the treatment. This includes not only the team members providing direct patient care but also those indirectly involved such as the client service team and management team.

Granted, those not providing direct care do not need to have the same level of knowledge and skills that the doctors and technicians need. However, if they understand the basics of common diseases, the benefits of prevention and treatment, and the fundamental process of providing care, the support team can better communicate with clients, vendors, and other veterinary professionals. Together the support team can help provide a united front in the care of the pet.

The medical team (doctors, technicians, and assistants) need to have a stronger grasp of medical terminology to effectively communicate a patient's medical needs. Although it may seem onerous to learn and use, the use of a common language allows the medical team to communicate easily and efficiently. The ability and discipline to use proper medical terminology can prevent delays in treatment due to confusion in communication. For example, in surgery, a doctor realizes that he or she needs a curved hemostatic forceps due to an unexpected hemorrhage. But instead of specifically asking for that specific item, he or she instead asks for a "clamp." Now, the surgical assistant must take time to first decipher that a "clamp" is a hemostatic forceps and then decide which type of forceps to retrieve and present to the doctor. If fortune is on their side, the assistant can read the doctor's mind and grab just the right instrument. However, the assistant may present a large Rochester Carmalt forceps, which may be too large in this case, delaying necessary treatment. In this scenario, delayed treatment results in continued hemorrhage and patient morbidity. Another example is the use of abbreviated words that are like other abbreviated words, such as "dex." For some, "dex" indicates dexamethasone, and for others, dexmedetomidine. Consider a patient in need of dexamethasone as an adjunct treatment for an Addisonian crisis, but instead of ordering 4 mg of dexamethasone intravenously, he or she asks for 4 mg of "dex" given intravenously. The technician may interpret this as 4 mg of dexmedetomidine intravenously, thus sedating an already compromised patient with what most would consider an excessively high dosage of sedative.

In addition to using proper terminology, using precise language is important. This includes objective measurements with appropriate units of measurement. In dentistry, often times records will indicate a patient has "deep periodontal pockets." This would indicate any periodontal probing depth greater than 3 mm in a dog. The prognosis and treatment for a 5-mm periodontal pocket of the palatal side of a maxillary canine tooth is very different from a 12-mm pocket of the same side. While one can be treated with closed root planing, the other may indicate an oronasal fistula and necessitate extraction.

Great communication is not solely using correct and precise words. It also includes a discussion of what is expected during a medical procedure. In dentistry, this typically includes general anesthesia, often on patients with comorbidities. If the anesthetist and doctor discuss that patient's likely anesthetic challenges, it helps the anesthetist prepare

BOX 15.1	Anesthetic Risk Assessment
Anesthetic Status	**Description**
1	Patient without systemic illness
2	Patient with mild systemic illness
3	Patient with moderate systemic illness but is still active
4	Patient with severe systemic illness
5	Moribund patient who will not survive without surgery

Modified from the American Society of Anesthesiologists. asahq.org. https://www.asahq.org/standards-and-practice-parameters/statement-on-asa-physical-status-classification-system.

to address the complications and helps instill confidence. Ultimately, delays in care are reduced. A common tool used in discussing anesthetic concerns is an anesthetic risk assessment (ARA). An *ARA* typically has five levels of risk with one being the lowest risk and five being the highest. Variations exist, but a typical *ARA* is summarized in Box 15.1.

In the same way, discussing expectations during the procedure helps the procedural assistant anticipate needed instruments and materials. Finally, the team should be detailed in discussions of the immediate Postoperative needs of the patient. These needs include administering medications upon recovery, ensuring the oral cavity is clean of debris, verifying the completion of all procedures, and providing specific instructions regarding extubation of the patient.

Check off lists are a tool which, when used correctly, can reduce the risk of forgetting crucial parts of a surgical procedure and assure clear communication between team members during surgical procedures. Ultimately, medical complications are reduced. A *check off list* consists of a list of procedural needs that are read off by one party and verbally confirmed by a second party that the need is met before moving onto the next phase of the procedure. This two-party confirmation assures that steps are not missed. The author uses a list with three specific timelines: preoperative, intraoperative, and postoperative needs. Preoperative needs include acknowledgment that preoperative diagnostics were assessed, anesthetic concerns addressed, and all involved understood what procedures will be performed. Intraoperative needs include updates on the procedure along with anesthetic updates. Postoperative needs include immediate postoperative care and nursing instructions, confirmation that all procedures were performed, and any concerns with equipment or instruments that need to be addressed.

The concept of using a procedural check-off was not developed by the author. The credit for this belongs to Atul Gawande, MD, MPH who describes the process of developing procedural checklists in *The Checklist Manifesto*.

CLIENT COMMUNICATION

Effective communication with the pet owner includes helping them understand the disease process and treatment options, set expectations, and prepare them for their role in treatment. Educating pet owners on the disease their pet is experiencing and the treatment options available is not only ethically important but can also help persuade them to accept treatment for their pet. Previously in this text, the importance of using medical terminology was stressed. The use of medical terminology needs to be slightly altered when speaking with pet owners. In most instances, they are not medical professionals and are not familiar with terms used in the veterinary community. This does not mean that medical terminology cannot be used, but some terms may need to be explained or altered. For example, substituting the term "gums" for "gingiva" is completely acceptable when speaking with pet owners. Conversely, some terms do not fully convey the severity of the situation, such as "pulling a tooth" compared to "surgical extraction of a tooth." Ultimately, we must communicate with our clients in a way that informs them, while not marginalizing the situation and the way this is performed may vary between clients and situations.

Included in conversations about the disease process should be why the disease has occurred (or may occur if discussing prevention), risk factors involved with the disease, expectations if the disease is not treated, reasonable treatment options, and common complications. All of these, along with discussion about anesthesia expectations, are a part of *informed consent*.

One of the major roadblocks to have our clients accept recommendations for dental procedures is their fear of general anesthesia. Taking time to explain the anesthetic process and the safety measures in place to reduce the risk of anesthetic mishaps can help reassure them that general anesthesia is in their pet's best interest. However, we must carefully choose appropriate candidates, protocols, and understand that anesthesia safety is not guaranteed. Each of these factors should be discussed with the pet owner. It is acceptable to discuss the *ARA* with pet owners, making sure to explain it in terms that are comprehendible. This is also an opportunity to discuss what steps are being taken to decrease risk to their pet, including patient monitoring, supportive care, and how common anesthetic challenges (such as hypotension and hypothermia) are addressed. This part of client communication often provides peace of mind to pet owners.

Once a pet is scheduled for a dental procedure, explicit instructions regarding how to prepare for the day are necessary. These include fasting instructions, when to give previously prescribed medications, and how to prepare the home for the pet's return. As well, documentation should be included in the medical records that show these steps were made and that the pet owner acknowledges these.

The day of the pet's procedure should include updates regarding diagnostic findings and updates to the care plan. If additional pathology was found during the examination, the pet owner should be informed of what the finding was and treatment options before proceeding to treatment. This can prevent frustration and conflict later. It is extremely important that the pet owner understand that he or she should be available for updates during the day. In case the clients cannot be contacted, it is advised that the clients acknowledge if they would rather have their pet recovered from anesthesia without additional treatments performed or to have the doctor use his or her judgment regarding the best treatment. Note that the latter choice may still lead to client disappointment and later challenges.

Postoperatively, the client should be informed of what to expect for recovery immediately and in the following weeks, aftercare instructions including feeding and activity limitations, when to start medications, and needed follow-up. It is best to verbally discuss these to give the client an opportunity to ask questions and to provide a written or electronic summary.

Finally, thorough client education helps manage expectations. Preemptive discussions of complications and financial matters help prevent hard conversations in the future. Of course, human nature dictates that some clients will still push back on these matters. But with documented discussions regarding expectations (noted in consent forms and medical records), the team can be confident that they have done their due diligence.

Client communication also includes discussions regarding preventative care. These should be part of the discussion with every pet owner during dental procedures and wellness appointments. Included in these discussions should be periodontal disease prevention and prevention of fractured teeth. A more detailed discussion of preventative periodontal care are discussed elsewhere in the text. Included in verbal communication is visual communication such as demonstrations with models. Models can be used to demonstrate brushing and how to recognize periodontal disease. Skulls can be used but may be objectional to some pet owners. Regarding prevention of fractured teeth, keeping examples of appropriate chew toys is a great tool to demonstrate to clients what their pet can chew. In no way can an exhaustive list be made, but representative items can be shown.

INTERHOSPITAL COMMUNICATION

When communicating between hospitals, using common medical language and organized medical records can help assure continuity of care for veterinary patients. Documents including all diagnostic results, radiographs, complete SOAP format records, and a summary of the disease process the patient is referred for are all valuable.

Again, using currently accepted terminology is recommended. If this discipline is maintained during medical record keeping, additional effort is not required when transferring records between hospitals. One can rest assured, in the case of dental terminology, updated lists of current nomenclature are available to the public at https://avdc.org/avdc-nomenclature/.

MEDICAL RECORDS

The use of problem-oriented medical records in a SOAP format, including a master problem list is one of the more common and effective methods of medical record keeping in veterinary medicine.

SOAP format medical records organize the record into four parts: subjective, objective, assessment, and plan. The subjective portion includes the presenting complaint and pertinent medical history provided by the client. As these pieces typically cannot be measured, quantified, or otherwise objectively described, they are listed as subjective. Anything that can be quantified and accurately described is listed in the objective portion. This includes vital signs and descriptions of abnormalities, including their grading. Examples include grading of a systolic heart murmur and description of an oral mass including location, texture, color size, and number. The assessment demonstrates the training of thought of the clinician as he or she reaches a diagnosis, the possible treatment options, and the expected outcome. Finally, the plan is listed, which includes surgical procedures to be performed, prescribed medications, recommended home care, and expected follow-up. Although different styles of SOAP format medical records exist, each still includes these four pieces.

Once a diagnosis has been reached, it should be added to the master problem list. The *master problem list* includes the date the diagnosis was reached, the diagnosis itself, and the date it was resolved (if applicable). Even in a veterinary dental practice, other pertinent diseases should be listed as they may affect dental treatment outcomes. When diseases are resolved, they are kept on the list as inactive. Dental charts are described in additional detail elsewhere in the text. It should be noted that the dental chart includes portions of both the objective portion of the record and the plan.

Diagnostic images should be shared between hospitals regardless of whether a radiographic report has been provided. This will allow subsequent hospitals to track the progression of the disease and compare it to previous images when new pathology is noted. As labial mounting is the preferred method of presenting dental radiographs (see radiology chapter), there is no need to label the radiograph itself as what tooth is imaged. However, the date of the radiograph should be noted. If computed tomography images are to be sent, all images available should be sent as well to view the images. Individual CT images alone do not present the complete clinical picture.

In a referral situation, it is useful for the referring clinic to summarize the reason for referral, pertinent health history, and current medications. Although this information should be available in the medical records, a brief synopsis ensures the patient is being treated for the pathology it was referred for. Along the same lines, the referral clinic should summarize the care the patient received as well as send all records back to the primary care veterinarian.

Dental charts are a clear and efficient means to denote pathology, record treatment, and monitor the progression of treatment. Several variations of the dental chart exist. The type used is preferential, but the chart should be easily readable by colleagues and interpretable by outside parties if needed. Specific notes can be made via written word, abbreviations, or drawn illustrations.

Written words can be more descriptive, but with the limitation on space to write in a dental chart, conservation of verbiage is necessary. This makes abbreviations and drawn illustrations necessary. Abbreviations are an excellent tool for marking pathology if the reader knows what the abbreviation means. A master abbreviation list should be available to the reader. This has obvious limitations in that it requires more information to be inserted into the dental chart. An accepted list of abbreviations has already been developed by the American Veterinary Dental College. This list is consistently updated and available at https://avdc.org/wpfd_file/abbreviations/. If a master abbreviation list is not available, the abbreviations used are not understood by colleagues when records are shared between hospitals.

AVDC Abbreviations for Use in Case Logs
Equine and Small Animal

This list of abbreviations has been recommended by the Nomenclature Committee and approved by the AVDC Board. The list is in alphabetical order.

Anatomical items are shown in **black font**.

Conditions and diagnostic procedures appropriate for use in the Diagnosis column of a case log entry are shown in blue font.

Treatment procedure and related items suitable for inclusion in the Procedure column in the case log entry are shown in red font.

Note: Use of other abbreviations in AVDC case logs is not permitted—write out the whole word if it must be included in a case log entry.

For further information on the use of particular definitions, visit the Nomenclature page on the AVDC web site.

Abbreviation		Definition
A		**Alveolus**
AB		Abrasion
ABE		Alveolar bone expansion
ALV		Alveolectomy/alveoloplasty
ANO		Anodontia
AOS		Alveolar osteitis
AP		**Apex**
	AP/X	Apicoectomy
APN		Apexification
AT		Attrition
ATE		Abnormal tooth extrusion
B		Biopsy
	B/B	Bite biopsy
	B/CN	Core needle biopsy
	B/E	Excisional biopsy
	B/I	Incisional biopsy
	B/NA	Needle aspiration
	B/NB	Needle biopsy
	B/P	Punch biopsy
	B/S	Surface biopsy
BR		Bite registration
BRI		Bridge
BTH		Ball therapy
BUC		Buccotomy

Continued

Abbreviation		Definition
BUP		Bullous pemphigoid
C		**Canine**
CA		Caries
	CA/INF	Infundibular caries (equines)
	CA/INF/D	Distal infundibular caries
	CA/INF/M	Mesial infundibular caries
	CA/PER	Peripheral caries (in equines)
CB		Crossbite
	CB/C	Caudal crossbite
	CB/R	Rostral crossbite
CC		Calcinosis circumscripta
CEJ		**Cementoenamel junction**
CFL		Cleft lip
	CFL/R	Cleft lip repair
CFP		Cleft palate
	CFP/R	Cleft palate repair
CFS		Cleft soft palate
	CFS/R	Cleft soft palate repair
CFSH		Soft palate hypoplasia
	CFSH/R	Soft palate hypoplasia repair
CFSU		Unilateral cleft soft palate
	CFSU/R	Unilateral cleft soft palate repair
CFT		Traumatic cleft palate
	CFT/R	Traumatic cleft palate repair
CHO		Calvarial hyperostosis
CL		Chewing lesion
	CL/B	Chewing lesion (buccal mucosa/cheek)
	CL/L	Chewing lesion (labial mucosa/lip)
	CL/P	Chewing lesion (palatal mucosa/palate)
	CL/T	Chewing lesion (lingual/sublingual mucosa/tongue)
CMO		Craniomandibular osteopathy
COM		Commissurotomy
CON		**Condylar process of the mandible**
	CON/X	Condylectomy
COO		Condensing osteitis
COR		**Coronoid process of the mandible**
	COR/X	Coronoidectomy
CPL		Cheiloplasty/commissuroplasty
CR		**Crown**
	CR/A	Crown amputation
	CR/AC	**Anatomical crown**
	CR/C	Ceramic crown (full)
	CR/C/P	Ceramic crown (partial)
	CR/CC	**Clinical crown**
	CR/L	Crown lengthening
	CR/M	Metal crown (full)
	CR/M/P	Metal crown (partial)
	CR/P	Crown preparation
	CR/R	Resin crown (full)
	CR/R/P	Resin crown (partial)
	CR/RC	**Reserve crown**
	CR/PFM	Porcelain fused to metal crown (full)

	CR/PFM/P	Porcelain fused to metal crown (partial)
	CR/T	Temporary crown
	CR/XP	Crown reduction
CS		Culture/sensitivity
CT		Computed tomography
	CT/CB	Cone-beam CT
CTH		Chemotherapy
CU		Contact mucositis or contact mucosal ulceration
CUS		Contact ulcerative stomatitis
D		Diastema
	D/O	Open diastema
	D/ODY	Diastema odontoplasty (or widening)
	D/V	Valve diastema
DC		Diagnostic cast
	DC/D	Die
	DC/SM	Stone model
DI		Discharge
	DI/ND	Right nasal discharge
	DI/NS	Left nasal discharge
	DI/NU	Bilateral nasal discharge
	DI/OD	Right ocular discharge
	DI/OS	Left ocular discharge
	DI/OU	Bilateral ocular discharge
DMO		Decreased mouth opening
DP		Defect preparation (prior to filling a dental defect)
DT		**Deciduous tooth**
	DT/P	Persistent deciduous tooth
DTC		Dentigerous cyst
	DTC/R	Dentigerous cyst removal
E		**Enamel**
	E/D	Enamel defect
	E/H	Enamel hypoplasia
	E/HM	Enamel hypomineralization
	E/P	Enamel pearl
EM		Erythema multiforme
ENO		Enophthalmos
EOG		Eosinophilic granuloma
	EOG/L	Eosinophilic granuloma (lip)
	EOG/P	Eosinophilic granuloma (palate)
	EOG/T	Eosinophilic granuloma (tongue)
ER		Erosion
ESP		Elongated soft palate
	ESP/R	Elongated soft palate reduction
EXO		Exophthalmos
F		Flap
	F/AD	Advancement flap
	F/AP	Apically positioned flap
	F/CO	Coronally positioned flap
	F/EN	Envelope flap
	F/HI	Hinged (overlapping) flap
	F/IS	Island flap
	F/LA	Laterally positioned flap
	F/RO	Rotation flap
	F/TR	Transposition flap

Continued

Abbreviation		Definition
FB		Foreign body
	FB/R	Foreign body removal
FOD		Fibrous osteodystrophy
FOL		Folliculitis
FRE		Frenuloplasty (frenulotomy, frenulectomy)
FT		Fiberotomy
FX		Fracture (tooth or jaw; see T/FX for tooth fracture abbreviations)
	FX/R	Repair of jaw fracture
	FX/R/EXF	External skeletal fixation
	FX/R/IAS	Interarch splinting (between upper and lower dental arches)
	FX/R/IDS	Interdental splinting (between teeth within a dental arch)
	FX/R/IQS	Interquadrant splinting (between left and right upper or lower jaw quadrants)
	FX/R/MMF	Maxillomandibular fixation (other than muzzling and interarch splinting)
	FX/R/MZ	Muzzling
	FX/R/PL	Bone plating
	FX/R/WIR/C	Wire cerclage
	FX/R/WIR/OS	Intraosseous wiring
GC		Gingival curettage
GE		Gingival enlargement (in the absence of a histological diagnosis)
GF		Graft
	GF/B	Bone graft
	GF/C	Cartilage graft
	GF/CT	Connective tissue graft
	GF/F	Fat graft
	GF/G	Gingival graft
	GF/M	Mucosal graft
	GF/N	Nerve graft
	GF/S	Skin graft
	GF/V	Venous graft
GH		Gingival hyperplasia
GR		Gingival recession
GTR		Guided tissue regeneration
GV		Gingivectomy/gingivoplasty
HC		Hypercementosis
HS		Hemisection
HYP		Hypodontia
I1,2,3		**Incisor**
IM		Detailed imprint of hard and/or soft tissues (e.g., individual teeth or palate defect)
	IM/F	Full-mouth impression (i.e., imprints of teeth of upper and lower dental arches)
IMP		Implant
INF		**Infundibulum**
IOF		Intraoral fistula
	IOF/R	Intraoral fistula repair
IP		Inclined plane
	IP/AC	Acrylic inclined plane
	IP/C	Composite inclined plane
	IP/M	Metal (i.e., lab-produced) inclined plane
ITH		Immunotherapy
LAC		Laceration
	LAC/B	Laceration (cheek skin/buccal mucosa)
	LAC/G	Laceration (gingiva/alveolar mucosa)
	LAC/L	Laceration (lip skin/labial mucosa)

	LAC/O	Laceration (palatine tonsil/oropharyngeal mucosa)
	LAC/P	Laceration (palatal mucosa)
	LAC/R	Laceration repair
	LAC/T	Laceration (lingual/sublingual mucosa)
LE		Lupus erythematosus
LIN		**Tongue**
	LIN/X	Tongue resection
LIP		**Lip/cheek**
	LIP/X	Lip/cheek resection
LN		**Lymph node (regional, i.e., facial, mandibular, parotid, lateral and medial retropharyngeal)**
	LN/E	Lymph node enlargement
	LN/X	Lymph node resection
M1,2,3		**Molar**
MAL		Malocclusion
	MAL1	Class 1 malocclusion (neutroclusion; dental malocclusion with normal upper/lower jaw length relationship)
	MAL1/BV	Buccoversion
	MAL1/DV	Distoversion
	MAL1/LABV	Labioversion
	MAL1/LV	Linguoversion
	MAL1/MV	Mesioversion
	MAL1/PV	Palatoversion
	MAL2	Class 2 malocclusion (mandibular distoclusion; symmetrical skeletal malocclusion with the lower jaw relatively shorter than the upper jaw)
	MAL3	Class 3 malocclusion (mandibular mesioclusion; symmetrical skeletal malocclusion with the upper jaw relatively shorter than the lower jaw)
	MAL4	Class 4 malocclusion (asymmetrical skeletal malocclusion in a caudoventral, side-to-side or dorsoventral direction)
	MAL4/DV	Asymmetrical skeletal malocclusion in a dorsoventral direction
	MAL4/RC	Asymmetrical skeletal malocclusion in a rostrocaudal direction
	MAL4/STS	Asymmetrical skeletal malocclusion in a side-to-side direction
MAR		Marsupialization
MET		Metastasis
	MET/D	Distant metastasis
	MET/R	Regional metastasis
MMM		Masticatory muscle myositis
MN		**Mandible/mandibular**
	MN/FX	Mandibular fracture
MRI		Magnetic resonance imaging
MX		**Maxilla/maxillary**
	MX/FX	Maxillary fracture
N		**Nose/nasal/nasopharyngeal**
	N/EN	Rhinoscopy
	N/LAV	Nasal lavage
	N/NS	Naris stenosis
	N/NS/R	Naroplasty
	N/NPS	Nasopharyngeal stenosis
	N/NPS/R	Nasopharyngeal stenosis repair
	N/POL	Nasopharyngeal polyp
	N/SCC	Nasal SCC (check abbreviations under OM for other tumors)
OA		Orthodontic appliance
	OA/A	Orthodontic appliance adjustment
	OA/AR	Arch bar

Continued

Abbreviation		Definition
	OA/BKT	Bracket, button or hook
	OA/CMB	Custom-made OA/BKT
	OA/EC	Elastic chain, tube or thread
	OA/I	Orthodontic appliance installment
	OA/R	Orthodontic appliance removal
	OA/WIR	Orthodontic wire
OAF		Oroantral fistula
	OAF/R	Oroantral fistula repair
OC		Orthodontic counseling
ODY		Odontoplasty
OFF		Orofacial fistula
	OFF/R	Orofacial fistula repair
OLI		Oligodontia
OM		Oral/maxillofacial mass
	OM/AA	Acanthomatous ameloblastoma
	OM/AD	Adenoma
	OM/ADC	Adenocarcinoma
	OM/APN	Anaplastic neoplasm
	OM/APO	Amyloid-producing odontogenic tumor
	OM/CE	Cementoma
	OM/FIO	Feline inductive odontogenic tumor
	OM/FS	Fibrosarcoma
	OM/GCG	Giant cell granuloma
	OM/GCT	Granular cell tumor
	OM/HS	Hemangiosarcoma
	OM/LI	Lipoma
	OM/LS	Lymphosarcoma
	OM/MCT	Mast cell tumor
	OM/MM	Malignant melanoma
	OM/OO	Osteoma
	OM/OS	Osteosarcoma
	OM/MTB	Multilobular tumor of bone
	OM/PAP	Papilloma
	OM/PCT	Plasma cell tumor
	OM/PNT	Peripheral nerve sheath tumor
	OM/POF	Peripheral odontogenic fibroma
	OM/RBM	Rhabdomyosarcoma
	OM/SCC	Squamous cell carcinoma
	OM/UDN	Undifferentiated neoplasm
OMJL		Open-mouth jaw locking
	OMJL/R	Open-mouth jaw locking reduction
ONF		Oronasal fistula
	ONF/R	Oronasal fistula repair
OP		Operculectomy
OR		Orthodontic recheck
OS		Orthognathic surgery
OSN		Osteonecrosis
OSS		Osteosclerosis
OST		Osteomyelitis
PA		**Periapical**
	PA/A	Periapical abscess
	PA/C	Periapical cyst

	PA/G	Periapical granuloma
	PA/P	Periapical pathology (if a distinction between granuloma, abscess, or cyst cannot be made)
PCB		Post-and-core build-up
PCD		Direct pulp capping
PCI		Indirect pulp capping
PD		Periodontal disease
	PD0	Clinically normal
	PD1	Gingivitis only (without attachment loss)
	PD2	Early periodontitis (<25% attachment loss)
	PD3	Moderate periodontitis (25%–50% attachment loss)
	PD4	Advanced periodontitis (>50% attachment loss)
PDE		Acquired palate defect
	PDE/R	Acquired palate defect repair
PEC		Pericoronitis
PEO		Periostitis ossificans
PH		**Pulp horn (in equines numbered by the du Toit system)**
	PH/D	Pulp horn defect
PHA		**Pharynx**
	PHA/IN	Pharyngitis
PM1-4		**Premolar**
POB		Palatal obturator
PRO		Professional dental cleaning (scaling, polishing, irrigation)
PTY		Ptyalism
PU		**Pulp**
	PU/M	Mineralization of pulp
	PU/S	Pulp stone
PV		Pemphigus vulgaris
PYO		Pyogenic granuloma
R		Restoration (filling of a dental defect)
	R/A	Filling made of amalgam
	R/C	Filling made of composite
	R/CP	Filling made of compomer
	R/I	Filling made of glass ionomer
RAD		Radiography
	RAD/SG	Sialography
RBA		Retrobulbar abscess
RCR		Retained crown-root or clinical crown-reserve crown or clinical crown-reserve crown and root
RCT		Standard root canal therapy
	RCT/S	Surgical root canal therapy
RO		**Root**
	RO/AC	**Anatomical root**
	RO/CR	**Clinical root**
	RO/X	Root resection/amputation
RP		Root planing
	RP/C	Closed root planing
	RP/O	Open root planing
RPA		Retropharyngeal abscess
RR		Internal resorption
RTH		Radiotherapy
RTR		Retained root or reserve crown

Continued

Abbreviation		Definition
S		Surgery
	S/M	Partial mandibulectomy
	S/MB	Bilateral partial mandibulectomy (removal of parts of the left and right mandibles)
	S/MD	Dorsal marginal mandibulectomy (marginal mandibulectomy, mandibular rim excision)
	S/MS	Segmental mandibulectomy (removal of a full dorsoventral sement of a mandible)
	S/MT	Total mandibulectomy (removal of one entire mandible)
	S/P	Partial palatectomy
	S/X	Partial maxillectomy
	S/XB	Bilateral partial maxillectomy (removal of parts of the left and right maxillae and/or other facial bones)
SCI		Scintigraphy
SG		**Salivary gland**
	SG/ADC	Salivary gland adenocarcinoma (check abbreviations under OM for other tumors)
	SG/ADS	Sialadenosis
	SG/IN	Sialadenitis
	SG/MAR	Marsupialization
	SG/MUC/S	Sublingual sialocele
	SG/MUC/P	Pharyngeal sialocele
	SG/MUC/C	Cervical sialocele
	SG/NEC	Necrotizing sialometaplasia
	SG/RC	Mucous retention cyst
	SG/SI	Sialolith
	SG/X	Salivary gland resection
SHE		Shear mouth (increased occlusal angulation of equine cheek teeth)
SIN		**Sinus**
	SIN/CF	**Conchofrontal sinus**
	SIN/CF/F	Conchofrontal sinus flap
	SIN/CMX	**Caudal maxillary sinus**
	SIN/EN	Sinoscopy
	SIN/F	Sinus flap
	SIN/IN	Sinusitis (e.g., SIN/IN/RMX = rostral maxillary sinusitis)
	SIN/LAV	Sinus lavage
	SIN/MX/F	Maxillary sinus flap
	SIN/RMX	**Rostral maxillary sinus**
	SIN/SP	**Sphenopalatine sinus**
	SIN/TRP	Sinus trephination
	SIN/VC	**Ventral conchal sinus**
SR		Surgical repositioning
ST		Stomatitis
	ST/CS	Caudal stomatitis
SYM		**Mandibular symphysis**
	SYM/R	Mandibular symphysis repair
	SYM/S	Mandibular symphysis separation
T		**Tooth**
	T/A	Avulsed tooth
	T/CCR	Concrescence
	T/DEN	Dens invaginatus
	T/DIL	Dilaceration
	T/E	Embedded tooth

	T/EL	Tooth elongation (abnormal intraoral and/or periapical extension of the coronal and/or apical portions of the tooth; e.g., T/EL/CC = elongation of the clinical crown)
	T/FDR	Fused roots
	T/FUS	Fusion
	T/FX	Fractured tooth (see next seven listings for fracture types)
	T/FX/EI	Enamel infraction
	T/FX/EF	Enamel fracture
	T/FX/UCF	Uncomplicated crown fracture
	T/FX/CCF	Complicated crown fracture
	T/FX/UCRF	Uncomplicated crown-root facture
	T/FX/CCRF	Complicated crown-root fracture
	T/FX/RF	Root fracture
	T/GEM	Gemination
	T/I	Impacted tooth
	T/LUX	Luxated tooth
	T/MAC	Macrodontia
	T/MIC	Microdontia
	T/NE	Near pulp exposure
	T/NV	Nonvital tooth
	T/PE	Pulp exposure
	T/RI	Tooth reimplantation (for an avulsed tooth)
	T/RP	Tooth repositioning (for a luxated tooth)
	T/SN	Supernumerary tooth
	T/SR	Supernumerary root
	T/TRA	Transposition
	T/U	Unerupted tooth
	T/V	Vital tooth
	T/XP	Partial tooth resection
TMA		Trauma
	TMA/B	Ballistic trauma
	TMA/E	Electric trauma
	TMA/BRN	Burn trauma
	TMA/R	Trauma repair
TMJ		**Temporomandibular joint**
	TMJ/A	Temporomandibular joint ankylosis (true or false)
	TMJ/A/R	Temporomandibular joint ankylosis repair
	TMJ/D	TMJ dysplasia
	TMJ/FX	Temporomandibular joint fracture
	TMJ/FX/R	Temporomandibular joint fracture repair
	TMJ/LUX	TMJ luxation
	TMJ/LUX/R	Temporomandibular joint luxation reduction
TON		**Palatine tonsil**
	TON/IN	Tonsillitis
	TON/X	Tonsillectomy
TP		Treatment plan
TR		Tooth resorption
TRP		Trephination
TS		Trisection
TT		Temporal teratoma
US		Ultrasonography
VPT		Vital pulp therapy
X		Closed extraction of a tooth (without sectioning)

Continued

Abbreviation		Definition
XS		Closed extraction of a tooth (with sectioning)
	XS/ODY	Removal of interproximal crown tissue to facilitate transoral extraction of a tooth
XSS		Open extraction of a tooth
	XSS/APX/RPL	Extraction of a tooth after apicoectomy and repulsion
	XSS/BUC	Transbuccal extraction of a tooth after buccotomy
	XSS/BUC/ALV	Transbuccal extraction of a tooth after buccotomy and alveolectomy
	XSS/COM	Transbuccal extraction of a tooth after commissurotomy
	XSS/COM/ ALV	Transbuccal extraction of a tooth after commissurotomy and alveolectomy
	XSS/MIB	Extraction of a tooth via minimally invasive buccotomy (small incision made for introduction of straight instrumentation to elevate, section or drill into a cheek tooth for the purpose of facilitating its transoral extraction)
	XSS/RPL	Extraction of a tooth after repulsion
ZYG		**Zygoma (zygomatic arch)**
	ZYG/X	Zygomectomy

AVDC Nomenclature Introduction

NOMENCLATURE ADOPTED BY THE AVDC BOARD

Last updated 2023

American Veterinary Dental College (AVDC) has adopted the following items as standard nomenclature for use in College documents. Note that current abbreviations are in brackets if appropriate. All used with permission AVDC.

Note: equine specific terminology has been omitted

DEFINITIONS OF VETERINARY DENTISTRY, EQUINE DENTISTRY, AND BEAKOLOGY

Veterinary dentistry is a discipline within the scope of veterinary practice that involves professional consultation, evaluation, diagnosis, prevention, treatment (nonsurgical, surgical, or related procedures) of conditions, diseases, and disorders of the oral cavity and maxillofacial area and their adjacent and associated structures; it is provided by a licensed veterinarian, within the scope of the veterinarian's education, training, and experience, in accordance with the ethics of the profession and applicable law.

Equine dentistry is the practice of veterinary dentistry performed in equids (genus Equus: horses, asses, and zebras).

Beakology is the branch of science dealing with the anatomy, physiology, and pathology (including diagnosis and treatment of such pathology) of the beak and associated tissues of vertebrate animals that have beaks or beak-like structures.

DEFINITIONS OF ITEMS APPLYING TO MORE THAN ONE ORAL TISSUE OR DISEASE

Congenital: Of or relating to a disease, condition, or characteristic that is present at birth and may be inherited or result from an insult during pregnancy

Acquired: Of or relating to a disease, condition, or characteristic that develops after birth and is not inherited

Inherited: Of or relating to a disease, condition, or characteristic that results from the genetic make-up of the individual animal and may be present at birth or develop later in life

Culture/sensitivity (CS): Bacteria cultured in a medium and analyzed for sensitivity to antibiotics

Laceration (LAC): A tear or cut in the gingiva/alveolar mucosa **(LAC/G)**, tongue/sublingual mucosa **(LAC/T)**, lip skin/labial mucosa **(LAC/L)**, cheek skin/buccal mucosa **(LAC/B)**, palatal mucosa **(LAC/P)**, or palatine tonsil/oropharyngeal mucosa **(LAC/O)**; debridement and suturing of such

Chewing lesion (CL): Mucosal lesion resulting from self-induced bite trauma on the cheek **(CL/B)**, lip **(CL/L)**, palate **(CL/P)**, or tongue/sublingual region **(CL/T)**

Foreign body (FB): An object originating outside the body; removal of the foreign body is abbreviated with **FB/R**

Burn (TMA/BRN): Injury to the skin, mucosa, or other body parts caused by fire, heat, radiation, electricity, or a caustic agent

Ballistic trauma (TMA/B): Physical trauma sustained from a projectile that was launched through space, most commonly by a weapon such as a gun or a bow

Electric injury (TMA/E): Physical trauma to skin, mucosa, or other tissues when coming into direct contact with an electrical current

ANATOMY OF ORAL, DENTAL, AND RELATED STRUCTURES

Dental Anatomy

Pulp cavity: Space within the tooth

Pulp chamber: Space within the crown of a tooth

Root canal: Space within the root of a tooth

Apical foramen: Opening at the apex of a tooth, through which neurovascular structures pass to and from the dental pulp

Apical delta: Multiple apical foramina forming a branching pattern at the apex of a tooth reminiscent of a river delta when sectioned and viewed through a microscope; this occurs in some brachyodont teeth

Ameloblasts: Epithelial cells involved in the formation of enamel (amelogenesis)

Enamel (E): Mineralized tissue covering the crown of brachyodont teeth

Anatomic crown (CR/AC): That part of a tooth that is coronal to the cementoenamel junction (or anatomic root)

Clinical crown (CR/CC): That part of a tooth that is coronal to the gingival margin; also called erupted crown in equines

Anatomic root (RO/AR): That part of a tooth that is apical to the cementoenamel junction (or anatomic crown)

Clinical root (RO/CR): That part of a brachyodont tooth that is apical to the gingival margin

Cementoenamel junction: Area of a tooth where cementum and enamel meet

Reserve crown (CR/RC): The part of the crown of a hypsodont tooth that is apical to the gingival margin

Nomenclature and Numbering of Teeth

Incisor Teeth

The incisors will be referred to as (right or left) (maxillary or mandibular) first, second, or third incisors numbered from the midline.

Reference(s): Peyer B. *Comparative Odontology.* 1st ed. Chicago, IL: University of Chicago Press; 1968:1–347.

Nickel R, Schummer A, Seiferle E, et al. Teeth, general and comparative. In: *The Viscera of Domestic Mammals.* 1st ed. Berlin: Verlag Paul Parey; 1973:75–99.

Premolar Teeth in the Cat

In the cat, the tooth immediately distal to the maxillary **canine** is the second **premolar**, the tooth immediately distal to the mandibular canine is the third premolar.

Reference(s): Nickel R, Schummer A, Seiferle E, et al. Teeth, general and comparative. In: *The Viscera of Domestic Mammals.* 1st ed. Berlin: Verlag Paul Parey; 1973:75–99.

Tooth Numbering

The existence of the conventional anatomic names of teeth as well as the various tooth numbering systems is recognized. The correct anatomic names of teeth are (right or left), (maxillary or mandibular), (first, second, third, or fourth), (incisor, canine, premolar, and molar), as applicable, written out in full or abbreviated form. The modified Triadan system is presently considered to be the tooth numbering system of choice in veterinary dentistry; gaps are left in the numbering sequence where there are missing teeth (e.g., the first premolar encountered in the feline left maxilla is numbered 206, not 205. The two lower right premolars are 407 and 408, not 405 and 406).

The use of both anatomic names and the modified Triadan system is acceptable for recording and storing veterinary dental information. The use of anatomic names in publications is required by many leading journals and is recommended. It offers the advantage of veterinary dental publications being understandable to other health professionals and scientists with an interest in veterinary dentistry.

Reference(s): Floyd MR. The modified Triadan system: nomenclature for veterinary dentistry. *J Vet Dent.* 1991;8:18–19.

Comments:

In January 1972, the International Dental Federation adopted a new, two-digit, user-friendly nomenclature system for use in the human dental patient. This new system eliminated the plus and minus signs of the Haderup system and the brackets of the Winkel system. Following the acceptance of the new system for human dental nomenclature, Professor Dr. MedDent H. Triadan, a dentist at the University of Bern, Switzerland, introduced a similar system for animals. Owing to the fact that many animals, including his canine model, have more than nine teeth in a quadrant, the Triadan system for animals utilizes three digits instead of two digits.

ABBREVIATIONS ASSOCIATED WITH TEETH

Tooth (T): Hard structure embedded in the jaw; used for biting and chewing

Incisor (I): Incisor tooth

Canine (C): Canine tooth

Premolar (P): Premolar tooth

Molar (M): Molar tooth

Alveolus (A): Socket in the jaw for a tooth root or reserve crown (plural: alveoli)

Crown (C): Coronal portion of a tooth

Root (RO): Radicular portion of a tooth

Apex (AP): End of the root or reserve crown (plural: apices)

Generations of Teeth in Diphyodont Species
Primary Tooth Replaced by a Permanent (Secondary) Tooth

The **deciduous dentition** period is the period during which only deciduous teeth are present.

The **mixed dentition** period is the period during which both deciduous and permanent teeth are present.

The **permanent dentition** period is the period during which only permanent teeth are present.

Reference: Anonymous. In: *Nomina Anatomica Veterinaria.* 4th ed. Zurich and Ithaca, NY: World Association of Veterinary Anatomists; 1994.

Boucher CO, Zwemer TJ. *Boucher's Clinical Dental Terminology—A Glossary of Accepted Terms in All Disciplines of Dentistry.* 4th ed. St. Louis, MO: Mosby; 1993.

Evans HE. *Miller's Anatomy of the Dog.* 3rd ed. Philadelphia, PA: WB Saunders Co; 1993.

The term **"Persistent deciduous tooth"** is etymologically correct, although the term "retained deciduous tooth" is commonly used. The latter term, however, can be confused with an unerupted deciduous tooth.

Reference: Eisenmenger E, Zetner K. *Tierv§rztliche Zahnheilkunde.* 1st ed. Berlin: Verlag Paul Parey; 1982:44–50.

SURFACES OF TEETH AND DIRECTIONS IN THE MOUTH
Vestibular/Buccal/Labial

Vestibular is the correct term referring to the surface of the tooth facing the vestibule or lips; **buccal** and **labial** are acceptable alternatives.

Reference(s): Anonymous. In: *Nomina Anatomica Veterinaria*. 4th ed. Zurich and Ithaca, NY: World Association of Veterinary Anatomists; 1994.

Comment(s): The term "facial" specifically refers to the surfaces of the rostral teeth visible from the front. According to Dr. A.J. Bezuidenhout, a veterinary anatomist at Cornell University, "facial" is a bit of a misnomer. Traditionally "facial" has been used in human dentistry for the aspect of teeth visible from the front (i.e., incisors and canines).

Lingual/Palatal

Lingual: The surface of a mandibular or maxillary tooth facing the tongue is the lingual surface. Palatal can also be used when referring to the lingual surface of maxillary teeth.

Mesial/Distal

Mesial and **distal** are terms applicable to tooth surfaces. The **mesial** surface of the first incisor is next to the median plane; on other teeth, it is directed toward the first incisor. The **distal** surface is opposite to the mesial surface.

Rostral/Caudal

Rostral and **caudal** are the positional and directional anatomic terms applicable to the head in a sagittal plane in nonhuman vertebrates. **Rostral** refers to a structure closer to or a direction toward the most forward structure of the head. **Caudal** refers to a structure closer to or a direction toward the tail.

Anterior and *posterior* are synonymous terms used in human dentistry.

TEETH ABNORMALITIES AND RELATED PROCEDURES

Enamel Abnormalities

Abrasion (AB): Tooth wear caused by contact of a tooth with a nondental object

Attrition (AT): Tooth wear caused by contact of a tooth with another tooth

Erosion (ER): Demineralization of tooth substance owing to external acids

Caries (CA): Degradation of dental hard tissue caused by demineralization owing to acids released during bacterial fermentation of carbohydrates

Enamel defect (ED): Lesion affecting the structural integrity of enamel

Enamel hypoplasia (E/H): refers to inadequate deposition of enamel matrix. This can affect one or several teeth and may be focal or multifocal. The crowns of affected teeth can have areas of normal enamel next to areas of hypoplastic or missing enamel.

Enamel hypomineralization (E/HM): refers to inadequate mineralization of enamel matrix. This often affects several or all teeth. The crowns of affected teeth are covered by soft enamel that may be worn rapidly

Enamel infraction (T/FX/EI): Incomplete fracture (crack) of the enamel without loss of tooth substance

Enamel fracture (T/FX/EF): Fracture with loss of crown substance confined to the enamel

Tooth Formation Abnormalities

Persistent deciduous tooth (DT/P): A deciduous tooth that is present when it should have exfoliated

Supernumerary tooth (T/SN): Presence of an extra tooth (also called hyperdontia)

Hypodontia (HYP): Developmental absence of a few teeth

Oligodontia (OLI): Developmental absence of numerous teeth

Anodontia (ANO): Failure of all teeth to develop

Macrodontia (T/MAC): Tooth/teeth larger than normal

Microdontia (T/MIC): Tooth/teeth smaller than normal

Transposition (T/TRA): Two teeth that have exchanged position

Fusion (T/FUS): Combining of adjacent tooth germs and resulting in partial or complete union of the developing teeth; also called synodontia

Concrescence (T/CCR): Fusion of the roots of two or more teeth at the cementum level

Fused roots (T/FDR): Fusion of roots of the same tooth

Gemination (T/GEM): A single tooth bud's attempt to divide partially (cleft of the crown) or completely (presence of an identical supernumerary tooth); also called twinning

Supernumerary root (T/SR): Presence of an extra root

Dilaceration (T/DIL): Disturbance in tooth development, causing the crown or root to be abruptly bent or crooked

Dens invaginatus (T/DEN): Invagination of the outer surface of a tooth into the interior, occurring in either the crown (involving the pulp chamber) or the root (involving the root canal); also called dens in dente

Enamel pearl (E/P): Small, nodular growth on the root of a tooth made of enamel with or without a small dentin core and sometimes a covering of cementum

Unerupted tooth (T/U): Tooth that has not perforated the oral mucosa

Embedded tooth (T/E): Unerupted tooth covered in bone the eruption of which is compromised by lack of eruptive force

Impacted tooth (T/I): Unerupted or partially erupted tooth the eruption of which is prevented by contact with a physical barrier

Dentigerous cyst (DTC): Odontogenic cyst initially formed around the crown of a partially erupted or unerupted tooth; also called follicular cyst or tooth-containing cyst; removal is abbreviated as **DTC/R**

Folliculitis (FOL): Inflammation of the follicle of a developing tooth

Pericoronitis (PEC): Inflammation of the soft tissues surrounding the crown of a partially erupted tooth

Tooth Resorption

Tooth resorption is classified based on the severity of the resorption (**Stages 1–5**) and on the location of the resorption (**Types 1–3**).

The AVDC classification of tooth resorption is based on the assumption that tooth resorption is a progressive condition.

Tooth resorption (TR): Resorption of dental hard tissue

Internal resorption (RR): Tooth resorption originating within the pulp cavity

Stages of Tooth Resorption

Stage 1 (TR 1): Mild dental hard tissue loss (cementum or cementum and enamel)

Stage 2 (TR 2): Moderate dental hard tissue loss (cementum or cementum and enamel with loss of dentin that does not extend to the pulp cavity)

Stage 3 (TR 3): Deep dental hard tissue loss (cementum or cementum and enamel with loss of dentin that extends to the pulp cavity); most of the tooth retains its integrity

Stage 4 (TR 4): Extensive dental hard tissue loss (cementum or cementum and enamel with loss of dentin that extends to the pulp cavity); most of the tooth has lost its integrity

TR4a: Crown and root are equally affected.

Stage 4 (TR 4): Extensive dental hard tissue loss (cementum or cementum and enamel with loss of dentin that extends to the pulp cavity); most of the tooth has lost its integrity

TR4b: Crown is more severely affected than the root

Stage 4 (TR 4): Extensive dental hard tissue loss (cementum or cementum and enamel with loss of dentin that extends to the pulp cavity); most of the tooth has lost its integrity

TR4c: Root is more severely affected than the crown

Stage 5 (TR 5): Remnants of dental hard tissue are visible only as irregular radiopacities and gingival covering is complete

Types of Resorption Based on Radiographic Appearance

Type 1 (T1): On a radiograph of a tooth with type 1 (T1) appearance, a focal or multifocal radiolucency is present in the tooth with otherwise normal radiopacity and normal periodontal ligament space.

Type 2 (T2): On a radiograph of a tooth with type 2 (**T2**) appearance, there is narrowing or disappearance of the periodontal ligament space in at least some areas and decreased radiopacity of part of the tooth.

Type 3 (T3): On a radiograph of a tooth with type 3 (**T3**) appearance, features of both type 1 and type 2 are present in the same tooth. A tooth with this appearance has areas of normal and narrow or lost periodontal ligament space, and there is focal or multifocal radiolucency in the tooth and decreased radiopacity in other areas of the tooth.

Tooth Fracture Classification

The **Tooth Fracture (T/FX)** classification shown below can be applied for brachyodont and hypsodont teeth, which covers domesticated species and many wild species.

Fractures of teeth in some wild species may not fit into this classification because of differences in the tissues present in the teeth.

When used in AVDC case log entries, the **tooth fracture abbreviations** noted below are to be stated as T/FX/(specific abbreviation, e.g., [T/FX/CCF]).

Enamel infraction (T/FX/EI): Incomplete fracture (crack) of the enamel without loss of tooth substance

Enamel fracture (T/FX/EF): Fracture with loss of crown substance confined to the enamel

Uncomplicated crown fracture (T/FX/UCF): Fracture of the crown that does not expose the pulp

Complicated crown fracture (T/FX/CCF): Fracture of the crown that exposes the pulp

Uncomplicated crown-root fracture (T/FX/UCRF): Fracture of the crown and root that does not expose the pulp

Complicated crown-root fracture (T/FX/CCRF): Fracture of the crown and root that exposes the pulp

Root fracture (T/FX/RF): Fracture involving the root

Retained root or reserve crown (RTR): Presence of a root remnant or reserve crown remnant

Retained crown-root or clinical crown-reserve crown or clinical crown-reserve crown and root (RCR): Presence of a crown-root remnant (in brachyodont teeth), clinical crown-reserve crown remnant (in aradicular hypsodont teeth) or clinical crown-reserve crown and root remnant (in radicular hypsodont teeth)

Enamel infraction (EI): An incomplete fracture (crack) of the enamel without loss of tooth substance

Enamel fracture (EF): A fracture with loss of crown substance confined to the enamel

Uncomplicated crown fracture (UCF): A fracture of the crown1 that does not expose the pulp

Complicated crown fracture (CCF): A fracture of the crown1 that exposes the pulp:

Uncomplicated crown-root fracture (UCRF): A fracture of the crown and root that does not expose the pulp

Complicated crown-root fracture (CCRF): A fracture of the crown and root that exposes the pulp

Root fracture (RF): A fracture involving the root

ENDODONTIC TERMINOLOGY

Endodontics is a specialty in dentistry and oral surgery that is concerned with the prevention, diagnosis, and treatment of diseases of the pulp-dentin complex and their impact on associated tissues.

Apexogenesis: Physiologic formation of the apex of a vital tooth

Pulp (PU): Soft tissue in the pulp cavity

Odontoblasts: Cells of mesenchymal origin that line the outer surface of the pulp and the biological function of which is the formation of dentin (dentinogenesis)

Predentin: Unmineralized dentin matrix produced by odontoblasts

Dentin: Mineralized tissue surrounding the pulp and containing dentinal tubules that radiate outward from the pulp to the periphery

Primary dentin: Dentin produced until root formation is completed (e.g., dogs, cats) or the tooth comes into occlusion (e.g., horses)

Secondary dentin: Dentin produced after root formation is completed

Tertiary dentin: Dentin produced as a result of a local insult; can be reactionary (produced by existing odontoblasts) or reparative (produced by odontoblast-like cells that differentiated from pulpal stem cells as a result of an insult)

Sclerotic dentin: Transparent dentin characterized by mineralization of the dentinal tubules as a result of an insult or normal aging

Periapical (PA): Pertaining to tissues around the apex of a tooth, including the periodontal ligament and the alveolar bone

Fracture (FX): Breaking of a bone or tooth

Vital tooth (T/V): Tooth with vital pulp

Nonvital tooth (T/NV): Tooth with nonvital pulp or from which the pulp has been removed

Pulp stones (PU/S): Intrapulpal mineralized structures

Mineralization of the pulp (PU/M): Pulpal mineralization resulting in regional narrowing or complete disappearance of the pulp cavity

Hypercementosis (HC): Excessive deposition of cementum around the root or reserve crown of a tooth

Near pulp exposure (T/NE): Thin layer of dentin separating the pulp from the outer tooth surface

Pulp exposure (T/PE): Tooth with an opening through the wall of the pulp cavity uncovering the pulp

Tooth luxation (T/LUX): Clinically or radiographically evident displacement of the tooth within its alveolus

Tooth avulsion (T/A): Complete extrusive luxation with the tooth out of its alveolus

Periapical pathology (PA/P): Pertaining to disease around the apex of a tooth

Periapical cyst (PA/C): Odontogenic cyst formed around the apex of a tooth after stimulation and

proliferation of epithelial rests in the periodontal ligament (also known as a radicular cyst)

Periapical granuloma (PA/G): Chronic apical periodontitis with an accumulation of mononuclear inflammatory cells and an encircling aggregation of fibroblasts and collagen that on diagnostic imaging appears as a diffuse or circumscribed radiolucent lesion

Periapical abscess (PA/A): Acute or chronic inflammation of the periapical tissues characterized by a localized accumulation of suppuration

Osteosclerosis (OSS): Excessive bone mineralization around the apex of a vital tooth caused by low-grade pulp irritation (asymptomatic; not requiring endodontic therapy)

Condensing osteitis (COO): Excessive bone mineralization around the apex of a nonvital tooth caused by long-standing and low-toxic exudation from an infected pulp (requiring endodontic therapy)

Alveolar osteitis (AOS): Inflammation of the alveolar bone considered to be a complication after tooth extraction

Osteomyelitis (OST): Localized or wide-spread infection of the bone and bone marrow

Osteonecrosis (OSN): Localized or wide-spread necrosis of the bone and bone marrow

Phoenix abscess: Acute exacerbation of chronic apical periodontitis

Intraoral fistula (IOF): Pathologic communication between tooth, bone, or soft tissue and the oral cavity; use **IOF/R** for its repair

Orofacial fistula (OFF): Pathologic communication between the oral cavity and face; use **OFD/R** for its repair

Indirect pulp capping (PCI): Procedure involving the placement of a medicated material over an area of near pulp exposure

Direct pulp-capping (PCD): Procedure performed as part of vital pulp therapy and involving the placement of a medicated material over an area of pulp exposure

Vital pulp therapy (VPT): Procedure performed on a vital tooth with pulp exposure, involving partial pulpectomy, direct pulp capping, and access/fracture site restoration

Apexification (APN): Procedure to promote apical closure of a nonvital tooth

Standard (orthograde) root canal therapy (RCT): Procedure that involves accessing, debriding (including total pulpectomy), shaping, disinfecting, and obturating the root canal and restoring the access and/or fracture sites

Surgical (retrograde) root canal therapy (RCT/S): Procedure that involves accessing the bone surface (through mucosa or skin), fenestration of the bone over the root apex, apicoectomy, and retrograde filling

Apicoectomy (AP/X): Removal of the apex of a tooth; also called root end resection

Retrograde filling: Restoration placed in the apical portion of the root canal after apicoectomy

Tooth repositioning (T/RP): Repositioning of a displaced tooth

Interdental splinting (IDS): Fixation using intraoral splints between teeth within a dental arch (e.g., for avulsed or luxated teeth that underwent reimplantation or repositioning); if performed for jaw fracture repair, use FX/R/IDS

Operative Dentistry and Prosthodontic Terminology

Operative (or restorative) dentistry is a specialty in dentistry and oral surgery that is concerned with the art and science of the diagnosis, treatment, and prognosis of defects of teeth that do not require prosthodontic crowns for correction.

Prosthodontics (or dental prosthetics or prosthetic dentistry) is a specialty in dentistry and oral surgery that is concerned with the provision of suitable substitutes for the clinical crown of teeth or for one or more missing or lost teeth and their associated parts. Maxillofacial prosthetics is considered a subspecialty of prosthodontics, involving palatal obturators and maxillofacial prostheses to replace resected or lost tissues.

Odontoplasty (ODY): Surgical contouring of the tooth surface

Defect preparation (DP): Removal of dental hard tissue to establish in a tooth the biomechanically acceptable form necessary to receive and retain a defect restoration

Restoration (R): Anything that replaces lost tooth structure, teeth, or oral tissues, including fillings, inlays, onlays, veneers, crowns, bridges, implants, dentures, and obturators

Defect restoration: Filling made of amalgam **(R/A)**, glass ionomer **(R/I)**, composite **(R/C)**, or compomer **(R/CP)** within a prepared defect

Bridge (BRI): Fixed partial denture used to replace a missing or lost tooth by joining permanently to adjacent teeth or implants

Crown preparation (CR/P): Removal of enamel or enamel and dentin to establish on a tooth the biomechanically acceptable form necessary to receive and retain a prosthodontic crown

Temporary crown (CR/T): Provisional, short-term cap made of resin to protect a prepared crown until cementation of a prosthodontic crown

Full crown: Prosthodontic crown made of metal **(CR/M)**, resin **(CR/R)**, ceramic **(CR/C)**, or porcelain fused to metal **(CR/PFM)** that covers the tip and all sides of a prepared crown

Partial crown: Prosthodontic crown (e.g., three-quarter crown) made of metal **(CR/M/P)**, resin **(CR/R/P)**, ceramic **(CR/C/P)**, or porcelain fused to metal **(CR/PFM/P)** that covers part of a prepared crown

Implant (IMP): Titanium rod-shaped endosseous device to support intraoral prosthetics that resemble a tooth or group of teeth to replace one or more missing or lost teeth

Crown reduction (CR/XP): Partial removal of tooth substance to reduce the height or an abnormal extension of the clinical crown

Crown amputation (CR/A): Total removal of clinical crown substance

Post and core (PCB): Placing a post into the root canal of a tooth that had root canal therapy and build-up of a core made of filling material around the portion of the post that extends out from the pulp cavity

JAW AND TMJ ABNORMALITIES

Jaw and TMJ Anatomy

All mammals have two maxillas (or maxillae) and two mandibles. The adjective "maxillary" is often used in a wider sense (e.g., "maxillary fractures") to include other facial bones, in addition to the maxillary bone proper.

> **Reference(s):** Anonymous. In: *Nomina Anatomica Veterinaria*. 4th ed. Zurich and Ithaca, NY: World Association of Veterinary Anatomists; 1994.
>
> Evans HE. The skull. In: Evans HE, ed. *Miller's Anatomy of the Dog*. 4th ed. Philadelphia, PA: W.B. Saunders; 1993:128–166.
>
> Hildebrand M. *Analysis of Vertebrate Structure*. 4th ed. New York, NY: John Wiley & Sons; 1995.
>
> Nickel R, Schummer A, Seiferle E, et al. Teeth, general and comparative. In: *The Viscera of Domestic Mammals*. 1st ed. Berlin: Verlag Paul Parey; 1973:75–99.
>
> Verstraete FJM. Maxillofacial fractures. In: Slatter DH, ed. *Textbook of Small Animal Surgery*. 3rd ed. Philadelphia, PA: WB Saunders Co; 2003:2190–2207.

Incisive Bones

In domestic animals, the correct name for the paired bones that carry the maxillary incisors, located rostral to the maxillary bones, is the incisive bones, not the premaxilla.

> **Reference(s):** Anonymous. In: *Nomina Anatomica Veterinaria*. 4th ed. Zurich and Ithaca, NY: World Association of Veterinary Anatomists; 1994.

CLINICALLY RELEVANT TERMS RELATED TO THE MANDIBLE AND TEMPOROMANDIBULAR JOINT: ANATOMIC STRUCTURE COMMENTS

Mandible: All animals have two mandibles, not one; removing one entire mandible is a total mandibulectomy, not a hemimandibulectomy

Body of the mandible: The part that carries the teeth; often incorrectly referred to as horizontal ramus

Incisive part: The part that carries the incisors

Molar part: The part that carries the premolars and molars; premolar-molar part would probably have been more accurate

Alveolar margin: Often incorrectly referred to as alveolar crest

Ventral margin: Free ventral border

Mandibular canal: Contains a neurovascular bundle; often incorrectly referred to as the medullary cavity of the mandible

Mental foramens or foramina: Rostral, middle, or caudal mental foramina in the dog and cat

Ramus of the mandible: The part that carries the three processes; often incorrectly referred to as the vertical ramus

Angular process: Caudoventral process (in *Carnivora*)

Coronoid process: Process for the attachment of the temporal muscle

Condylar process: Consisting of mandibular head and mandibular neck; often incorrectly referred to as condyloid process

Mandibular head: Articular head of the condylar process

Mandibular neck: Neck of the condylar process

Mandibular notch: The notch on the caudal aspect, between the coronoid and condylar processes; not to be confused with the facial vascular notch

Mandibular angle: Angle between the body and ramus of the mandible.

Facial vascular notch: Shallow indentation on the ventral aspect of the mandible, rostral to the angular process (absent in carnivores)

Mandibular foramen: The entrance to the mandibular canal

Intermandibular joint (mandibular symphysis): Median connection of the bodies of the right and left mandibles (in adult Sus and Equus replaced by synostosis), consisting of intermandibular synchondrosis and intermandibular suture

Intermandibular synchondrosis: The smaller part of the intermandibular joint formed by cartilage

Intermandibular suture: The larger part of the intermandibular joint formed by connective tissue

Temporomandibular joint (TMJ): The area where the condylar process of the mandible articulates with the mandibular fossa of the temporal bone

Articular disk: A flat structure composed of fibro-cartilagenous tissue and positioned between the articular surfaces of the condylar process of the mandible and mandibular fossa of the temporal bone, separating the joint capsule in dorsal and ventral compartments; often incorrectly referred to as meniscus

Mandibular fossa: Concave depression in the temporal bone that articulates with the mandibular head

Retroarticular process: A projection of the temporal bone that protrudes ventrally from the caudal end of the zygomatic arch and carries part of the mandibular fossa

Reference(s): Anonymous. In: *Nomina Anatomica Veterinaria.* 4th ed. Zurich and Ithaca, NY: World Association of Veterinary Anatomists; 1994.

Scapino RP. The third joint of the canine jaw. *J Morphol.* 1965;116:23–50.

OTHER TERMS RELATING TO THE JAWS AND TMJ

Alveolar jugum (plural: alveolar juga): The palpable convexity of the buccal alveolar bone overlying a large tooth root

Reference(s): Anonymous. In: *Nomina Anatomica Veterinaria.* 4th ed. Zurich and Ithaca, NY: World Association of Veterinary Anatomists; 1994.

Evans HE. *Miller's Anatomy of the Dog.* 3rd ed. Philadelphia, PA: WB Saunders Co; 1993.

Dental arch: Referring to the curving structure formed by the teeth in their normal position; upper dental arch formed by the maxillary teeth, lower dental arch formed by the mandibular teeth

Jaw quadrant: Referring to the left or right upper or lower jaw

Interarch: Referring to the area between the upper and lower dental arches

Interquadrant: Referring to the area between the left and right upper or lower jaw quadrants

Jaw and Related Abbreviations

Mandible/mandibular (MN): Referring to the lower jaw

Maxilla/maxillary (MX): Referring to the upper jaw

Mandibular symphysis (SYM): Joint between the left and right mandibles (intermandibular joint)

Zygomatic arch (ZYG): Consisting of the zygomatic process of the temporal bone and the temporal process of the zygomatic bone; also called zygoma

JAW TRAUMA

Maxillary fracture (MX/FX): Fracture of the upper jaw (maxilla and other facial bones)

Mandibular fracture (MN/FX): Fracture of the lower jaw (mandible)

Symphyseal separation (SYM/S): Separation of the two mandibles in the mandibular symphysis; this includes parasymphyseal fractures where the fracture line is partly or completely paramedian to the symphysis; repair of symphyseal separation with wire (circumferential or interquadrant) and/or intraoral resin splinting is abbreviated with

Repair of a jaw fracture (FX/R): Used when any of the other abbreviations do not describe the jaw fracture repair technique applied

Maxillomandibular fixation (FX/R/MMF): Fixation that brings together the upper and lower jaws; use MMF for devices other than muzzles and splints

Muzzling (FX/R/MZ): Maxillomandibular fixation using a prefabricated or custom-made muzzle; also used in horses to prevent eating (e.g., postsedation)

Interarch splinting (FX/R/IAS): Maxillomandibular fixation using intraoral splints (commonly resin that can be reinforced with wire)

Interquadrant splinting (FX/R/IQS): Fixation using intraoral splints (commonly resin that can be reinforced with wire) between the left and right upper or lower jaw quadrants

Interdental splinting (FX/R/IDS): Fixation using intraoral splints (commonly resin that can be reinforced with wire) between teeth within a dental arch

Intraosseous wiring (FX/R/WIR/OS): Fixation using intraosseous wire

Bone plating (FX/R/PL): Fixation using bone plates

External skeletal fixation (FX/R/EXF): Fixation using pins or wires and extraoral splinting

Wire cerclage (FX/R/WIR/C): Fixation using circumferential wiring

Temporomandibular Joint Trauma and Other Conditions

Decreased mouth opening (DMO): Difficulty opening the mouth by the animal or decreased range of mouth opening upon oral examination

Temporomandibular joint fracture (TMJ/FX): Fracture of one or more bony structures forming the temporomandibular joint; surgical repair is abbreviated with TMJ/FX/R

Temporomandibular joint ankylosis (TMJ/A): Fusion between the bones forming the temporomandibular joint or those in close proximity, resulting in a progressive inability to open the mouth; removal of bone in ankylotic areas is abbreviated with TMJ/A/R

Temporomandibular joint luxation (TMJ/LUX): Displacement of the condylar process of the mandible; manual or surgical reduction of temporomandibular joint luxation is abbreviated with TMJ/LUX/R

Temporomandibular joint dysplasia (TMJ/D): Dysplasia of soft or hard tissues forming the temporomandibular joint

Open-mouth jaw locking (OMJL): Inability to close the mouth due to locking of the coronoid process of the mandible ventrolateral to the ipsilateral zygomatic arch; manual reduction of open-mouth jaw locking is abbreviated with OMJL/R

Zygomectomy (ZYG/X): Resection (usually partial) of the zygomatic arch

Coronoidectomy (COR/X): Resection (usually partial) of the coronoid process of the mandible

Condylectomy (CON/X): Resection of the condylar process of the mandible

PERIODONTAL ANATOMY AND DISEASE

Definitions of Stage, Grade, and Index

Stage: The assessment of the extent of pathologic lesions in the course of a disease that is likely to be progressive (e.g., stages of periodontal disease, staging of oral tumors)

Grade: The quantitative assessment of the degree of severity of a disease or abnormal condition at the time of diagnosis, irrespective of whether the disease is progressive (e.g., a grade 2 mast cell tumor based on mitotic figures)

Index: A quantitative expression of predefined diagnostic criteria whereby the presence and/or severity of pathologic conditions are recorded by assessing a numerical value (e.g., gingival index, plaque index)

STAGES OF PERIODONTAL DISEASE

The degree of severity of periodontal disease (PD) relates to a single tooth; a patient may have teeth that have different stages of periodontal disease.

Normal (PD0): Clinically normal; gingival inflammation or periodontitis is not clinically evident.

Stage 1 (PD1): Gingivitis only without attachment loss; the height and architecture of the alveolar margin are normal.

Stage 2 (PD2): Early periodontitis; less than 25% of attachment loss or, at most, there is a stage 1 furcation involvement in multirooted teeth. There are early radiologic signs of periodontitis. The loss of periodontal attachment is less than 25% as measured either by probing of the clinical attachment level or radiographic determination of the distance of the alveolar margin from the cementoenamel junction relative to the length of the root.

Stage 3 (PD3): Moderate periodontitis; 25% to 50% of attachment loss as measured either by probing of the clinical attachment level, radiographic determination of the distance of the alveolar margin from the cementoenamel junction relative to the length of the root, or there is a stage 2 furcation involvement in multirooted teeth.

Stage 4 (PD4): Advanced periodontitis; more than 50% of attachment loss as measured either by probing of the clinical attachment level, or radiographic determination of the distance of the alveolar margin from the cementoenamel junction relative to the length of the root, or there is a stage 3 furcation involvement in multirooted teeth.

Reference(s): Wolf HF, Rateitschak EM, Rateitschak KH, et al. *Color Atlas of Dental Medicine: Periodontology.* 3rd ed. Stuttgart: Georg Thieme Verlag; 2005.

Furcation Involvement and Mobility Index
Furcation Index

Stage 1 (F1): Furcation 1 involvement exists when a periodontal probe extends less than halfway under the crown in any direction of a multirooted tooth with attachment loss.

Stage 2 (F2): Furcation 2 involvement exists when a periodontal probe extends greater than halfway under the crown of a multirooted tooth with attachment loss but not through and through.

Stage 3 (F3): Furcation exposure exists when a periodontal probe extends under the crown of a multirooted tooth, through and through from one side of the furcation out the other.

Tooth Mobility Index
Stage 0 (M0): Physiologic mobility up to 0.2 mm.

Stage 1 (M1): The mobility is increased in any direction other than axial over a distance of more than 0.2 mm and up to 0.5 mm.

Stage 2 (M2): The mobility is increased in any direction other than axial over a distance of more than 0.5 mm and up to 1.0 mm.

Stage 3 (M3): The mobility is increased in any direction other than axial over a distance exceeding 1.0 mm or any axial movement.

Gingival and Periodontal Pathology

Gingivitis: Inflammation of gingiva

Periodontitis: Inflammation of nongingival periodontal tissues (i.e., the periodontal ligament and alveolar bone)

Gingival recession (GR): Root surface exposure caused by apical migration of the gingival margin or loss of gingiva.

Gingival enlargement (GE): Clinical term, referring to overgrowth or thickening of gingiva in the absence of a histologic diagnosis

Gingival hyperplasia (GH): Histologic term, referring to an abnormal increase in the number of normal cells in a normal arrangement and resulting clinically in gingival enlargement

Abnormal tooth extrusion (ATE): Increase in clinical crown length not related to gingival recession or lack of tooth wear

Alveolar bone expansion (ABE): Thickening of alveolar bone at labial and buccal aspects of teeth

Periodontal Treatment

Professional oral care includes mechanical procedures performed in the oral cavity.

Professional dental cleaning (PRO) refers to scaling (supragingival and subgingival plaque and calculus removal) and polishing of the teeth with power/hand instrumentation performed by a trained veterinary health care provider under general anesthesia. See also AVDC Position Statements on Dental Health Care Providers and on Non-Professional Dental Scaling.

Periodontal therapy refers to the treatment of diseased periodontal tissues that include professional dental cleaning as defined above and one or more of the following: root planing, gingival curettage, periodontal flaps, regenerative surgery, gingivectomy/gingivoplasty, and local administration of antiseptics/antibiotics.

Home oral hygiene refers to measures taken by pet owners that are aimed at controlling or preventing plaque and calculus accumulation.

Gingival curettage (GC): Removal of damaged or diseased tissue from the soft tissue lining of a periodontal pocket

Root planing (RP): Removal of dental deposits from and smoothing of the root surface of a tooth; it is closed (**RP/C**) when performed without a flap or open (**RP/O**) when performed after creation of a flap

Gingivectomy (GV): Removal of some or all gingiva surrounding a tooth

Gingivoplasty (GV): A form of gingivectomy performed to restore physiological contours of the gingiva

Guided tissue regeneration (GTR): Regeneration of tissue directed by the physical presence and/or chemical activities of a biomaterial; often involves placement of barriers to exclude one or more cell types during healing of tissue

Crown lengthening (CR/L): Increasing clinical crown height by means of gingivectomy/gingivoplasty, apically positioned flaps, post and core build-up, or orthodontic movement

Frenuloplasty (frenulotomy, frenulectomy) (FRE): Reconstructive surgery or excision of a frenulum

Hemisection (HS): Splitting of a tooth into two separate portions

Trisection (TS): Splitting of a tooth into three separate portions

Partial tooth resection (T/XP): Removal of a crown-root segment with endodontic treatment of the remainder of the tooth

Root resection/amputation (RO/X): Removal of a root with maintenance of the entire crown and endodontic treatment of the remainder of the tooth

Flap Surgery

Flap (F): A sheet of tissue partially or totally detached to gain access to structures underneath or to be used in repairing defects; can be classified based on the location of the donor site (local or distant), attachment to donor site (pedicle, island, or free), tissue to be transferred (e.g., mucosal, mucoperiosteal, cutaneous, myocutaneous), tissue thickness (partial-thickness or full-thickness), blood supply (random pattern or axial pattern), and direction and orientation of transfer (envelope, advancement, rotation, transposition, and hinged).

Location of Donor Site

Local flap: Harvested from an adjacent site
Distant flap: Harvested from a remote site

Attachment to Donor Site

Pedicle flap: Attached by tissue through which it receives its blood supply
Island flap (F/IS): Attached by a pedicle made up of only the nutrient vessels
Free flap: Completely detached from the body; it has also been suggested that a free flap be termed a graft

Tissue to Be Transferred

Mucosal flap: Containing mucosa
Mucoperiosteal flap: Containing mucosa and underlying periosteum
Cutaneous (or skin) flap: Containing epidermis, dermis, and subcutaneous tissue
Myocutaneous flap: Containing skin and muscle
Gingival flap: Containing gingiva
Alveolar mucosa flap: Containing alveolar mucosa
Periodontal flap: Containing gingiva and alveolar mucosa
Labial flap: Containing lip mucosa
Buccal flap: Containing cheek mucosa
Sublingual flap: Containing sublingual mucosa
Palatal flap: Containing palatal mucosa
Pharyngeal flap: Containing pharyngeal mucosa

Tissue Thickness

Partial-thickness (or split-thickness) flap: Consisting of a portion of the original tissue thickness

Full-thickness flap: Having the original tissue thickness

Blood Supply

Random pattern flap: Randomly supplied by nonspecific arteries

Axial pattern flap: Supplied by a specific artery

Direction and Orientation of Transfer

Envelope flap (F/EN): Retracted away from a horizontal incision; there is no vertical incision

Advancement (or sliding) flap (F/AD): Carried to its new position by a sliding technique in a direction away from its base

Rotation flap (F/RO): A pedicle flap that is rotated into a defect on a fulcrum point

Transposition flap (F/TR): Flap that combines the features of an advancement flap and a rotation flap

Hinged flap (F/HI): Folded on its pedicle as though the pedicle was a hinge; also called a turnover or overlapping flap

Apically positioned flap (F/AP): Moved apical to its original location

Coronally positioned flap (F/CO): Moved coronal to its original location

Mesiodistally or distomesially positioned flap: Moved distal or mesial to its original location along the dental arch; also called a laterally positioned flap (**F/LA**)

ORAL PATHOLOGY: INFLAMMATORY DISEASES, TUMORS, OTHER ABNORMALITIES

Oral Inflammation

Note that a definitive diagnosis of inflammation often cannot be made based on physical examination findings alone.

Oral and oropharyngeal inflammation is classified by location:

Gingivitis: Inflammation of gingiva

Periodontitis: Inflammation of nongingival periodontal tissues (i.e., the periodontal ligament and alveolar bone)

Alveolar mucositis: Inflammation of alveolar mucosa (i.e., mucosa overlying the alveolar process and extending from the mucogingival junction without obvious demarcation to the vestibular sulcus and to the floor of the mouth)

Sublingual mucositis: Inflammation of mucosa on the floor of the mouth

Labial/buccal mucositis: Inflammation of lip/cheek mucosa

Caudal mucositis: Inflammation of mucosa of the caudal oral cavity bordered medially by the palatoglossal folds and fauces, dorsally by the hard and soft palate, and rostrally by alveolar and buccal mucosa

Feline stomatitis (FST): A condition in the cat characterized by inflammation of the oral mucosa, often affecting the area immediately lateral to the palatoglossal folds (caudal stomatitis, ST/CS) with or without inflammation of other oral mucosa (i.e., gingiva, alveolar mucosa, labial/buccal mucosa, sublingual mucosa, and/or lingual mucosa); it commonly presents during the chronic stage, with or without (often proliferative) inflammation extending into mucosa of the oropharynx

Contact mucositis and contact mucosal ulceration (CU): Lesions in susceptible individuals that are secondary to mucosal contact with a tooth surface bearing the responsible irritant, allergen, or antigen. They have also been called "contact ulcers" and "kissing ulcers"

Palatitis: Inflammation of mucosa covering the hard and/or soft palate

Glossitis: Inflammation of mucosa of the dorsal and/or ventral tongue surface

Osteomyelitis (OST): Inflammation of the bone and bone marrow

Cheilitis: Inflammation of the lip (including the mucocutaneous junction area and skin of the lip)

Tonsillitis (TON/IN): Inflammation of the palatine tonsil

Pharyngitis (PHA/IN): Inflammation of the pharynx

AUTOIMMUNE CONDITIONS AFFECTING THE MOUTH

Pemphigus vulgaris (PV): Autoimmune disease characterized histologically by intraepithelial blister formation (after breakdown or loss of intercellular adhesion), biochemically by evidence of circulating autoantibodies against components of the epithelial desmosome–tonofilament complexes, and clinically by the presence of vesiculobullous and/or ulcerative oral and mucocutaneous lesions

Bullous pemphigoid (BUP): Autoimmune disease characterized histologically by subepithelial clefting (separation at the epithelium–connective tissue interface), biochemically by evidence of circulating autoantibodies against components of the basement membrane, and clinically by the presence of erythematous, erosive, vesiculobullous, and/or ulcerative oral lesions

Lupus erythematosis (LE): Autoimmune disease characterized histologically by basal cell destruction, hyperkeratosis, epithelial atrophy, subepithelial and perivascular lymphocytic infiltration, and vascular dilation with submucosal edema; biochemically by the evidence of circulating autoantibodies against various cellular antigens in both the nucleus and cytoplasm; and clinically by the presence of acute lesions (systemic **LE**) to skin, mucosa and multiple organs or chronic lesions (discoid **LE**) mostly confined to the skin of the face and mucosa of the oral cavity

Masticatory muscle myositis (MMM): Autoimmune disease affecting the temporal, masseter, and medial and lateral pterygoid muscles of the dog. The term masticatory myositis is an acceptable alternative

ORAL TUMORS

The AVDC Nomenclature Committee is working with human oral pathologists, veterinary pathologists, and veterinary oncologists to develop a set of names for specific tumor types that will be acceptable for standard use in veterinary dental patients.

Abbreviations to be used in AVDC case logs are shown in blue in brackets.

The term "epulis" (plural = "epulides") is a general term referring to a gingival mass lesion of any type. Examples of epulides include the following: focal fibrous hyperplasia, peripheral odotogenic fibroma, acanthomatous ameloblastoma, nonodontogenic tumors, pyogenic granulomas, and reactive exostosis.

Types of Neoplasms Occurring in Oral Tissues (Listed in Alphabetical Order)

Acanthomatous ameloblastoma (OM/AA): A typically benign, but aggressive, histologic variant of a group of epithelial odontogenic tumors known collectively as ameloblastomas that have a basic structure resembling the enamel organ (suggesting derivation from ameloblasts); the acanthomatous histologic designation refers to the central cells within nests of odontogenic epithelium that are squamous and may be keratinized rather than stellate

Adenoma (OM/AD): Benign epithelial tumor in which the cells form recognizable glandular structures or in which the cells are derived from glandular epithelium

Adenocarcinoma (OM/ADC): An invasive, malignant epithelial neoplasm derived from glandular tissue of either the oral cavity, nasal cavity, or salivary tissue (major or accessory)

Amyloid-producing odontogenic tumor (OM/APO): A benign epithelial odontogenic tumor characterized by the presence of odontogenic epithelium and extra-cellular amyloid

Anaplastic neoplasm (OM/APN): A malignant neoplasm the cells of which are generally undifferentiated and pleomorphic (displaying variability in size, shape, and pattern of cells and/or their nuclei)

Cementoma (OM/CE): A benign odontogenic neoplasm of mesenchymal origin, consisting of cementum-like tissue deposited by cells resembling cementoblasts

Feline inductive odontogenic tumor (OM/FIO): A benign tumor unique to adolescent and young adult cats that originates multifocally within the supporting connective tissue as characteristic, spherical condensations of fibroblastic connective tissue associated with islands of odontogenic epithelium; has also been incorrectly called inductive fibroameloblastoma

Fibrosarcoma (OM/FS): An invasive, malignant mesenchymal neoplasm of fibroblasts; a distinct histologically low-grade, biologically high-grade variant is often found in the oral cavity

Giant cell granuloma (OM/GCG): A benign, tumor-like growth consisting of multinucleated giant cells within a background stroma on the gingiva (peripheral giant cell granuloma) or within bone (central giant cell granuloma); also called giant cell epulis

Granular cell tumor (OM/GCT): A benign tumor of the skin or mucosa with uncertain histogenesis, most commonly occurring on the tongue; also called myoblastoma

Hemangiosarcoma (OM/HS): A malignant neoplasm of vascular endothelial origin characterized by extensive metastasis; it has been reported in the gingiva, tongue, and hard palate

Lipoma (OM/LI): A benign mesenchymal neoplasm of lipocytes

Lymphosarcoma (OM/LS): A malignant neoplasm defined by a proliferation of lymphocytes within solid organs such as the lymph nodes, tonsils, bone marrow, liver, and spleen; the disease also may occur in the eye, skin, nasal cavity, oral cavity, and gastrointestinal tract; also known as lymphoma

Malignant melanoma (OM/MM): An invasive, malignant neoplasm of melanocytes or melanocyte precursors that may or may not be pigmented (amelanotic); also called melanosarcoma

Mast cell tumor (OM/MCT): A local aggregation of mast cells forming a nodular tumor, having the potential to become malignant; also called mastocytoma

Multilobular tumor of bone (OM/MTB): A potentially malignant and locally invasive neoplasm of bone that more commonly affects the mandible, hard palate, and flat bones of the cranium with a multilobular histologic pattern of bony or cartilaginous matrix surrounded by a thin layer of spindle cells that gives it a near pathognomonic radiographic "popcorn ball" appearance; also called multilobular osteochondrosarcoma, multilobular osteoma, multilobular chondroma, chondroma rodens, and multilobular osteosarcoma

Odontoma (OM/OD): Odontogenic tumor that contains varying proportions of odontogenic epithelium, papillary ectomesenchyme, and dental hard matrices. It is rare in veterinary species, is typically found in younger animals, and generally manifests as unilateral and focal lesion. The compound odontoma (OM/ODD) is well differentiated, often containing recognizable tooth-like structures (denticles) with enamel, dentin, cementum, and pulp, whereas the complex odontoma (OM/ODX) is less organized, usually containing a scrambled mix of odontogenic epithelium and dental hard matrices (mostly dentin or osteodentin) embedded in a fibrovascular stroma typically lacking overt features of ectomesenchyme of the dental papilla. Because the proliferative potential of the compound odontoma is limited, some investigators consider it to be a hamartomatous malformation (hamartoma) rather than a true neoplasm.

Osteoma (OM/OO): A benign neoplasm of bone consisting of mature, compact, or cancellous bone

Osteosarcoma (OM/OS): A locally aggressive malignant mesenchymal neoplasm of primitive bone cells that have the ability to produce osteoid or immature bone

Papilloma (OM/PAP): An exophytic, pedunculated, cauliflower-like benign neoplasm of epithelium; canine papillomatosis is thought to be caused by infection with canine papillomavirus in typically young dogs; severe papillomatosis may be recognized in older immunocompromised dogs

Peripheral nerve sheath tumor (OM/PNT): A group of neural tumors arising from Schwann cells or perineural fibroblasts (or a combination of both cell types) of the cranial nerves, spinal nerve roots, or peripheral nerves; they may be classified as histologically benign or malignant

Peripheral odontogenic fibroma (OM/POF): A benign mesenchymal odontogenic tumor associated with the gingiva and believed to originate from the periodontal ligament; characterized by varying amounts of inactive-looking odontogenic epithelium embedded in a mature, fibrous stroma, which may undergo osseous metaplasia; historically has been referred to as fibromatous epulis or—when bone or tooth-like hard tissue present within the lesion—ossifying epulis

Plasma cell tumor (OM/PCT): A proliferation of plasma cells, commonly occurring on the gingiva or dorsum of the tongue; also called plasmacytoma

Rhabdomyosarcoma (OM/RBM): A malignant neoplasm of skeletal muscle or embryonic mesenchymal cells

Squamous cell carcinoma (OM/SCC): An invasive, malignant epithelial neoplasm of the oral epithelium with varying degrees of squamous differentiation

Undifferentiated neoplasm (OM/UDN): A malignant neoplasm the cells of which are generally immature and lack distinctive features of a particular tissue type

Diagnostic and Nonsurgical Treatment Procedures

Biopsy (B): Removal of tissue from a living body for diagnostic purposes. The term has also been used to describe the tissue being submitted for evaluation

Guided biopsy (B/G): Using computed tomography or ultrasonography to guide an instrument to the selected area for tissue removal

Surface biopsy (B/S): Removal of tissue brushed, scraped, or obtained by an impression smear from the intact or cut surface of the tissue in question

Needle aspiration (B/NA): Removal of tissue by application of suction through a hollow needle attached to a syringe

Needle biopsy (B/NB): Removal of tissue by puncture with a hollow needle

Core needle biopsy (B/CN): Removal of tissue with a large hollow needle that extracts a core of tissue

Bite biopsy (B/B): Removal of tissue by closing the opposing ends of an instrument

Punch biopsy (B/P): Removal of tissue by a punch-type instrument

Incisional biopsy (B/I): Removal of a selected portion of tissue by means of surgical cutting

Excisional biopsy (B/E): Removal of the entire tissue in question by means of surgical cutting

Radiotherapy (RTH): Use of ionizing radiation to control or kill tumor cells; also called radiation therapy

Chemotherapy (CTH): Use of cytotoxic antineoplastic drugs (chemotherapeutic agents) to control or kill tumor cells

Immunotherapy (ITH): Use of the immune system to control or kill tumor cells

Radiography (RAD): Two-dimensional imaging of dental, periodontal, oral, and maxillofacial structures using an X-ray machine and radiographic films, sensor pads, or phosphor plates

Computed tomography (CT): A method of medical imaging that uses computer-processed X-rays to produce tomographic images or "slices" of specific areas of the body; digital geometry processing is used to generate three-dimensional images of an object of interest from a large series of two-dimensional

X-ray images taken around a single axis of rotation

Cone-beam CT (CT/CB): Variation of traditional CT that rotates around the patient, capturing data using a cone-shaped X-ray beam

Magnetic resonance imaging (MRI): A method of medical imaging that uses the property of nuclear magnetic resonance to image nuclei of atoms inside the body

Ultrasonography (US): A method of medical imaging of deep structures of the body by recording the echoes of pulses of ultrasonic waves directed into the tissues and reflected by tissue planes where there is a change in density

Scintigraphy (SCI): A method of medical imaging that uses radioisotopes taken internally (e.g., by mouth, injection, and inhalation); the emitted radiation is captured by external detectors (gamma cameras) to form two-dimensional images

Surgical Treatment Procedures for Oral Tumors

Surgery (S): Branch of medicine that treats diseases, injuries, and deformities by manual or operative methods

Buccotomy (BUC): Incision through the cheek (e.g., to gain access to an intraoral procedure)

Cheiloplasty/commissuroplasty (CPL): Reconstructive surgery of the lip/lip commissure

Commissurotomy (COM): Incision through the lip commissure (e.g., to gain access to an intraoral procedure)

Partial mandibulectomy (S/M): Surgical removal (en block) of part of the mandible and surrounding soft tissues

Dorsal marginal mandibulectomy (S/MD): A form of partial mandibulectomy in which the ventral border of the mandible is maintained; also called marginal mandibulectomy or mandibular rim excision

Segmental mandibulectomy (S/MS): A form of partial mandibulectomy in which a full dorsoventral segment of the mandible is removed

Bilateral partial mandibulectomy (S/MB): Surgical removal of parts of the left and right mandibles and surrounding soft tissues

Total mandibulectomy (S/MT): Surgical removal of one mandible and surrounding soft tissues

Partial maxillectomy (S/X): Surgical removal (en block) of part of the maxilla and/or other facial bones and surrounding soft tissues

Bilateral partial maxillectomy (S/XB): Surgical removal of parts of the left and right maxillae and/or other facial bones and surrounding soft tissues

Partial palatectomy (S/P): Partial resection of the palate

OTHER ORAL PATHOLOGY

Chewing lesion (CL): Mucosal lesion resulting from self-induced bite trauma on the cheek (**CL/B**), lip (**CL/L**), palate (**CL/P**), or tongue/sublingual region (**CL/T**)

Eosinophilic granuloma (EOG): Referring to conditions affecting the lip/labial mucosa (**EOG/L**), hard/soft palate (**EOG/P**), tongue/sublingual mucosa (**EOG/T**), and skin that are characterized histopathologically by the presence of an eosinophilic infiltrate

Pyogenic granuloma (PYO): Inflammatory proliferation at the vestibular mucogingival tissues of the mandibular first molar tooth (in the cat probably owing to malocclusion and secondary traumatic contact of these tissues by the ipsilateral maxillary fourth premolar tooth)

Erythema multiforme (EM): Typically drug-induced hypersensitivity reaction characterized by erythematous, vesiculobullous, and/or ulcerative oral and skin lesions

Calcinosis circumscripta (CC): Circumscribed areas of mineralization characterized by deposition of calcium salts (e.g., in the tip of the tongue)

Retrobulbar abscess (RBA): Abscess behind the globe of the eye

Retropharyngeal abscess (RPA): Abscess behind the pharynx

Craniomandibular osteopathy (CMO): Disease characterized by cyclical resorption of normal bone and excessive replacement by immature bone along mandibular, temporal, and other bone surfaces in immature and adolescent dogs

Calvarial hyperostosis (CHO): Disease characterized by irregular, progressive proliferation, and thickening of the cortex of the bones forming the calvarium in adolescent dogs

Fibrous osteodystrophy (FOD): Disease characterized by the formation of hyperostotic bone lesions, in which deposition of unmineralized osteoid by hyperplastic osteoblasts and production of fibrous connective tissue exceed the rate of bone resorption; usually caused by primary or secondary hyperparathyroidism; resulting in softened, pliable, and distorted bones of the face ("rubber jaw," "bighead," or "bran disease")

Periostitis ossificans (PEO): Periosteal new bone formation in immature dogs, manifesting clinically as (usually) unilateral swelling of the mid to caudal body of the mandible and radiographically as two-layered (double) ventral mandibular cortex

TONGUE, LIPS, PALATE, PHARYNX, NOSE, FACE, SALIVARY GLANDS, AND LYMPH NODES

Anatomy of the Tongue, Lips, Cheek, and Palate

Tongue (LIN): Fleshy muscular organ in the mouth used for tasting, licking, swallowing, articulating, and thermoregulation; use **LIN/X** for tongue resection

Lip/cheek (LIP): Fleshy parts that form the upper and lower edges of the opening of the mouth/side of the face below the eye; use **LIP/X** for lip/cheek resection

Lip avulsion (LIP/A): A traumatic separation of the lip from the underlying connective tissue; use LIP/A/R for lip avulsion repair

Hard palate: The part of the palate supported by bone

The **midline of the hard palate** is not a symphysis but is formed by the interincisive suture, the median palatine suture of the palatine processes of the maxillary bones, and the median suture of the palatine bones.

Reference(s): Anonymous. In: *Nomina Anatomica Veterinaria*. 4th ed. Zurich and Ithaca, NY: World Association of Veterinary Anatomists; 1994. Evans HE. *Miller's Anatomy of the Dog*. 3rd ed. Philadelphia, PA: WB Saunders Co; 1993.

Palatine rugae: Transverse ridges of mucosa on the hard palate

Incisive papilla: Elevation of mucosa at the rostral end of the median line of junction of the halves of the palate, concealing the orifices of the incisive ducts

Soft palate: The caudal part of the palate that is not supported by bone

Abnormalities of the Palate

Palate defect (PDE): Acquired communication between the oral and nasal cavities along the hard or soft palate; surgical repair is abbreviated **PDE/R**

Cleft lip (CFL): Congenital longitudinal defect of the upper lip or upper lip and most rostral hard palate (regardless of location); surgical repair is abbreviated **CFL/R**

Cleft palate (CFP): Congenital longitudinal defect in the midline of the hard and soft palate; surgical repair is abbreviated **CFP/R**

Cleft soft palate (CFS): Congenital longitudinal defect in the midline of the soft palate only; surgical repair is abbreviated **CFS/R**

Unilateral soft palate defect (CFSU): Congenital longitudinal defect of the soft palate on one side only; surgical repair is abbreviated **CFSU/R**

Soft palate hypoplasia (CFSH): Congenital decrease in length of the soft palate; surgical lengthening of the soft palate is abbreviated **CFSH/R**

Traumatic cleft palate (CFT): Acquired longitudinal defect in the midline of the hard and/or soft palate resulting from trauma; surgical repair is abbreviated **CFT/R**

Oronasal fistula (ONF): Acquired communication between the oral and nasal cavities along the upper dental arch; surgical repair is abbreviated **ONF/R**

Oroantral fistula (OAF): Acquired communication between the oral cavity and maxillary sinus in pigs, ruminants, and equines (also called oromaxillary fistula in equines); surgical repair is abbreviated **OAF/R**

Elongated soft palate (ESP): Congenital increase in length of the soft palate; surgical reduction of the soft palate is abbreviated **ESP/R**

Palatal obturator (POB): Prosthetic device for temporary or permanent closure of palate defects

ANATOMY OF THE NOSE, PHARYNX, TONSIL, AND FACE

Palatine tonsil (TON): Tonsil related to the lateral attachment of the soft palate

Tonsillar fossa: Depression containing the palatine tonsil

Semilunar fold: Mucosal fold from the ventrolateral aspect of the soft palate, forming the medial wall of the tonsillar fossa

Pharynx (PHA): Throat caudal to the oral cavity and divided into nasopharynx and oropharynx

Fauces: The fauces are defined as the lateral walls of the oropharynx that are located medial to the palatoglossal folds. The areas lateral to the palatoglossal fold, commonly involved in feline stomatitis, are not the fauces.

Reference(s): Anonymous. In: *Nomina Anatomica Veterinaria*. 4th ed. Zurich and Ithaca, NY: World Association of Veterinary Anatomists; 1994.

Evans HE. *Miller's Anatomy of the Dog*. 3rd ed. Philadelphia, PA: WB Saunders Co; 1993.

Nose/nasal (N): Referring to the part of the face or facial region that contains the nostrils and nasal cavity

SALIVARY GLAND ABNORMALITIES AND DIAGNOSTIC PROCEDURES

Ptyalism (PTY): Excessive flow of saliva; also called hypersalivation

Sublingual sialocele (SG/MUC/S): Mucus extravasation phenomenon manifesting in the sublingual region; also called **ranula**

Pharyngeal sialocele (SG/MUC/P): Mucus extravasation phenomenon manifesting in the pharyngeal region

Cervical sialocele (SG/MUC/C): Mucus extravasation phenomenon manifesting in the intermandibular or cervical region

Mucus retention cyst (SG/RC): Intraductal mucus accumulation with duct dilation resulting from obstruction of salivary flow (e.g., owing to a sialolith)

Sialadenitis (SG/IN): Inflammation of a salivary gland

Sialadenosis (SG/ADS): Noninflammatory, nonneoplastic enlargement of a salivary gland; also called **sialosis**

Necrotizing sialometaplasia (SG/NEC): Squamous metaplasia of the salivary gland ducts and lobules with ischemic necrosis of the salivary gland lobules; also called **salivary gland infarction**

Salivary gland adenocarcinoma (SG/ADC): Adenocarcinoma arising from salivary glandular or ductal tissue; use abbreviations under **OM** for other salivary gland tumors.

Sialocele (or salivary mucocele): Clinical term indicating a swelling that contains saliva and includes mucus extravasation phenomenon and mucus retention cyst

Mucus extravasation phenomenon: Accumulation of saliva that leaked from a salivary duct into subcutaneous or submucosal tissue and consequent tissue reaction to saliva

Sialolithiasis (SG/SI): Condition characterized by the presence of one or more sialoliths, a calcareous concretion or calculus (stone) in the salivary duct or gland

Sialography (RAD/SG): Radiographic technique where a radiopaque contrast agent is infused into the ductal system of a salivary gland before imaging is performed

Salivary gland resection (SG/X): Surgical removal of a salivary gland

Marsupialization (MAR): Exteriorization of an enclosed cavity by resecting a portion of the cutaneous or mucosal wall and suturing the cut edges of the remaining wall to adjacent edges of the skin or mucosa, thereby creating a pouch; use **SG/MAR** for marsupialization of a sublingual or pharyngeal sialocele

LYMPH NODES

Lymph node (LN): Lymphoid tissue that produces lymphocytes and has a capsule; filters lymph fluid, as afferent lymph vessels enter the node and efferent lymph vessels leave the node

Tonsil (TON): Lymphoid tissue that produces lymphocytes but lacks a capsule; not filtering lymph fluid, as there are no afferent lymph vessels

Lymph node enlargement (LN/E): Palpable or visual enlargement of a lymph node

Regional metastasis (MET/R): Neoplastic spread to regional lymph node(s) confirmed by biopsy

Distant metastasis (MET/D): Neoplastic spread to distant sites confirmed by biopsy or diagnostic imaging

Lymph node resection (LN/X): Surgical removal of a lymph node

OCCLUSAL ABNORMALITIES

Normal Occlusion

Ideal occlusion can be described as perfect interdigitation of the upper and lower teeth. In the dog, the ideal tooth positions in the arches are defined by the occlusal, interarch, and interdental relationships of the teeth of the archetypal dog (i.e., wolf). This ideal relationship with the mouth closed can be defined by the following:

Maxillary incisor teeth are all positioned rostral to the corresponding mandibular incisor teeth.

The crown cusps of the mandibular incisor teeth contact the cingulum of the maxillary incisor teeth.

The mandibular canine tooth is inclined labially and bisects the interproximal (interdental) space between the opposing maxillary third incisor tooth and canine tooth.

The maxillary premolar teeth do not contact the mandibular premolar teeth.

The crown cusps of the mandibular premolar teeth are positioned lingual to the arch of the maxillary premolar teeth.

The crown cusps of the mandibular premolar teeth bisect the interproximal (interdental) spaces rostral to the corresponding maxillary premolar teeth.

The mesial crown cusp of the maxillary fourth premolar tooth is positioned lateral to the space between the mandibular fourth premolar tooth and the mandibular first molar tooth.

Normal occlusion in cats is similar to dogs.

Maxillary incisor teeth are labial to the mandibular incisor teeth, with the incisal tips of the mandibular incisors contacting the cingula of the maxillary incisors or occluding just palatal to the maxillary incisors.

Mandibular canine teeth fit equidistant in the diastema between the maxillary third incisor teeth and the maxillary canine teeth, touching neither.

The incisor bite and canine interdigitation form the dental interlock.

Each mandibular premolar tooth is positioned mesial to the corresponding maxillary premolar tooth.

The maxillary second premolar tooth points in a space between the mandibular canine tooth and third premolar tooth.

The subsequent teeth interdigitate, with the mandibular premolars and first molar being situated lingual to the maxillary teeth.

The buccal surface of the mandibular first molar tooth occludes with the palatal surface of the maxillary fourth premolar tooth.

The maxillary first molar tooth is located distopalatal to the maxillary fourth premolar tooth.

Malocclusion (MAL) is any deviation from normal occlusion described above.

Malocclusion may be caused by abnormal positioning of a tooth or teeth (dental malocclusion) or by asymmetry or other deviation of bones that support the dentition (skeletal malocclusion).

The diagnosis for a patient with malocclusion is abbreviated as MAL (malocclusion) 1 or 2 or 3 or 4 (= malocclusion class designation)/specific malocclusion abbreviation and tooth or teeth number(s).

Example: MAL1/CB/R202 for a dog with class 1 malocclusion and a rostral crossbite of the left maxillary second incisor.

If multiple teeth have the same malocclusion, include the tooth numbers with a comma in between (e.g., MAL1/CB/R202,302).

Dental Malocclusions

Neutroclusion: Class 1 Malocclusion (MAL1)

A normal rostrocaudal relationship of the maxillary and mandibular dental arches with malposition of one or more individual teeth

Distoversion (MAL1/DV) describes a tooth that is in its anatomically correct position in the dental arch, but which is abnormally angled in a distal direction.

Mesioversion (MAL1/MV) describes a tooth that is in its anatomically correct position in the dental arch, but which is abnormally angled in a mesial direction.

Linguoversion (MAL1/LV) describes a tooth that is in its anatomically correct position in the dental arch, but which is abnormally angled in a lingual direction.

Palatoversion (MAL1/PV) describes a tooth that is in its anatomically correct position in the dental arch, but which is abnormally angled in a palatal direction.

Labioversion (MAL1/LABV) describes an incisor or canine tooth that is in its anatomically correct position in the dental arch, but which is abnormally angled in a labial direction.

Buccoversion (MAL1/BV) describes a premolar or molar tooth that is in its anatomically correct position in the dental arch, but which is abnormally angled in a buccal direction.

Crossbite (CB) describes a malocclusion in which a mandibular tooth or teeth have a more buccal or labial position than the antagonist maxillary tooth. It can be classified as rostral or caudal:

In **rostral crossbite (CB/R)**, one or more of the mandibular incisor teeth is labial to the opposing maxillary incisor teeth when the mouth is closed; similar to posterior crossbite in human terminology.

In **caudal crossbite (CB/C)**, one or more of the mandibular cheek teeth is buccal to the opposing maxillary cheek teeth when the mouth is closed; similar to posterior crossbite in human terminology.

SKELETAL MALOCCLUSIONS

Symmetrical Skeletal Malocclusions

Mandibular Distoclusion: Class 2 Malocclusion (MAL2)

An abnormal rostrocaudal relationship between the dental arches in which the mandibular arch occludes caudal to its normal position relative to the maxillary arch.

Mandibular mesioclusion: Class 3 Malocclusion: (MAL3)

An abnormal rostrocaudal relationship between the dental arches in which the mandibular arch occludes rostral to its normal position relative to the maxillary arch.

Asymmetrical Skeletal Malocclusions

Maxillomandibular Asymmetry: Class 4 Malocclusion (MAL4)

Asymmetry in a rostrocaudal, side-to-side, or dorsoventral direction:

Maxillomandibular asymmetry in a rostrocaudal direction (**MAL4/RC**) occurs when mandibular mesioclusion or distoclusion is present on one side of the face while the contralateral side retains normal dental alignment.

Maxillomandibular asymmetry in a side-to-side direction (**MAL4/STS**) occurs when there is a loss of the midline alignment of the maxilla and mandible.

Maxillomandibular asymmetry in a dorsoventral direction (**MAL4/DV**) results in an open bite, which is defined as an abnormal vertical space between opposing dental arches when the mouth is closed.

The expression "wry bite" is a layman term that has been used to describe a wide variety of unilateral occlusal abnormalities. Because "wry bite" is nonspecific, its use is not recommended.

Management of Malocclusion

Orthodontics is a specialty in dentistry and oral surgery that is concerned with the prevention, interception, and correction of malocclusion.

Preventive orthodontics is concerned with the client's education, the development of the dentition and maxillofacial structures, the diagnostic procedures undertaken to predict malocclusion, and the therapeutic procedures instituted to prevent the onset of malocclusion. Preventive procedures are undertaken in anticipation of the development of a problem. Examples of preventive procedures include:

- Client education about timetables on exfoliation of deciduous teeth and eruption of permanent teeth
- Fiberotomy (severing of gingival fibers around a permanent tooth to prevent its relapse after corrective orthodontics)
- Operculectomy (surgical removal of an operculum to enable eruption of a permanent tooth)
- Extraction of a tooth that could pose a risk to development of malocclusion

Interceptive orthodontics is concerned with the elimination of a developing or established malocclusion. Interceptive procedures are typically undertaken in the growing patient. Examples of interceptive procedures include:

- Crown reduction of a permanent tooth in malocclusion
- Extraction of a tooth in malocclusion

Corrective orthodontics is concerned with the correction of malocclusion without loss of the maloccluded tooth or part of its crown. This is accomplished by means of tooth movement. Examples of corrective procedures include:

- Surgical repositioning of a tooth
- Orthognathic surgery to treat skeletal malocclusion
- Passive movement of a tooth using an inclined plane
- Active movement of a tooth using an elastic chain

Treatment plan (TP): Written document that outlines the progression of therapy (advantages, disadvantages, costs, alternatives, outcome, and duration of treatment)

Impression (IM): Detailed imprint of hard and/or soft tissues that is formed with specific types of impression materials

Full-mouth impression (IM/F): Imprints of the dentition and/or surrounding soft tissues of the upper and lower dental arches

Diagnostic cast (DC): Positive replica created by pouring a liquid material into an impression or placing an impression into a liquid material; once the material has hardened, the cast is removed and used to study and to plan treatment; also called die (**DC/D**) when made from an impression of a particular tooth/area of interest or stone model (**DC/SM**) when made from a full-mouth impression

Bite registration (BR): Impression used to record a patient's occlusion, which is then used to articulate diagnostic casts

Fiberotomy (FT): Severing gingival fibers around a permanent tooth to prevent its relapse after corrective orthodontics

Operculectomy (OP): Surgical removal of an operculum to enable eruption of a permanent tooth

Surgical repositioning (SR): Repositioning of a developmentally displaced tooth

Orthognathic surgery (OS): Surgical procedure to alter relationships of dental arches; typically performed to correct skeletal malocclusion

Bracket/button/hook (OA/BKT): Device made of metal or plastic that is bonded to the tooth surface and aids in the attachment of wires or elastics; use **OA/CMB** if custom made

Elastic chain/tube/thread (OA/EC): Orthodontic elastics used to move teeth

Orthodontic wire (OA/WIR): Metal wire with "memory" used to move teeth

Arch bar (OA/AR): Device attached to one dental arch to move individual teeth in between the device's attachments

Orthodontic appliance (OA): Device attached to a tooth or teeth to move a tooth or teeth

Orthodontic appliance adjustment (OA/A): Abbreviation used at the time of adjustment of the orthodontic appliance

Orthodontic appliance installation (OA/I): Abbreviation used at the time of installation of the orthodontic appliance

Orthodontic appliance removal (OA/R): Abbreviation used at the time of removal of the orthodontic appliance

Orthodontic counseling (OC): Client communication on the genetic basis, diagnosis, and treatment of malocclusion and the legal and ethical implications of orthodontics

Ball therapy (BTH): Removable orthodontic device in the form of a ball or cone-shaped rubber toy (e.g., to passively move linguoverted mandibular canine teeth)

Inclined plane (IP): Fixed orthodontic device made of acrylic (**IP/A**), composite (**IP/C**), or metal (**IP/M**) with sloping planes (e.g., to passively move linguoverted mandibular canine teeth)

Orthodontic recheck (OR): Examination of a patient treated with an orthodontic appliance.

Oral Surgery

Tooth Extraction-Related Terminology

Closed extraction (X or XS): Extraction of teeth without flap creation; **X** is used when closed extraction is performed without tooth sectioning; **XS** is used when closed extraction is performed with tooth sectioning or removal of interproximal crown tissue

Open extraction (XSS): Extraction of teeth after flap creation and alveolectomy

Alveolectomy (ALV): Removal of some or all of the alveolar bone

Alveoloplasty (ALV): A form of alveolectomy performed to restore physiologic contours or achieve smooth contours of the alveolar bone

Palate, Pharynx, and Nasal Surgery

Naroplasty (NAS/R): Surgical correction of stenotic nares

Tonsillectomy (TON/X): Surgical resection of the palatine tonsil

Grafts and Related Terminology

Transplantation: Act or process of transferring something from one part or individual to another

Transplant: Something transferred from one part or individual to another

Graft (GF): Nonliving material or living tissue used for implantation or transplantation to replace a diseased part or compensate for a defect

Gingival graft (GF/G): Gingiva or gingiva-like tissue (e.g., from the hard palate) used to replace gingiva in a gingival defect

Connective tissue graft (GF/CT): Connective tissue from a keratinized mucosa (e.g., from the hard palate) placed in a gingival defect and which is partially or completely covered with gingiva and/or alveolar mucosa in the recipient bed

Mucosal graft (GF/M): Mucosa used to take place of a removed piece of mucosa or cover a mucosal defect

Bone graft (GF/B): A surgical procedure by which bone or a bone substitute is used to take the place of a removed piece of bone or bony defect

Cartilage graft (GF/C): Cartilage used to take the place of a removed piece of bone or fill a bony defect

Skin graft (GF/S): Skin used to take place of a removed piece of skin/mucosa or skin/mucosa defect

Venous graft (GF/V): A vein used to take place of a removed segment of artery/vein or arterial/venous defect

Nerve graft (GF/N): A nerve used to take place of a removed segment of nerve or nerve defect

Fat graft (GF/F): Adipose tissue used to provide volume to a defect or to prevent ingrowth of other tissues into the defect

Autograft: Tissue transferred from one area to another area of the animal's own body

Isograft: Tissue transferred between genetically identical animals

Allograft: Tissue transferred between genetically dissimilar animals of the same species

Xenograft: Tissue transferred between animals of different species

Particulate graft: A graft containing equally or variably sized particles

Full-thickness graft: A graft consisting of the full thickness of a tissue

Partial-thickness (split-thickness) graft: A graft consisting of a portion of the thickness of a tissue

Mesh graft: A type of partial-thickness graft in which multiple small incisions have been made to increase the stretching and flexibility of the graft

Composite graft: A graft composed of at least two different tissues (e.g., skin-muscle-and-bone graft)

Implant (IMP): Something inserted into or applied to living tissue

Implantation: The act or process of inserting something into or applying something to living tissue

BIBLIOGRAPHY

Adrian AI, Balke M, Lynch R, Fink L. Radiographic outcome of the endodontic treatment of 55 fractured canine teeth in 43 dogs (2013–2018). *J Vet Dent.* 2022;39(3):250–256.

Alterman JB, Huff JF. Guided tissue regeneration in four teeth using a liquid polymer membrane: a case series. *J Vet Dent.* 2016;33(3):185–194.

Bell CM, Edstrom E, Shope B, et al. Characterization of oral pathology in cats affected by patellar fracture and dental anomaly syndrome (PADS). *J Vet Dent.* 2023;40(4):284–297.

Booij-Vrieling HE, de Vries TJ, Schoenmaker T, et al. Everts, Osteoclast progenitors from cats with and without tooth resorption respond differently to 1,25-dihydroxyvitamin D and interleukin-6. *Res Vet Sci.* 2012;92(2):311–316.

Booij-Vrieling HE, Tryfonidou MA, Riemers FM, Penning LC, Hazewinkel HAW. Inflammatory cytokines and the nuclear vitamin D receptor are implicated in the pathophysiology of dental resorptive lesions in cats. *Vet Immunol Immunopathol.* 2009;132(2–4):160–166.

Crossley DA. Tooth enamel thickness in the mature dentition of domestic dogs and cats: preliminary study. *J Vet Dent.* 1995;12(3):111–113.

Feigin K, Bell C, Shope B, Henzel S, Snyder C. Analysis and assessment of pulp vitality of 102 intrinsically stained teeth in dogs. *J Vet Dent.* 2022;39(1):21–33.

Ford KR, Anderson JG, Stapleton BL, et al. Medical management of canine chronic ulcerative stomatitis using cyclosporine and metronidazole. *J Vet Dent.* 2023;40(2):109–124.

Hale FA. Localized intrinsic staining of teeth due to pulpitis and pulp necrosis in dogs. *J Vet Dent.* 2001;18(1):14–20.

Harvey C, Serfilippi L, Barnvos D. Effect of frequency of brushing teeth on plaque and calculus accumulation, and gingivitis in dogs. *J Vet Dent.* 2015;32(1):16–21.

Heaton M, Wilkinson J, Gorrel C, Butterwick R. A rapid screening technique for feline odontoclastic resorptive lesions. *J Small Anim Pract.* 2004;45(12):598–601.

Hernández SZ, Negro VB, de Puch G, Saccomanno DM. Morphology of the cementoenamel junction in permanent teeth of dogs: a scanning electron microscopic study. *J Vet Dent.* 2020;37(3):159–166.

Krug W, Losey J. Area of desensitization following mental nerve block in dogs. *J Vet Dent.* 2011;28(3):146–150.

Kuntsi-Vaattovaara H, Verstraete FJ, Kass PH. Results of root canal treatment in dogs: 127 cases (1995–2000). *J Am Vet Med Assoc.* 2002;220(6):775–780.

Lawal FM, Adetunji A. A comparison of epidural anaesthesia with lignocaine, bupivacaine and a lignocaine-bupivacaine mixture in cats. *J S Afr Vet Assoc.* 2009;80(4):243–246.

Lee DB, Arzi B, Kass PH, Verstraete FJM. Radiographic outcome of root canal treatment in dogs: 281 teeth in 204 dogs (2001–2018). *J Am Vet Med Assoc.* 2022; 260(5):535–542.

Luotonen N, Kuntsi-Vaattovaara H, Sarkiala-Kessel E, Junnila JJT, Laitinen-Vapaavuori O, Verstraete FJM. Vital pulp therapy in dogs: 190 cases (2001–2011). *J Am Vet Med Assoc.* 2014;244(4):449–459.

Martel DP, Fox PR, Lamb KE, Carmichael DT. Comparison of closed root planing with versus without concurrent doxycycline hyclate or clindamycin hydrochloride gel application for the treatment of periodontal disease in dogs. *J Am Vet Med Assoc.* 2019;254(3):373–379.

Martin-Flores M, Scrivani PV, Loew E, Gleed CA, Ludders JW. Maximal and submaximal mouth opening with mouth gags in cats: implications for maxillary artery blood flow. *Vet J.* 2014;200(1):60–64.

Reiter AM, Lyon KF, Nachreiner RF, Shofer FS. Evaluation of calciotropic hormones in cats with odontoclastic resorptive lesions. *Am J Vet Res.* 2005;66(8):1446–1452.

Snyder LBC, Snyder CJ, Hetzel S. Effects of buprenorphine added to bupivacaine infraorbital nerve blocks on isoflurane minimum alveolar concentration using a model for acute dental/oral surgical pain in dogs. *J Vet Dent.* 2016;33(2):90–96.

Soltero-Rivera M, Vapniarsky N, Rivas IL, Arzi B. Clinical, radiographic and histopathologic features of early-onset gingivitis and periodontitis in cats (1997–2022). *J Feline Med Surg.* 2023;25(1).

Strøm PC, Arzi B, Lommer MJ, et al. Radiographic outcome of root canal treatment of canine teeth in cats: 32 cases (1998–2016). *J Am Vet Med Assoc.* 2018;252(5):572–580.

Verstraete FJ, Kass PH, Terpak CH. Diagnostic value of full-mouth radiography in cats. *Am J Vet Res.* 1998;59(6):692–695.

Verstraete FJ, Kass PH, Terpak CH. Diagnostic value of full-mouth radiography in dogs. *Am J Vet Res.* 1998;59(6):686–691.

Verstraete FJ, Terpak CH. Anatomical variations in the dentition of the domestic cat. *J Vet Dent.* 1997;14(4):137–140. Erratum in: *J Vet Dent.* 1998;15(1):34.

Abrasion   Wear of the teeth not from normal tooth-on-tooth contact.

Absorbent points   Tightly rolled, tapered paper used for drying a pulp canal after it has been prepared (debrided) and irrigated.

Acanthomatous ameloblastoma   Proliferating epithelial cells of dental origin. Although classified as benign, these epulides tend to invade bone, which makes dental radiographic evaluation and aggressive surgery important.

Alginate   An irreversible hydrocolloid impression material in dentistry for making impressions of jaws in the preparation for orthodontic appliances.

Alveolar mucosa   The less densely keratinized gingival tissue covering the bone.

Alveolar mucositis   Inflammation of alveolar mucosa (i.e., mucosa overlying the alveolar process and extending from the mucogingival junction without obvious demarcation to the vestibular sulcus and to the floor of the mouth).

Alveolar process   The tooth socket made of bundle bone and trabecular bone.

Ameloblasts   Cells that take part in forming dental enamel.

Amelogenesis imperfecta   An abnormality of enamel formation, including genetic and/or developmental enamel formation and maturation abnormalities such as enamel hypoplasia and enamel hypomineralization.

Anaerobic bacteria   Bacteria that do not require oxygen to survive.

Anatomic system   A numbering system used for medical record annotation in which the correct anatomic names of teeth are written out in full or abbreviated form.

Anionic detergent   A class of detergents (soap) having a negatively charged surface-active ion such as sodium alkylbenzene sulfonate. The detergent works by destroying the cell walls of bacteria.

Anisognathic jaw relationship   Naturally unequal jaw relationship in which the upper dental arch is slightly wider than the lower.

Ankylosis   Fusion of two hard tissue structures such as joints or tooth to alveolar process.

Anodontia   The absence of teeth.

Antiseptic   Any substance that inhibits the growth of bacteria.

Apex   The pointed end of a cone-shaped part or the end of a tooth root where blood vessels and nerves enter the tooth.

Apical   Toward the apex of the tooth.

Apical delta   Terminus of the root canal of cats and dogs made of dozens of formina as compared to the apical foramen of primates.

Apicoectomy   Excision of the apical portion of the root of a tooth through an opening in overlying tissues of the jaw.

Aradicular hypsodont   A tooth that grows continuously throughout life.

Arkansas stone   A sharpening stone used for the final sharpening of an instrument that is already close to sharpness.

Atraumatic malocclusion   Malposition of the teeth caused by hereditary factors or by nutritional or other atraumatic changes in teeth, temporomandibular joints (TMJs), mandibular symphysis, or bone that result in improper tooth alignment.

Attrition   The wearing away of a tooth, resulting from the friction of teeth against each other.

American Veterinary Dental College (AVDC)   Certifying organization authorized by the American Veterinary Medical Association to board certify veterinary dentists.

Anesthetic risk assessment (ARA)   Anesthetic risk assessment. A five-point scale used to assess perceived risk of anesthetic complications for a particular patient.

Avulsion   Complete displacement of the tooth from the socket.

Barbed broach   Instrument useful in the removal of intact pulp. It can also be used to remove from the root canal absorbent points, cotton pellets, separated file tips, and other foreign material such as dirt, gravel, and grass.

Biofilm   An aggregate of bacterial colonies protected by a polysaccharide complex.

Bisecting-angle technique   A radiographic technique obtained by visualizing an imaginary line that bisects the angle formed by the X-ray film and the structure being radiographed.

Blind intubation   Placing an endotracheal tube into the trachea without being able to visualize the epiglottis. Usually performed in rabbits and other small mammals.

Bone augmentation   A procedure in which bone is "built" using a synthetic material or natural graft.

Bone necrosis   Cellular death of the bone.

Brachycephalic   Having a short wide head. Characteristic of some breeds (e.g., Boxers, Pugs, Bulldogs, and Persian cats).

Brachyodont   A tooth with a true distinction between crown and root structure, with a root that does not grow once the tooth erupts.

Buccal   The direction toward the outside of the teeth, usually toward the cheeks.

Buccotomy   A full-thickness incision through the skin, mucosa, and subcutaneous tissue to allow for direct visualization and the ability to treat cheek teeth.

Buccoversion   A premolar or molar tooth that is in its anatomically correct position in the dental arch but which is abnormally angled in a buccal direction.

Bupivacaine   A local anesthetic commonly used in dentistry. It is most commonly used at a concentration of 0.5% solution or 5 mg/mL.

Calcium hydroxide   A compound used topically in solution or lotions; in dentistry used to encourage deposition of secondary dentin.

Calculus   Mineralized deposits of calcium phosphate and carbonate, with organic matter, deposited on tooth surfaces. May initiate caries and periodontal disease.

Calculus removal forceps   A dental instrument that allows for quick removal of large pieces of calculus.

Calicivirus   A virus that causes disease in cats. It is one of the two important viral causes of respiratory infection in cats and may be a trigger leading to feline chronic ulcerative gingivostomatitis.

Canine tooth   The long, pointed tooth in the interdental space between incisors and cheek teeth; there is one in each jaw on both sides.

Caries   Cavities. Loss of dental hard tissue due to acidic decay from byproducts of bacterial metabolism.

Carnassial tooth   Lay terminology to describe a shearing tooth. The upper P4 and lower M1 in the dog and cat.

Carnivore   Any animal, particularly mammals of the order Carnivora, that primarily eats flesh. Includes cats, dogs, bears, etc.

Caudal crossbite   A malocclusion in which one or more of the mandibular cheek teeth is buccal to the opposing maxillary cheek teeth when the mouth is closed.

Caudal mucositis   Inflammation of mucosa of the caudal oral cavity, bordered medially by the palatoglossal folds and fauces, dorsally by the hard and soft palate, and rostrally by alveolar and buccal mucosa.

Caudal stomatitis   The painful inflammation and ulceration extending into the tissues of the lateral palatine folds.

Cementoenamel junction   The tooth location where the enamel and the cementum meet.

Cementum   The bonelike connective tissue that attaches the periodontal ligament to the tooth.

Check off list   Tool containing a list of steps necessary to complete a procedure designed to be read by one member of a team and verbally confirmed by a second.

Cheek pouch impaction   A condition in which food is impacted in the cheek pouches, causing mild buccal irritation or stomatitis. Treatment consists of the removal of the impacted material, and in severe cases, antibiotic therapy may be warranted.

Cheek retractors   Single-bladed instruments that retract the cheek on a single-side or double-bladed instruments with a spring wire that spreads both buccal folds at the same time.

Cheilitis   Inflammation of the lip (including the mucocutaneous junction area and skin of the lip).

Chemical plaque control   Usage of products to reduce plaque via antiseptic action or other nonmechanical means.

Chlorhexidine   An antiseptic with antibacterial, antifungal, and some antiviral activity.

Cingulum   A ledge on the palatal side of the maxillary incisors.

Class I malocclusion   Overall normal occlusion except that one or more teeth are out of alignment.

Class II malocclusion   A malocclusion occurring when the mandible is shorter than normal. This may cause the adult canines and incisors to penetrate the hard palate, and irritation and ulceration of the hard palate may result.

Class III malocclusion   A malocclusion that has several forms and may be caused by the mandible being too long (mandibular prognathism). As a result, the mandibular incisors occlude labial to the maxillary incisors.

Class IV malocclusion   A malocclusion with asymmetry between the left and right sides.

Closed extraction   Dental extraction performed without raising a mucogingival flap and exposing bone.

Closed periodontal debridement   Procedure performed with hand instruments and an ultrasonic device to remove plaque, calculus, and debris from a periodontal pocket.

Closed position   The position obtained when the face of the curette is facing the foot surface when inserted into the pocket.

Computerized radiology   Form of digital radiography using a light-sensitive phosphor plate and scanner to create a radiograph.

Cone beam tomography   Type of computed tomography (CT) which uses a cone-shaped fan of radiation to produce a three-dimensional image. This is superior for bone and hard tissue but has limitations with soft-tissue imaging.

Conical stone   A sharpening stone that is used to provide a final sharpening to the instrument by working on its face.

Contact dermatitis   Delayed hypersensitivity reaction that develops 24–72 hours after contact with a substance.

Contact mucositis (also contact mucosal ulceration)   Lesions in susceptible individuals that are secondary to mucosal contact with a tooth surface bearing the responsible irritant, allergen, or antigen. They have also been called "contact ulcers" and "kissing ulcers."

Coronal   The direction toward the crown.

Cranial mandibular osteopathy   An inherited condition in which nonneoplastic bone forms in the region of the TMJ and occasionally extends into the mandible. It occurs primarily in West Highland white terriers and occasionally in other breeds.

Crestal bone loss   Form of horizontal bone loss where the coronal peak of alveolar bone is lost. Often the first sign of periodontitis.

Crossbite   A malocclusion in which a mandibular tooth or teeth have a more buccal or labial position than the antagonist maxillary tooth. It can be classified as rostral or caudal.

Curette   A dental instrument used for the removal of calculus both supragingivally and subgingivally.

Dental bur   A type of cutter used in a dental handpiece.

Dental composites   Tooth restorative materials made of a resin, filler, and coupling agent. Typically designed to cosmetically replace lost enamel and dentin.

Dental models   A manufactured copy of dentition made for orthodontic evaluation and treatment as well as for the manufacture of restorative crowns.

Dentigerous cyst   A cyst in which all or part of a tooth is in the cyst. It causes a local swelling of the jaw which may be visible externally.

Dentin   One of the hard tissues of the teeth that constitutes most of its bulk. It lies between the pulp cavity, the enamel within the crown, and the cementum within the root.

Dentinal bridge   New dentin formed between pulp capping material and pulp.

Dentinal tubules   Minute channels in the dentin of a tooth, which extend from the pulp cavity to the cementum or the enamel.

Diastema   A space or cleft (e.g., the space in the dental arch between the incisors and canines and cheek teeth).

Digital radiology (DR)   Radiology system utilizing a digital sensor directly wired to a computer.

Dilacerated root   An abnormally formed root.

Dilaceration   An abnormally shaped root resulting from trauma during tooth development.

Direct pulp-capping   A procedure, similar to vital pulpectomy, performed aseptically after purposeful or accidental iatrogenic pulpal exposure.

Disclosing solution   A solution that selectively stains all soft debris, pellicle, and bacterial plaque on teeth.

Distal   The portion farthest from the center of the dental arch.

Distoversion   A type of Class I malocclusion in which a tooth is in its anatomically correct position in the dental arch but which is abnormally angled in a distal direction.

Dolichocephalic Having a narrow, long head. Characteristic of some breeds (e.g., Collie, Borzoi, Greyhound, and Siamese cats).

Edentulous The absence of teeth.

Enamel The covering of the crown of the tooth and the hardest tissue in the body. It does not contain living cells.

Enamel hypomineralization Inadequate mineralization of enamel matrix.

Enamel hypoplasia A defect in tooth enamel production.

Endodontic abscess A localized collection of pus in a cavity formed by the disintegration of tissue. It frequently results from some form of trauma that has exposed the pulp and resulted in devitalization of the tooth.

Endodontic therapy Treatment of the dental pulp, including saving vital pulp, removing live or dead pulp, and preventing or treating infection.

Endodontics Dental specialty dealing with the treatment of conditions inside the tooth.

Endoscopic intubation Intubation using an otoscope with an endotracheal tube or intravenous (IV) catheter. This form of intubation calls for the use of an ear cone in a size appropriate for the size and depth of the animal's oral cavity. This form of intubation is primarily used with rats, hamsters, gerbils, chinchillas, and smaller rodents and lagomorphs.

Endotracheal intubation The insertion of a tube into the trachea. The purpose of intubation varies with the location and type of tube inserted; generally, the procedure is performed to maintain an open airway and for the administration of anesthetics or oxygen.

Epithelial attachment The epithelium attaching the gingiva to the tooth.

Ergonomics The science of designing the workplace so that operators remain in the most neutral positions possible.

Exodontics The branch of dentistry dealing with extraction of teeth.

Explorer A hand instrument used to detect plaque and calculus. It is also used to explore for cavities and check for exposed pulp chambers.

Extraction forceps An exodontic instrument used to grasp the tooth and remove it from the socket.

Eye shield A shield worn over the eyes that protects the wearer from either bacterial spray or, if filtered, intense light from light-curing units that may cause permanent retinal damage.

Feline orofacial pain syndrome (FOPS) A pain disorder of cats with behavioral signs of oral discomfort and tongue mutilation. It occurs mainly in Burmese cats and is thought to be caused by damage to the nerves of the peripheral nervous system possibly involving central and/or ganglion processing of sensory trigeminal information.

Feline stomatitis Also known as feline chronic gingivitis and stomatitis, painful immune-mediated inflammation of the oral cavity that is likely related to calicivirus.

Fibrosarcoma A sarcoma occurring in the mandible or maxilla that may create fleshy, protruding, firm masses that are sometimes friable.

File Instrument used to clean the root canal and remove dead or infected tissues. The term file is also used to describe instruments used in occlusal equilibration.

File separation Term used to describe the breakage of an endodontic file within a root canal.

Fistula Any abnormal, tube-like passage within body tissue.

Flat stone A stone used for sharpening dental equipment.

Floating Creating a level occlusal surface.

Four-handed dental charting The process of two individuals performing the oral examination with one probing and examining each tooth and the oral cavity while the other records the findings.

Free gingiva Portion of the gingiva not directly attached to the tooth that forms the gingival wall of the sulcus.

Frenula Small folds of integument or mucous membrane that limit the movements of an organ or part.

Full-coverage metal crowns A metal crown used to protect the surface of the endodontically treated tooth from further injury and to provide renewed height, shape, and function of severely deformed, fractured teeth.

Furcation The area in which the roots join the crown.

Fusion The joining of two developing teeth that have different tooth buds.

Gemination A tooth in which a tooth bud has partially divided in the attempt to form two teeth.

Gingiva The gums consisting of the mucosal tissue that lies over the alveolar bone.

Gingival hyperplasia The proliferation of gingival cells resulting in gingiva growing larger than it should.

Gingivectomy Surgical excision of all loose, infected, and diseased gingival tissue to eradicate periodontal infection and reduce the depth of the gingival sulcus.

Gingivitis Inflammation of the gingiva most often caused by bacterial plaque.

Gingivoplasty Surgical remodeling of the gingiva.

Glass ionomers A dental restorative material used for a base layer with composites to fill teeth.

Glossitis Inflammation of mucosa of the dorsal and/or ventral tongue surface.

Glucose oxidase Found in some toothpastes. Helps form the antibacterial hypothiocyanite ion.

Gram-positive aerobic bacteria Bacteria that resist decolorization by alcohol in Gram's method of staining. They require oxygen to survive.

Granuloma A tumor-like mass or nodule of granulation tissue.

Guided tissue regeneration Periodontal surgery used to reestablish lost periodontal bone by preventing the migration of epithelial tissue into a pocket.

Gutta-percha The coagulated latex used as a dental cement and in splints. It is the most popular core material used by veterinary practitioners.

Halitosis Bad breath.

Handle The part of the hand instrument that is grasped. Handles come in a variety of round, tapered, and hexagonal shapes.

HAZCOM The Federal Hazard communication standard (also known as HCS). Enforced by the Occupational safety and health administration (OSHA) of the United States Department of Labor, HAZCOM is based on employees' rights and their "need to know" identities of hazardous substances to which they may be exposed in the work environment.

Herbivore Animals that subsist in their natural state entirely by eating plants and plant products.

Heterodont dentition Having teeth of different shapes such as molars, incisors, etc.

High-speed handpiece   A handpiece used for cutting teeth in extractions and making access holes into the teeth in root canal therapy.

Hypodontia   Having fewer than the normal amount of teeth.

Iatrogenic   Resulting from the activity of a medical professional.

Iatrogenic pulpal exposure   The exposure of pulp induced by a medical professional.

Impacted tooth   A nonerupted or partially erupted tooth that is prevented from erupting further by any structure.

Impression tray   A receptacle or device that is used to carry impression material to the mouth, confine the material in apposition to the surfaces to be recorded, and to control the impression material while it sets to form the impression.

Incisors   The front teeth of either jaw.

India stone   A sharpening stone used for "coarse" sharpening of an overly dull instrument or for changing the plane of one or more of the sides of the instrument.

Indirect pulp-capping   A restorative procedure performed when the preparation of a carious lesion does not penetrate the pulp but is perilously close (0.5 mm) to it.

Inferior alveolar nerve block   A regional nerve block in which all of the teeth of the mandible on the side of infiltration as well as adjacent bone and soft tissue are blocked.

Infiltration blocks   A method of local anesthesia. Rather than blocking an entire quadrant, infiltration blocks only block the area where the infiltration has been administered.

Informed consent   Documentation discussing risks and expected outcome of a procedure with client certifying that they understand all presented.

Infraorbital block   A regional nerve block in which the infraorbital nerve is infiltrated as it exits the infraorbital canal.

Interceptive orthodontics   The process of extracting primary teeth to prevent orthodontic malocclusions.

Intermediate plexus   A middle zone of the periodontal membrane situated between the cemental group of fibers attached to the root of the tooth and the alveolar group of fibers attached to the alveolar bone.

Interproximal area   The area between adjoining teeth.

Intrinsic staining   Staining of the tooth from products within the pulp or dentin.

Intubation   The insertion of a tube, as into the larynx. The purpose of intubation varies with the location and type of tube inserted; generally, the procedure is done to allow for drainage, to maintain an open airway, or for the administration of anesthetics or oxygen.

Irrigation   The washing of a wound by a stream of water or other fluid.

Junctional epithelium   The epithelium that lies at the base of the gingival sulcus.

Labial   The direction toward the outside of the teeth, usually toward the lips.

Labioversion   An incisor or canine tooth that is in its anatomically correct position in the dental arch but which is abnormally angled in a labial direction.

Lactoperoxidase   A chemical that, when combined with glucose oxidase, produces the hypothiocyanite ion, which is the same ion produced naturally in saliva to help inhibit bacterial growth.

Lagomorph   A member of the order Lagomorpha. Includes the domestic rabbit, hare, and cottontail.

Lamina dura   A radiographic term referring to the dense cortical bone forming the wall of the alveolus. It appears radiographically as a bony white line next to the dark line of the periodontal space.

Lingual   In a direction toward the tongue. Pertains to the mandibular teeth.

Linguoversion   A mandibular tooth that is in its anatomically correct position in the dental arch but which is abnormally angled in a lingual direction.

Local antibiotic therapy   The application of antibiotics directly into the periodontal pockets after root planing or periodontal debridement. Has been known as perioceutic therapy.

Locking cotton pliers   A tool used to pick up paper points or gutta-percha without contaminating the container or points; also known as college pliers.

Low-speed handpiece   A handpiece used for polishing with prophy angles and for performing other dental procedures with contra-angles.

Luxation   Partial displacement of the tooth from the socket.

Minimal alveolar concentration (MAC)   Minimal alveolar concentration. Amount of inhalant anesthetic required to maintain a proper depth of anesthesia.

Major palatine nerve block   Nerve block placed over the major palatine nerve foramen used to anesthetize the mucosa of the hard palate.

Malignant melanoma   A tumor occurring on any site in the oral cavity: gingiva, buccal mucosa, hard and soft palates, and tongue. The tumor is locally invasive and highly metastatic to the lungs, regional lymph nodes, and bone.

Mandible   The lower jaw. In the dog and cat, the lower jaw consists of two mandibles that meet at the mandibular symphysis.

Mandibular symphysis   Joint between the left and right mandible of dogs and cats and many carnivores.

Master problem list   Part of the medical record including the date of a noted problem and date of resolution if applicable.

Material safety data sheet (MSDS)   A form with data regarding the properties of a particular substance. The MSDS provides workers with procedures for handling or working with a particular substance in a safe manner.

Maxilla   The upper jaw. The upper jaw of the dog and cat are made of paired maxillae and incisive bones.

Maxillary block   A regional nerve block in which both the maxillary nerve (rostrally becomes the infraorbital nerve) and the sphenopalatine nerve or ganglia are anesthetized. It is placed caudal and adjacent to the maxilla.

Maxillary brachygnathism   A malocclusion in which the maxilla is too short and the mandible appears to be normal length.

Maxillary-mandibular asymmetry   Skeletal malocclusions that can occur in a rostrocaudal, side-to-side, or dorsoventral direction.

Mechanical plaque control   Removal of plaque with a device such as a toothbrush, fingerbrush, or cotton-tipped applicator.

Medication-related osteonecrosis of the jaws (MRONJ)   Condition, often associated with alendronate usage in cats, in which the jaw bones have focal or multifocal regions of bone necrosis.

Mesaticephalic   A skull with the cranium and nasal cavity about equal lengths. Seen in a majority of dog breeds.

Mesial   Situated in the middle; median; nearer the center of the dental arch.

Mesioversion   A type of Class I malocclusion in which a tooth that is in its anatomically correct position in the dental arch is abnormally angled in a mesial direction.

Middle mental block   A regional nerve block in which the inferior alveolar nerve within the mandibular canal via the middle mental foramen is anesthetized.

Modified pen grasp   The preferred method for holding hand instruments in which the instrument is held with the thumb and index finger. The instrument rests on the index finger, and the middle, ring, and little fingers are extended. The middle, ring, and little fingers are then placed alongside the index finger.

Molars   The cheek teeth that are not preceded by premolars.

Monofluorophosphate (MFP) fluoride   MFP fluoride is the form of fluoride most commonly found in over-the-counter products.

Mucogingival junction   The line of demarcation where the attached gingiva and alveolar mucosa meet.

Mucositis   The painful inflammation and ulceration of the mucosal tissues lining the digestive tract.

Multiplanar reconstruction (MPR)   Tool used with CT in which a structure can be viewed in three dimensions by simultaneously studying images made in three tangential fields.

Neutral position   Sitting with the knees slightly below the hips, the back straight, the elbows at a 90-degree angle, and the thumbs relaxed at the top of the hand.

Occlusal equilibration   Creating a level occlusal surface.

Occlusion   The way the teeth fit together. Dogs and cats have sectorial occlusion, which means chewing occurs on the sides of the teeth.

Odontoblasts   Cells that line the pulp chamber and produce dentin.

Odontoma   A mass of cells that have enamel, dentin, cementum, and small tooth-like structures.

Odontoplasty   The process of recontouring a tooth surface, which is not limited to leveling an occlusal surface.

Oligodontia   Having few teeth.

Omnivore   Animals that eat both plant and animal foods.

Open extraction   Dental extraction performed with the aid of a mucoginval flap.

Open position   The position obtained when the curette is moved over the calculus and repositioned so that the cutting surface is under the calculus ledge.

Oral medicine   Dental specialty dealing with the effects of cancer and other medical conditions on the mouth.

Oronasal fistula   An abnormal opening between the oral and nasal cavities.

Orthodontics   The correction of dental malocclusions.

OSHA   Occupational Safety and Health Administration.

Osteomyelitis   Inflammation of the bone and bone marrow.

Palatal   The direction toward the inside of the maxillary tooth.

Palatine rugae   Raised ridges of the hard palatal mucosa

Palatitis   Inflammation of mucosa covering the hard and/or soft palate.

Parallel technique   A radiographic technique indicated to evaluate the caudal mandibular teeth and nasal cavity.

Patency   The condition of being open.

Pedodontics   Dental specialty dealing with the treatment of dental disease in puppies and kittens.

Pellicle   Substrates such as glycoproteins to form a layer on the tooth, which allow for bacterial attachment.

Periapical lucency   Radiolucent structure of the periapical tissues thatmay indicate endodontic inflammation.

Pericorontitis   Periodontal inflammation due to a tooth not fully erupting.

Periodontal abscess   A localized collection of pus in a cavity formed by the disintegration of tissue.

Periodontal debridement   The treatment of gingival and periodontal inflammation. Its goal is the mechanical removal of surface irritants while maintaining soft tissue and allowing it to return to a healthy, noninflamed state.

Periodontal disease   An inflammation and infection of the tissues surrounding the tooth, collectively called the periodontium.

Periodontal ligament   Ligament that connects the tooth root to the alveolar process with minor connections between roots and from the gingiva to the root.

Periodontal pockets   An area of diseased gingival attachment, characterized by loss of attachment and eventual damage to the tooth's supporting bone.

Periodontal probe   An instrument in dentistry primarily used to measure pocket depths around the tooth in order to establish the state of health of the periodontium.

Periodontal therapy   Treatment of diseased periodontal tissues.

Periodontics   Dental specialty dealing with the treatment of conditions in the surrounding tooth structure (*perio* means around, and *dontics* means tooth).

Periodontitis   Inflammation of nongingival periodontal tissues (i.e., the periodontal ligament and alveolar bone).

Periodontium   The attachment apparatus of the tooth to the jaw made of the gingiva, alveolar bone, cementum, and periodontal ligament.

Periosteal elevator   An instrument used to lift the gingiva away from the bone during periodontal surgery.

Periostitis ossificans   A benign lesion seen in young breed dogs that will spontaneously resolve with age.

Perio-to-endo lesion   A localized collection of pus in a cavity formed by the disintegration of tissue. These abscesses are some of the most commonly detected facial or jaw abscesses. They occur owing to extension of periodontal disease apically to enter the pulp of the tooth.

Peripheral odontogenic fibroma   Fibroma characterized by the presence of a tumor in the tissues of the gingiva; it contains primarily fibrous tissues and has been known as fibromatous epulis.

Persistent deciduous teeth   Deciduous teeth that did not exfoliate and may cause orthodontic and periodontic abnormalities by possibly displacing the adult teeth.

Pharyngitis   Inflammation of the pharynx.

Phosphor plate   Used in computed radiography. Often polyester plate with a radiosensitive phosphor used in place of dental film.

Piezoelectric ultrasonic scaler   An ultrasonic scaler that uses crystals in the handpiece to pick up the vibration. These units have a wide, back-and-forth tip motion.

Pigtail explorer   A curved explorer that allows the operator to easily avoid touching the parts of the tooth that are not being explored.

Plaque   A mass adhering to the enamel surface of a tooth, composed of a mixed colony of bacteria.

Plugger   An instrument with blunted tips used to obtain vertical (apical) compaction.

Pocket A space resulting from the gingiva separating from the tooth owing to inflammation.

Porcelain-fused-to-metal crowns A cosmetically pleasing crown with a metal shell on which is fused a veneer of porcelain. It is used to protect the surface of the endodontically treated tooth from further injury and to provide renewed height, shape, and function of severely deformed, fractured teeth.

Power scaler A scaler that converts electric or pneumatic energy into a mechanical vibration. When the power scaler is placed against the calculus, the vibration shatters it, freeing it from the tooth surface.

Premolars Cheek teeth present in both generations found between the molars and the canines.

Preventative orthodontics Extraction to reduce the risk of future pathology such as extracting crowded teeth to prevent periodontitis.

Professional dental cleaning Dental scaling and polishing under general anesthesia.

Prophy angles Attachments on slow-speed or electric motor handpiece that are used to polish teeth.

Prophy cup The rubber cup used on the prophy angle for polishing teeth.

Prophy paste The paste used for polishing teeth.

Prophylaxis Prevention of or protective treatment for disease. Often used interchangeable but incorrectly to describe cleaning the teeth in dogs and cats.

Prosthodontics Dental specialty dealing with the process of restoring the tooth to normal health.

Pseudopocket A pocket, adjacent to a tooth, resulting from gingival hyperplasia or swelling, and the periodontal membrane and alveolar bone are normal.

Pull stroke A hand instrument technique for the removal of calculus.

Pulp Blood vessels, nerves, and connective tissues that support the odontoblastic cells lining the pulp chamber and root canal.

Pulpectomy Removal of dental pulp.

Pyogenic granuloma Inflammatory lesion, often found in cats, due to repetitive oral trauma typically from biting soft tissues.

Rasps Instruments used to level an abnormally uneven occlusive table of the teeth.

Reamer Instrument used to clean the root canal and remove dead or infected tissues. Reamers are used in a twisting, auger-like motion that delivers filings from the depth of the canal to the access site.

Regional nerve block A method of local anesthesia in which local anesthetic is placed on a major nerve (as opposed to an infiltration block).

Repetitive motion disorder A family of muscular conditions that result from repeated motions performed in the course of normal work or daily activities.

Resective osseous surgery Periodontal surgery in which bone is removed to prevent or treat disease.

Restorative dentistry Restoring the form and function of damaged teeth.

Retrograde intubation Intubation in which a needle is inserted through the midventral neck region between two of the tracheal rings and directed toward the head. The needle is stopped as soon as it penetrates the trachea. This type of intubation can be used on all sizes of rodents and lagomorphs, but it can be traumatic and irritating to the trachea.

Root canal sealant Cements or pastes used to seal the apical one-third of the root, dentinal tubules that radiate from the walls of the canal, and apical delta.

Root planing The traditional method of periodontal therapy. The objective of root planing is the removal of calculus and cementum from the root surface and the creation of a clean, smooth, glasslike root surface. In this treatment, everything, including cementum, is removed from the root surface.

Root scaling Mechanical removal of root deposits without removing cementum.

Rostral crossbite A malocclusion in which one or more of the mandibular incisor teeth is labial to the opposing maxillary incisor teeth when the mouth is closed.

Rotary scaler A type of scaler that is discouraged because it can easily damage the tooth. Also, the burs must be replaced often because they become dull very quickly.

Scaler A dental instrument used for scaling calculus from the crown surface. These instruments are particularly useful in removing calculus from narrow but deep fissures such as that located on the buccal surface of the fourth premolar.

Scissors bite Normal occlusion in dogs and cats, in which the mandibular (lower) teeth come into contact with the palatal side (inside) of the maxillary (upper) teeth.

Scurvy Disease caused by a nutritional deficiency of ascorbic acid (vitamin C).

Shank The part of the hand instrument that joins the working end with the handle.

Sharps Needles, scalpel blades, broken ampoules; anything in a hospital or clinic that has been used on patients and that may be contaminated with infectious material; to be discarded into special containers for disposal without any risk to disposal personnel.

Short finger stop technique Method of holding dental surgical instruments in which the index finger is kept near the working end of the instrument to reduce the risk of iatrogenic trauma if the instrument were to slip.

Same lingual opposite buccal (SLOB) rule SLOB rule used to identify roots that are laying side by side.

Slobbers A condition in which excess salivation results in moist dermatitis.

SOAP format medical records Medical records organized as subjective, objective, assessment, and plan.

Sodium hypochlorite An irrigating solution that helps break down and remove organic material. Bleach.

Sonic scaler An ultrasonic scaler that operates at 6000 cycles per second with a 0.5-mm amplitude and an elliptic, figure-of-eight motion.

Spearing canines A lay term used to describe mesioversion of the maxillary canine teeth.

Spreader An instrument with a tapered, round shaft, and pointed tip used to compress gutta-percha laterally and force sealant into dentinal tubules.

Squamous cell carcinoma A histologically distinct form of cancer arising in a variety of locations in the mouth. The cell's type is from the epithelium, and the appearance varies, but generally it is a nodular, gray-to-pink, irregular mass that invades the bone and causes tooth mobility.

Stannous fluoride   The most bactericidal fluoride. It is stable at a pH of 6.5.

Stethoscope-aided intubation   Intubation in which an endotracheal tube is attached to a standard clinical stethoscope using an appropriate adapter.

Stomatitis   Inflammation of the mucous lining of any of the structures in the mouth; in clinical use the term should be reserved to describe widespread oral inflammation (beyond gingivitis and periodontitis) that may also extend into submucosal tissues (e.g., marked caudal mucositis extending into submucosal tissues may be termed *caudal stomatitis*).

Subgingival scaling   Removal of tartar from the teeth beneath the free margin of gingival tissue.

Sublingual   The structures and surfaces beneath the tongue.

Sublingual mucositis   Inflammation of mucosa on the floor of the mouth.

Substantivity   The ability of chlorhexidine, parachlorometaxylenol, and triclosan to stick to surfaces.

Sulcus   The potential space between the surface of the tooth and the epithelium lining the free gingiva.

Superior alveolar block   Nerve block used to anesthetize the maxillary teeth performed by placing the needle and local anesthetic past the infraorbital foramen and into the canal.

Supernumerary teeth   Teeth in excess of the regular number; extra teeth.

Supragingival scaling   Removal of tartar from the teeth on the side of the gingival margin toward the dental crown.

Surgical root canal therapy   Endodontic therapy in which the root apex is surgically removed and filled with a root-end filling material.

Tartar   A yellowish film formed of calcium phosphate and carbonate, food particles, and other organic matter that is deposited on the teeth by the saliva.

Temporomandibular joint   The hinge joint of the jaw that connects the mandible to the temporal bone.

Terminal shank   The part of the shank that is closest to the working end of the hand instrument.

Thiols   Volatile sulfur compounds created by periodontal pathogens that create halitosis and tissue damage.

Three-way syringe   Part of the dental unit that creates a water spray and an air spray. The water spray is used for irrigating a tooth surface and clearing away prophy paste, tooth shavings, and other debris. The air spray can be used to dry the field.

Tongue entrapment   A condition in which the tongue is "pinned" in the intermandibular space because of mandibular cheek teeth growing to meet at the midline.

Tongue retractors   Instruments with a single, flat blade used to move the tongue away from the area to be inspected or treated.

Tonsillitis   Inflammation of the palatine tonsil.

Tooth abrasion   Wear of teeth not associated with normal tooth-to-tooth contact.

Tooth elongation   Abnormal intraoral and/or periapical extension of the coronal and/or apical portion of the tooth.

Tooth luxation   Incomplete traumatic displacement of a tooth from the alveolar process.

Tooth resorption   A process by which all or part of a tooth structure is lost from demineralization by odontoclasts. This has been documented in most mammalian species.

Torque   Ability to overcome resistance to movement.

Tracheotomy intubation   Intubation in which a tracheotomy is performed by making a longitudinal skin incision over the trachea midway between the larynx and thoracic inlet. A stab incision is made between two of the tracheal rings, and the endotracheal tube is passed into the trachea and then anchored with umbilical tape, which is tied to the tube and then around the animal's neck to prevent accidental extubation.

Traumatic malocclusion   Malposition of the teeth resulting from injury to the teeth resulting in broken crowns, which may cause overgrowth of the opposing tooth because of the lack of normal attrition.

Triadan system   A numbering system used for medical record annotation in which three numbers are used to identify each tooth. The first number identifies the quadrant (remember that there are four) of the mouth. The second and third numbers identify the tooth, which is always represented by two numbers.

Turbine   The internal portion of the high-speed handpiece that spins at an extremely high speed.

Ultrasonic ferroceramic rod   An ultrasonic device that vibrates at 42,000 cycles per second. All sides of the tip are equally active.

Ultrasonic instrument   Dental instrument that converts energy from a power source into a sound wave.

Ultrasonic metal strips/stacks   Ultrasonic devices that vibrate at 18,000, 25,000, and 30,000 cycles per second. The amplitude of tip movement is between 0.01 and 0.05 mm, which is extremely narrow.

Ultrasonic scaler   A type of scaler used to quickly remove smaller deposits of supragingival calculus.

Vertical releasing incision   Incision made into the gingiva and often mucosa in a coronal to apical direction to aid in creating a three- or four-cornered mucoperiosteal flap.

Vestibular   In a direction toward the lips and/or cheeks.

Veterinary oral health council (VOHC)   Established by the AVDC in 1997, the VOHC sets testing protocols for products. If product testing is approved, the product is awarded the VOHC seal of acceptance.

Vital pulp therapy   A procedure performed to maintain tooth vitality. It may be required when injury or iatrogenic action causes exposure of the pulp.

Vital pulpotomy   Removal of exposed, contaminated pulp, and disinfection of remaining pulp and access site. This procedure is indicated for recent fractures to preserve healthy dental pulp.

Working end   The part of the hand instrument that comes in contact with the tooth.

Working length   The distance from endodontic access to the apical terminus of a root.

ANSWERS TO WORKSHEETS

CHAPTER 1 WORKSHEET ANSWERS

1. mesaticephalic, brachycephalic, dolichocephalic
2. mandibular symphysis, temporomandibular joint
3. 28, 42
4. enamel
5. odontoblasts
6. gingiva, alveolar process, periodontal ligament, cementum
7. sulcus
8. periodontal ligament
9. $2 \times (3/3I, 1/1C, 4/4P, 2/3M) = 42$
10. $2 \times (3/3I, 1/1C, 3/2P, 1/1M) = 30$
11. first, second, third maxillary incisors, maxillary canine tooth, first maxillary premolar
12. second, third, and fourth mandibular premolars, first and second mandibular molars
13. maxillary fourth premolar
14. 100, 200, 300, 400
15. canine, first molar
16. 205, 407
17. four-handed dental charting
18. palatine rugae

CHAPTER 2 WORKSHEET ANSWERS

1. preventative orthodontics, interceptive orthodontics
2. West Highland terriers
3. I
4. gingivitis
5. periodontitis, periodontal disease
6. abrasion
7. attrition
8. enamel hypoplasia
9. endodontics
10. or endodontic therapy
11. irreversible pulpitis
12. luxation
13. tooth resorption

14. oronasal fistula
15. gingival hyperplasia
16. peripheral odontogenic fibroma
17. CCUS
18. acanthomatous ameloblastoma
19. squamous cell carcinoma
20. symphyseal separation

CHAPTER 3 WORKSHEET ANSWERS

1. Working end
2. two
3. Supragingival
4. Area-specific
5. toe
6. Dull, sharp
7. 75; 80
8. Electric or pneumatic
9. Magnetostrictive, piezoelectric
10. crystals
11. 30–40
12. water
13. 300,000 to 400,000
14. 5000 to 20,000
15. Single-use

CHAPTER 4 WORKSHEET ANSWERS

1. OSHA
2. Their own safety
3. Chemical, physical, biologic, ergonomic
4. Bacteria
5. Handwashing
6. Cold
7. Immediately
8. Material safety data sheets
9. Sterile
10. Life

CHAPTER 5 WORKSHEET ANSWERS

1. Supervising veterinarian
2. 0.5, 5
3. 2.0
4. Distal, third
5. Caudally, infraorbital
6. Mandibular, lingual, or medial
7. Third, first
8. Aspirate
9. Lingual, inferior alveolar
10. Buprenorphine, epinephrine
11. Middle mental
12. Sodium
13. Ropivacaine
14. Infiltration
15. 25 or 27

CHAPTER 6 WORKSHEET ANSWERS

1. inflammation, infection
2. pellicle
3. pink, bleeding
4. 1
5. 5
6. 3
7. causative link
8. halitosis
9. thiols
10. tooth mobility
11. renal and gastrointestinal disease
12. biofilm
13. 5
14. specific plaque hypothesis
15. saliva, calculus

CHAPTER 7 WORKSHEET ANSWERS

1. Calculus forceps
2. Water flow
3. Light
4. Modified
5. Oxygenates
6. Sanos, Oravet

7. Oscillating
8. Disclosing solution
9. Closed
10. Oral speculums

CHAPTER 8 WORKSHEET ANSWERS

1. before
2. demonstrator
3. daily
4. chlorhexidine
5. plaque, calculus
6. polyphosphates
7. supervision
8. 6–8
9. False
10. zinc ascorbate

CHAPTER 9 WORKSHEET ANSWERS

1. root planing
2. disrupting
3. 100
4. cementum
5. local antibiotic therapy
6. A special applicator
7. False
8. crosshatch
9. 1
10. True

CHAPTER 10 WORKSHEET ANSWERS

1. Stomatitis
2. 30
3. alveolar bone expansion
4. feline oral pain syndrome
5. one
6. extraction
7. bisphosphonates
8. patellar fracture and dental anomaly syndrome
9. Burmese
10. I

CHAPTER 11 WORKSHEET ANSWERS

1. lead safety aprons, screens, safe distance
2. six, 90–135
3. A patient who cannot undergo general anesthesia
4. 2
5. the mandibular molars
6. bisecting-angle technique
7. foreshortening
8. 45, 45
9. hard tissue
10. CR

CHAPTER 12 WORKSHEET ANSWERS

1. home care
2. authorization
3. veterinarians
4. extraction forceps
5. multirooted
6. T
7. open
8. short finger stop technique
9. iatrogenic fracture
10. inflammation

CHAPTER 13 WORKSHEET ANSWERS

1. gingivectomy
2. endodontic therapy
3. pulp death
4. root canal therapy
5. hand
6. length, width
7. pluggers
8. MTA
9. apicoectomy
10. endostops

CHAPTER 14 WORKSHEET ANSWERS

1. aradicular hypsodont, aradicular hypsodont, brachyodont
2. heterodont, incisor, premolar, molar, canine
3. intermediate plexus
4. anisognathic jaw relationship
5. guinea pigs, chinchillas
6. enamel, guinea pig.
7. first molar teeth, Mustelidae.
8. Traumatic, atraumatic.
9. guinea pig, cheek teeth
10. slobbers
11. 0
12. inferior alveolar vessels, bleeding
13. upper lip
14. sterile
15. 4

Note: Page numbers followed by "*f*" indicate figures, "*t*" indicate tables, and "*b*" indicate boxes.